1 MONTH OF
FREE
READING

at
www.ForgottenBooks.com

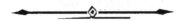

By purchasing this book you are eligible for one month membership to ForgottenBooks.com, giving you unlimited access to our entire collection of over 1,000,000 titles via our web site and mobile apps.

To claim your free month visit:

www.forgottenbooks.com/free13167

ISBN 978-0-483-00094-0
PIBN 10013167

THE

Canadian Journal

OF

Medicine and Surgery

A JOURNAL PUBLISHED MONTHLY IN THE INTEREST OF
MEDICINE AND SURGERY

J. J. CASSIDY, M.D., EDITOR.

VOL. XVi.

JULY TO DECEMBER, 1904

BUSINESS MANAGER

W. A. YOUNG, M.D., L.R.G.P.LOND

145 COLLEGE ST., TORONTO, CAN.

1904

Correspondence.   PAGE

"Neurasthenia in Some of its Relations to
Insanity." 215

Use Antitoxin as Early as Possible... 216

Editorials.

A Glance at the Atlantic City Meeting of
the American Medical Association . .   42

American Surgery Seen through French
Eyes............. 279

A New Prison Inspector.................... 341

Cawthra Mulock's Gift 339

Diseases Affecting Women on the Farm in
Ontario................................. 45

Editorial Notes. 51, 143, 206, 286, 342, 413

Honor Conferred on Dr. William Osler.... 205

Medical Editors at Atlantic City 44

New Researches in Diphtheritic Paralysis 200

Oliphant Nicholson's Views on the Treatment of Puerperal Eclampsia.......... 408

Our Report of the Ontario Medical Association 41

Personals·............... 56, 148, 211, 292, 346, 418

Quack Advertisements.................. ... 197

Raising the Matriculation Standard of the
College of Physicians and Surgeons of
Ontario 141

Something About Maternal Milk in England and France....................... 48

Strangulation or Inhibition 137

The Imperial Cancer Research Fund 282

The Passenger Car Ventilation System of
the Pennsylvania Railroad 333

The Vancouver Meeting of the Canadian
Medical Association 284

"These are All Honorable Men"........... 410

The Surgical Treatment of Gout.......... 405

Toronto's New Medical Library............ 202

What Should be the Conduct of Sanitarians
towards Patients with Venereal Diseases?................................. 337

News of the Month.

Canadian Medical Association 149

Items of Interest........ 60, 154, 217, 294, 351, 427

Opening Lecture of the Medical Faculty of
Toronto University 347

Medical Science Advance.... 420

Pan-American Medical Congress 423

The Gynecological Importance of Prolapsed Kidney.......................... 424

The Mississippi Valley Medical Association 348

The M. J. Breitenbach Company vs Siegel,
Cooper Company and Thomas H. Mc-
Innerney 59

The Royal and Imperial State Infirmary,
Vienna....... ....

The Sanitarium Built at Weston..........

The Wellcome Physiological Research
Laboratories at the St. Louis Exposition, 1904 ....

Typhoid Fever............................

Obituaries.

Death of Dr. C. W. Chaffee ....

Death of Dr. Ernest Wills, of Calgary,
N.W.T ....

Death of Dr. Reginald Henwood. ....

Dr. A. E. Mallory's Death.................

Original Contributions.

A Case of Gastroschisis or Fissura Abdominalis. By Joseph H. Peters, M.D.,
Hamilton, Ont..... 1

Acute Bronchitis. By R. J. Smith, M.D.,
Chicago, Ill..... ....

Address in Medicine. By R. E. McKechnie,
M.D., Vancouver, B.C............. .....

An Extraordinary Anemia—Report of a
Case. By F. V. Trebilcock, M.D.,
Enniskillen.............................

Chest Examinations: A System of Recording Observations. By J. H. Elliott,
M.B.....................................

Complications of Fractures and Amputations. By Thomas H. Manley, Ph.D.,
M.D, New York.......................

Neurasthenia in Some of Its Relations to
Insanity. By Campbell Meyers, M.D.,
Toronto................................

President's Address. By J. F. W. Ross
M.D., Toronto.........................

President's Address. By Simon J. Tunstall, B.A., M.D., Vancouver, B.C......

Report of a Case of Bilateral, Congenital
Dislocation of the Hip Treated by the
Lorenz Bloodless Method—A Brief Re-
view of the present Status of the Lorenz
Method. By H. P. H. Galloway, M.D. 1

The Arid Climates. By J. Frank McConnell, M.D., Las Cruces, Mex co........

The Diagnosis of Modified Smallpox (so-
called). By Charles A. Hodgetts, M.D.,
L.R.C.P. (Lond.).......................   1

The Medical Society ; Its Place and Equipment. By John Hunter, M.D. ·.........

The Surgical Treatment of Complete Descent of the Uterus. By E. C. Dudley,
M.D., Chicago ....

Thoughts on Cancer. By the Hon. Sir Wm.
Hingston, F.R.C.S., Montreal..........

Urinary Antisepsis in Gonorrheal Urethritis. By E. Reinhardt, M.D., New York. 3

School Hygiene. PAGE

Contagious and School Work in New York 136

Inheritance and Education............ 213

Report No. 1. of the Committee on Epidemics to the Ontario Provincial Board of Health 13

The Degeneration of the National Physique. 19

The Nuremberg Congress................. 212

Selected Articles.

A New Chloroform Inhaler 37

A Note on the Treatment of Sciatica...... 328

An Oration Delivered by Dr. W. P. C. Barton in 1821. With Explanatory Note. By William Pepper, M.D......20, 182

Jamaica, a Land Never Touched by Frost. 329

Local Anesthesia. By Horatio C. Wood, M.D., LL.D........ 31

Martindale Goods now Procurable in Toronto 400

Points on Endometritis.................... 396

Progress in the Treatment of Eczema. By Prof. Kromayer, Berlin............... 173

Proprietaries 397

The Importance of Careful General Preparation of the Patient for Surgical Operation.............................. 404

The Vivisection Problem : Two Views.... 319

Why I Give Preference to Buffalo Lithia over other Mineral Waters..... 401

Proceedings of Societies.

Ontario College of Physicians and Surgeons......... 126

The Great West and the Vancouver Meeting of the Canadian Medical Association 244

The Ontario Medical Association Convention 95

Physician's Library.

Abbott's Alkaloidal Digest. By W. C. Abbott, M.D..................... 74

A Clinical Study of Blood-Pressure. By Theodore C. Janeway, M.D........... 222

A Guide to the Clinical Examination of the Blood for Diagnostic Purposes. By Richard C. Cabot, M.D............... 73

A Guide to Urine Testing for Nurses and Others. By Mark Robinson, L.R.C.P. 76

A Hand-Book of Pathological Anatomy and Histology. By Francis Delafield, M.D., LL.D., and T. Mitchell Prudden, M.D., LL.D 357

A Hand-Book of Surgery. By Frederic R. Griffith, M.D....................... . 429

A Manual of Nursing. By Reynold Webb Wilcox, M.A., M.D., LL.D............ 74

A Manual of the Practice of Medicine. By Frederick Taylor, M.D., F.R.C.P 368

A Manual of Practical Medical Electricity, the Rontgen Rays, Finsen Light, Radium and its Radiations and High Frequency Current. By Dawson Turner, B.A., M.D..................... 2

Appleton's Medical Dictionary. By Frank P. Foster, M.D......................... 3

A Practical Treatise on Diseases of the Skin. By Jas. Nevins Hyde, A.M., M.D., and Frank Hugh Montgomery, M.D 3

A Practical Treatise on Genito-Urinary and Venereal Diseases and Syphilis. By Robert W. Taylor, A.M., M.D..... 2

A Practical Treatise on Medical Diagnosis for Students and Physicians. By John H. Musser, M.D.....................

A Reference Hand-Book of the Medical Sciences. By Albert H. Buck, M.D... 3

Aseptic and Antiseptic Preparations, and Treatment of Emergencies and Abdominal Operations. By Geo. Wackerhagen, M.D.. ... .

A System of Practical Surgery. By Prof. E. von Bergmann, M.D., Prof. P. von Bruns, M.D., and Prof. J. von Mikulics, M.D 219, 3

A System of Physiologic Therapeutics. Edited by Solomon Solis Cohen, A.M., M.D.......................................

A System of Practical Surgery. Edited by William T. Bull, M.D., and Carlton P. Flint M.D................................

A Text-Book of Alkaloidal Therapeutics. By W. J. Waugh, M.D., and W. A. Abbott, M.D............................ 2

A Text-Book of the Diseases of Women. By Charles B. Penrose, M.D., Ph.D.... 3

A Text-Book of Histology. By Frederick R. Bailey, A.M., M.D.................. 4

A Text-Book of Materia Medica. By Robert A. Hatcher, Ph.G., M.D., and Torald Sollmann, M.D................. 3

A Text-Book of Mechano-Therapy. By Axel V. Grafstrom, B.Sc., M. D........ 2

A Treatise on Obstetrics for Students and Practitioners. By Edward P. Davis, A.M., M.D 3

A Text-Book of Pathology for Practitioners and Students. By Joseph McFarland, M.D 3

A Text-Book of Physiological Chemistry. By Charles E. Simon, M.D..... 43

A Text-Book of Physiology. By Isaac Ott, A.M., M.D........ ....; 7

A Text-Book of Human Physiology. By Albert P. Brubaker, A.M., M.D........ 36

Blakiston's Quiz Compends. By W. T. St. Clair, A.M....\ 4

Atlas and Epitome of Diseases of the Mouth, Pharynx, and Nose By Dr. L. Grunwald, of Munich.. 22

Cap'n Eri. By Joseph C. Lincoln . . 221
Case Teaching in Surgery. By Herbert L.
    Burrell, M.D., and John Bapst Blake,
    M.D... 75
Commoner Diseases of the Eye: How to
    Detect and How to Treat Them. By
    Casey A. Wood, C M., M D., and
    Thomas A. Woodruff, M.D 72
Diseases of the Eye. By L. Webster Fox,
    A.M., M D............................... 72
Diseases of the Gall-Bladder and Bile-
    Ducts, Including Gall-Stone. By A.
    W. Mayo Robson, F.R.C.S.... 67
Diseases of the Intestines and Peritoneum.
    By Dr. Hermann Nothnagel............ 295
Diseases of the Nervous System. By F.
    Savary Pearce, M.D 435
Diseases of the Stomach and Their Surgical
    Treatment. By A. W. Mayo Robson,
    F.R.C.S., and B. G. A. Moynihan, M.S.,
    London, F.R.C.S 228
Elementary Practical Physiology. By
    John Thornton, M.A.. 434
Encyclopedia Medica. Edited by Chalmers
    Watson, M.D 429
Epilepsy and its Treatment. By William
    P. Spratling, M.D..... 225
Essentials of Anatomy. By Charles B.
    Nancrede, M.D 436
Essentials of Materia Medica, Thera-
    peutics and Prescription Writing. By
    Henry Morris, M.D 430
Essentials of Nervous Diseases and In-
    sanity; Their Symptoms and Treat-
    ment. By John C. Shaw, M.D 432
Fatigue. Edited by Prof. J. McKeen Cat-
    tell, M A.. Ph.D., and F. E. Beddard,
    M.A.. F.R.S 227
Graves' Disease, With and Without Ex-
    ophthalmic Goitre. By William
    Hanna Thompson, M.D., LL.D... 297
Guide to the Examination of the Throat,
    Nose and Ear. By Wm. Lamb, M.D. . 432
Insanity in Every-day Practice. By E. G.
    Younger, M.D 223
International Clinics. Edited by A. O. J.
    Kelly, M.D. 220, 436
Kirke's Hand-Book of Physiology. By
    Frederick C. Busch, B.S., M.D 371
Lectures on Clinical Psychiatry. By Dr.
    Emil Kraepelin 433
Lectures to General Practitioners on the
    Diseases of the Stomach and Intestine's
    By Boardman Reed, M.D........ 367
Malignant Disease of the Larynx—Carci-
    noma and Sarcoma. By Philip De
    Santi, F.R.C.S...................... 437
Manual of Materia Medica and Pharmacy.
    By E. Stanton Muir, Ph.G., V.M.D... 67
Medical Electricity. By H. Lewis Jones,
    M.A., M.D............................ 430
Medical Laboratory Methods and Tests.
    By Herbert French, M.A., M.D. 75
Medical Monograph Series. By Wyatt
    Wingrave 371
Medical Jurisprudence, Insanity and
    Toxicology. By Henry C. Chapman,
    M.D.............................. .... 228, 370

Modern Ophthalmology. By James Moores
    Ball, M.D..... ..:.... 29
Obstetric and Gynecologic Nursing. By
    Edward P. Davis, A.M., M.D 2
Old Gorgon Graham. By George Horace
    Lorimer 4:
Practical Materia Medica for Nurses. By
    Emily A. M. Stoney .... 3(
Progressive Medicine. By Hobart Amory
    Hare, M.D .... 1.
Radiotherapy and Phototherapy. By
    Charles Warrenuc Allen, M.D.. ...... 3.
Regional Minor Surgery. By Geo. Gray
    Van Schaick.......... 4
Rontgen Ray Diagnosis and Therapy. By
    Carl Beck. M.D......................
Small Hospitals: Establishment and Main-
    tenance. By A. Worcester, A:M.. M.D. 2
Special Diagnosis of Internal Medicine. By
    Dr. Wilhelm v. Leuhe..... .... 1.
Text-Book of Nervous Diseases and Psychi-
    atry. By Chas. L. Dana, A.M., M.D... 3
Text-Book of Human Physiology. By Dr.
    L. Landois.... 4
The Art of Compounding. By Wilbur L.
    Scoville, Ph.G.. . ... 4.
The Bacteriology of Every-Day Practice.
    By J. Odery Symes, M.D............ .
The Doctor's Recreation Series. By Chas.
    Wells Moulton.................. 218, 297, 3
The Man Who Pleases and the Woman
    Who Charms. By John A. Cone .....
The Nutrition of the Infant. By Ralph
    Vincent, M.D........................... 4
The Physician's Visiting List for 1905...... 4
The Practical Application of the Roentgen
    Rays in Therapeutics and Diagnosis.
    By Wm. Allen Pusey, A.M., M.D...... 4
The Practice of Medicine. By James
    Tyson, M.D............................. 3
The Practical Medicine Series of Year
    Books. By Gustavus P. Head, M.D.
    .... 69, 156, 2
The Principles and Practice of Gynecology
    for Students and Practitioners. By
    E. C. Dudley, A.M., M.D................ 3
The Principles of Hygiene. By D. H.
    Bergey, A.M., M.D..................... 3
The Seaboard Magazine.................... 2
The Surgical Treatment of Bright's Dis-
    ease. By George M. Edebohls, A.M.,
    M.D., LL.D.............................. 3
The Utero-Ovarian Artery; or, The Genital,
    Vascular Circle. By Byron Robinson,
    B.S., M.D. 3
The Urine and Clinical Chemistry of the
    Gastric Contents, the Common Poisons
    and Milk. By J. W. Holland, M.D.... 3
Tuberculosis and Acute General Miliary
    Tuberculosis. By Dr. G. Cornet, of
    Berlin........ ....../............... 2

The Canadian
Journal of Medicine and Surgery

A JOURNAL PUBLISHED MONTHLY IN THE INTEREST OF
MEDICINE AND SURGERY

VOL. XVI.   TORONTO, JULY, 1904.   NO. 1.

Original Contributions.

PRESIDENT'S ADDRESS.*

BY J. F. W. ROSS, M.D., TORONTO.

Gentlemen,—There are pinnacles to which we reach, only to be hurled down from the dizzy height into the valley below, to be hidden from the rude storms of the world where peace and quiet and easy-going hum-drum pervades the spot, while the green grass grows under the feet. This is the well-known valley of the "Have-beens." Hills have only two sides, one going up and the other going down, and when one has reached such honor as you have conferred upon me, he has climbed the up-side and must begin to descend. One is elated with the honor, but grieved with a retrospect of all that led up to it; one is pleased with the evidence of the good-will of his fellows—and a better lot of fellows never lived in any profession—but subdued with that soul-shaking feeling that youth is fleeting and age approaching. Each man naturally looks forward to the day upon which he may occupy the presidential chair, but when the day comes he would give much to be able to postpone the honor for another ten years. And now it is time for the past-presidents to move up and make room for me; but I do not intend to be placed upon the shelf, if health and strength remain. We all like to mingle with youth, but unfortunately youth and age were never meant to mix. Charles Kingsley has aptly put it:

> "When all the world is old, lad,
> And all the trees are brown;
> And all the sport is stale, lad,
> And all the wheels run down;

---

* Delivered at meeting of Ontario Medical Association, June, 1904.

4

Creep home and take your place there
  The spent and maimed among ;
God grant you find a face there
  You loved, when all was young."

It is a satisfaction, in dealing with the awful miseries of life, to know that others suffer, that suffering and death are the accompaniments of life, and from this springs much of the beautiful sympathy that is witnessed by our profession. We have a grand work to do. Charles Dickens has put it in the words of the doctor's wife, where she says, " We are not rich in the bank, but we have always prospered, and we have quite enough. I never walk with my husband but I hear the people bless him. I never go into a house of any degree but I hear his praises or see them in grateful eyes. I never lie down at night but I know that in the course of that day he has alleviated pain and soothed some fellow-creature in the time of need. I know that from the beds of those who were past recovery, thanks have often gone up in the last hour for his patient ministration. Is not this to be rich ?"

The young doctor must have as his main master faculty-sense-common-sense, and he must have a real turn for the profession. A great divine has said, " The grace of God can do much, but it canna gie a man common-sense." The danger of the present day is that the mind gets too much of too many things. A young medical student may have, as one author puts it, zeal, knowledge, ingenuity, attention, a good eye, a steady hand; he may be an accomplished anatomist, histologist, analyst, and yet with all the lectures and all the books and other helps of his teachers, he may be beaten in treating a whitlow or a colic by the nurse in the wards, or the old country doctor who was present at his birth. The prime qualifications for a doctor have been given by Dr. Brown in the words, Capax, Perspicax, Sagax, Efficax. Capax—room for the reception and proper arrangement of knowledge. Perspicax—a keen and accurate perception. Sagax—the power of judging, ability to choose and reject. Efficax—the will to do and a knowledge of the way to do it; the power to use the other three qualities.

The doctor must have a discerning spirit. There is a nick of time, or in other words, a presence of mind, and this he must have, or as Dr. Chalmers has said, " Power and promptitude." " Has he wecht, he has promptitude, has he power. He has power, has he promptitude, and moreover has he a discerning spirit." The doctor must be as a general in the field or the pilot in a storm. I often think he belongs to no one in particular, but is public property. His time is never his own. His children see little of him, and he leads a sort of Bohemian life—restless, active, thoughtful, worried, much beloved and occasionally cordially hated. He should be Bohemian in his tastes if he wishes for refinement to soften his manners and make him less of a wild beast. Art and literature, however, help to make noble only what is already noble, but such hobbies elevate and improve the mind and lift it above the rut of every-day life. A good education is a first essential. It is not necessary that everybody should know everything, but it is more to the purpose that every man when his turn comes should be able to do some one thing. "The boy who teaches himself natural history by actual bird nesting is healthier and happier, better equipped in body and mind for the battle of life, than the nervous, interesting, feverish boy with the big head and thin legs—the wonder of his class." It is well to have a pursuit as well as a study.

The doctor should marry, but his wife should be kept out of his work. Goldsmith said, "I was ever of opinion that the honest man, who married and brought up a large family, did more service than he who continued single and only talked of population." By marriage a man's sympathies are extended and his views of life are broadened. A touching picture of the refining influence of sorrow has been given us by Dr. Brown, the author of "Rab and His Friends," in speaking of his father. He says: "A child, the image of himself, lovely, pensive, and yet ready for any fun, with a keenness of affection, that perilled everything on being loved, who must cling to some one, and be clasped, made for a garden, not for the rough world, the child of his old age. This peculiar meeting of opposites was very marked. She was stricken with sudden illness. Her mother was gone, and so she was to her father the flower he had the sole keeping of, and his joy in her wild mirth, watching her childish moods of sadness, as if a shadow came over her young heaven, were themselves something to watch. She sunk at once and without pain, her soul quick and unclouded, and her little forefinger playing to the last with her father's curls, her eyes trying in vain to brighten his. The anguish, the distress, was intense; in its essence, permanent. He went mourning and looking for her all his days." But the affection, we learn, softened and refined him and made him better fitted for his work. His son tells us further, that "his affectionate ways with his students were often very curious. He contrived to get at their hearts and find out all their family and local specialities in a sort of shorthand way, and he never forgot them in after life." And such attentions are valued throughout life, and the clay is moulded and figured, and ornamented, enriched and burned in the fire and fitted for the battle of life. And the defective articles must be rejected, and the broken articles may, perhaps, be mended, but they are never the same again, and perhaps we would be better without them. Our ranks must be kept clean. We must have a good, healthy professional growth, and in Ontario, I am glad to say, that such exists. The regular who adopts the methods of the quack, is a much more dangerous individual than the quack himself. But we have others, who are by no means quacks, who unfortunately lack discernment, and who do not mean to do the harm that they certainly occasion. Our duty is to relieve and not to cause suffering. Some surgical procedures of the present day require severe criticism. Surgeons may be too conservative or not conservative enough. A few years ago we had an epidemic of the former, and now we are suffering from a plague of the latter. We are able to do so much that we are apt to do more than we should. I hope that the few dangerous individuals will soon be quarantined, so that the death rate and the cripple rate may diminish, and the epidemic be checked. The epidemic has been spreading and has assumed large proportions, and seems to affect chiefly young and middle-aged, nervous women. Men with exposed organs appear to be fairly free from its ravages.

But as a profession in general we have been making great strides. The State is being saved from the enormous losses incident to great epidemics, and the medical profession is out of pocket, as a consequence. It does not appear that proper efforts have been made to reimburse the doctors. We are asked to do what our friends the lawyers would take good care not to do, without a proper arrangement for the payment of a proper fee. We are asked to register births, to register deaths, to notify regarding infectious diseases, and to attend to the poor without remuneration. These are not charities. We are assisting and defending the commonwealth, and the commonwealth should pay us, and we should organize and agitate with this end in view. Unless such matters are attended to and a new method of payment of members of the profession is adopted, the numbers entering must be considerably reduced. In China the doctor is paid for keeping the family in good health. In Canada, we, as a profession, protect the people from dangerous diseases, but the services are not paid for, and are scarcely recognized. A few officials take all the fees. Our real charity is not among the really needy, but among the apparently well-to-do. A proper revision of the relations of medical and surgical fees to one another is much needed, and a ruling of the Association on the ethics of commissions is required. A special committee of this Association should be appointed to investigate these matters and submit a report at our next meeting.

It has been said that knowledge is no barren cold essence, but it is alive with the colors of the earth and sky and is radiant with light and stars. "If we endeavor to follow along the lines of experimental investigation of natural phenomena, we must obtain a fondness for the impartiality and truth which such a study incites," says Draper. "We will thus dedicate our days to the good of the human race, so that in the fading light of life's evening we may not, on looking back, be forced to acknowledge how insignificant and useless are the objects that we have pursued."

A paragraph that has greatly interested me by way of retrospect, is the following: "In olden times the surface of the Continent of Europe was for the most part covered with pathless forests; here and there it was dotted with monasteries and towns. There were low-lying districts, sometimes hundreds of miles in extent, that spread agues far and wide. In Paris and in London, the two largest cities, the houses were built of wood and daubed with clay, and the roofs were thatched with straw or reeds. There were no windows, and very few had wooden floors until after the introduction of the saw-mill, and such a thing as a carpet was unknown. A little straw scattered here and there in the room was the covering used for the floor. As there were no windows, the smoke of the ill-fed, cheerless fire escaped, Indian wigwam-wise, through a hole in the roof. It is needless to say that in such habitations there was but little protection from the weather. No attempt was made at drainage, and the putrefying garbage and rubbish were thrown out of the doors. Men, women and children slept in the same apartment and not unfrequently with domestic animals as companions, and, as a consequence, neither modesty nor morality could be maintained. The bed was usually a bag of straw and a wooden log for a pillow. Personal cleanliness was unknown, and great officers of the State, even dignitaries so high as the Archbishop of Canterbury, swarmed with vermin. Perfumes were largely used to conceal personal impurity. Many of the citizens clothed themselves in leather, a garment that with its ever-accumulating impurity lasted for many years. If a man could procure fresh meat once a week for his dinner he was considered to be in easy circumstances. Not only was there no house drainage but there was no street sewerage. There were no pavements or street lamps. After nightfall the shutters were thrown open and the slops were unceremoniously emptied down, to the discomfiture of the wayfarer tracking his path through the narrow streets with his lantern in his hand." What a picture for us to criticise in the present day. And yet we scarcely realize all the hard work, ignorance, bigotry, persecution and glorious self-denial that have given us what we have to-day in our Western civilization. Much progress has been due to the work of societies, such as that grand old society, The Royal Society of London. As University men and as educationalists, knowing as we do that our present-day conditions are due to the dissemination of knowledge, we should organize and promote similar societies and see to it that they hold as prominent a place in the community as the churches. It was by the Royal Society that Harvey's discovery of the circulation of the blood was first accepted. The same society gave so much encouragement to vaccination that Queen Caroline submitted her own children to the operation. All scientific observers are satisfied that Queen Caroline was right and the Royal Society was right. Then it was demonstrated that scurvy, the curse of long sea voyages, could be cured by the use of vegetable substances. We follow along and find jails and buildings ventilated and illuminated with gas. Cities were lit up and made much more habitable. If we expect to have progress, we must rally around our educational institutions and see to it that they are well provided with the means required to carry on, efficiently and well, the work of scientific investigation, and that they are untrammelled by the views of either Church or State, remembering always that the slogan of the twentieth century is " Knowledge is power." If this is done, man cannot lapse again into the dark days of the dismal centuries, when pestilences were looked upon as the visitations of God and not as we know them to be, the consequences of filth and wretchedness, easily prevented by personal and municipal cleanliness. In the twelfth century it was found necessary to pave the streets of Paris, as the stench from them was unbearable. Dysenteries and spotted fever, that had been prevalent, diminished, and a sanitary condition was soon established that approached to that of the Moorish cities of Spain that had been paved for centuries. But alas! for backsliding. Many of the Spanish cities have been allowed to lapse into an unsanitary condition, and the evidences of Spanish sanitation, as I saw it in Cuba, were not calculated to excite enthusiasm. Under the control of Western civilization and the proper application of knowledge, matters have been changed. When it was decided that plagues were not a visitation of God, quarantine was established. Nothing has protected the human race to greater extent than the establishment of proper quarantine. When anesthetics were first introduced, their use in labor was discouraged, as it was believed that women should not escape the curse denounced against them in Genesis. Now anesthetics are, I hope, very universally used to prevent the awful agonies of labor, by an enlightened, educated, scientific and humane profession. The very best evidence that can be brought forward to emphasize the benefits to mankind of improved methods of living has been obtained from the British Government reports of life insurance transactions, carried out in the seventeenth and again, a hundred years later, in the eighteenth century. " In 1693 the British Government borrowed money by selling annuities on lives from infancy upwards, on the basis of the average longevity. The contract was profitable. Ninety-seven years later, another tontine, or scale of annuities on the basis of the same expectation of life as in the previous century, was issued. These latter annuitants, however, lived so much longer than their predecessors that it proved to be a very costly loan for the Government. It was found that while 10,000 of each sex in the first tontine died under the age of twenty-eight, 5,772 males and 6,416 females in the second tontine died at the same age one hundred years later;" or in other words, 20,000 died in the first period and only 12,188 in the second period of one hundred years later, a very greatly diminished mortality, all conditions being identical except the improvements wrought by improved sanitation.

Once fairly introduced, discovery and invention have unceasingly advanced at an accelerated pace. Each continually reacted on the other, continually they sapped supernaturalism. The diffusion of knowledge by the newspapers and reviews has immensely increased the power of the press. Where ignorance reigns, crime is prevalent. In such cities as Naples, where the education laws, such as we have in Ontario, either do not exist or are not enforced, the streets are filled with street arabs, who are a nuisance and a menace to society, growing up in squalor, ignorance and filth. In our Western civilization such a condition of affars cannot exist, and I trust never will exist. The intellectual enlightenment, surrounding scientific activity, has imparted innumerable and invaluable blessings to the human race. Science is not confined to any one nation, but is cosmopolitan. We are living in an age of electric progress. The marvels of electric force have been studied and utilized for the great benefit of mankind. To-day the mummified remains of an Egyptian King, Amenophis II., who died 1436 B.C., are viewed in the original tomb with the aid of the rays of the electric light. The almost universal use of the electric light aids our work very materially. The telegraph and telephone are to be found in the very heart of Darkest Africa! The discovery of the achromatic microscope has rendered us great assistance in studving the nature of disease, and the X-ray has enabled us to pierce what was before impenetrable gloom. The harvest is ready, but not riper than it has been for centuries, but there are more enlightened and better educated and better equipped workers in the field. There is very much to be done, and we must be constantly up and doing. I say this particularly to the young and enthusiastic. The foundation of our knowledge as modern doctors is science, and the superstructure must be built upon scientific lines.

Hospitals are needed, not such as those that were first established, but modern, properly equipped and up-to-date institutions, with modern, up-to-date methods. Many hospitals have been erected through the munificence of individuals in the towns throughout our country. Every town of any size should have its hospital. Such institutions are not intended to do the work of the larger ones in larger centres, but there is a certain amount of work that can never reach the larger centres that can be done very satisfactorily in small hospitals properly equipped and served by a properly educated profession. Assistance from the larger fields of observation can be obtained when required and under improved conditions such aid will be of greater service.

Our prisons have been improved. Our younger criminals have been cared for. Our insane have been kept off the streets. Our poor are being looked after, and now health and comfort go hand in hand. The true function of our study and deliberation is to prevent rather than to cure disease, and we are fulfilling our functions. But yet death reigns everywhere and at all times, and in all places, and we know it. But he is not the stalking giant that he was. He has been marvellously reduced in stature. Our medical press requires considerable regeneration. The articles published are not censored as rigidly as they should be. Much that is written and published is incomplete, speculative, and inaccurate, and hence misleading. Our journals should be purely scientific publications, and not the hot-beds for the propagation of unstable theories. Looking back is not always a pleasant pastime, but there is a definite certainty about it that does not belong to the future. All that has been printed is liable at any time to be reviewed.

And now in closing, let me say that during the year that has passed, a much' desired amalgamation has been effected between two of our greatest educational institutions, Trinity and Toronto Universities. At first the task looked like a hopeless one, but owing to the good feeling existing between the rival faculties, it was finally achieved. Our province stands high in the banking world, in the musical world, and in the educational world. I was gratified to hear our Provincial University so well spoken of in the Motherland, and even in Egypt. The medical faculty of the University of Toronto, as now constituted, with its ever-increasing facilities, stands second to none, in Canada, at least; and the work accomplished, as evidenced by the standing obtained by our students abroad, is of a very high order.

Fathered by this Association is an institution intended to be a guardian and repository of our archives. We must be prepared to preserve our records for the use and assistance of those who come after us. A calamity befell the world when the Alexandrian Library was burned, and a calamity would befall the profession of this province if the books, collected under the name of the Ontario Medical Library, should meet with a similar fate. We are about to occupy new premises, but we need more money to carry on the good work. This is not a municipal matter but a provincial and professional need, and I hope that many of the out-of-town members of this Association will assist us. Such an institution to do the work well must be liberally endowed.

Three trustees have been appointed, and through the generosity of the members of the profession of Toronto, of our good friend, Prof. Wm. Osler, of Mr. George Gooderham, of Mr. E. B. Osler, Mr. Timothy Eaton and the executors of the estate of the late H. A. Massey, ten thousand dollars are already in sight.

I desire to thank this Association for the great honor it has conferred upon me, and to thank those who have organized and arranged this meeting.

I feel sure that the hope and desire of every member of this vigorous twenty-four-year-old Association is that it may long be spared to unite, to teach, and to guide the medical profession of this our great province.

ACUTE BRONCHITIS.

BY R. J. SMITH, M.D., CHICAGO, ILL.

WHILE this is one of the most common diseases at this time of the year, and often follows a mild course, receiving but little attention either from the patient or the physician, it very frequently becomes very serious and even threatens a fatal issue. Many cases of tuberculosis no doubt result from what was in the beginning thought to be but a mild " cold on the chest." Others, neglected or perfunctorily treated with little attention to hygiene, develop into pneumonia. Many of the so-called mild attacks are the forerunners of that *bete noir* of the family physician— chronic bronchitis.

In spite of the frequency of this disease, it is still treated empirically by the most advanced authors, and by the great majority of practicians; in other words, there has been found no " specific." Each case must be treated individually, each case is a law " unto itself."

As it is often the expression of a constitutional state, especially in those recurring cases which arise on the least exposure to damp, cold weather, non-elimination is always an important factor in the causation. Autotoxemia is a predisposing cause. The rheumatic diathesis often shows itself by frequent attacks of acute bronchitis; and these frequently follow by extension from an antecedent coryza, pharyngitis or laryngitis.

As preventive treatment, the hygiene of the body should be especially attended to at the change in the seasons, and a course of free elimination should be given. Proper clothing should be worn and too early change from heavy to light restricted.

The medicinal treatment of the acute attack of a simple bronchitis is directed against the inflammatory element, and the nerve irritation producing cough, often digestive disturbances.

For this purpose, aconitine amorphous, 1-134 grain, should be given every fifteen minutes to every half-hour or hour, until the fever is reduced. This occurs when the congestion and inflammation are relieved. The dose should then be continued at longer intervals until the patient recovers.

For the cough, morphine hydrobromate 1-67 grain may be given, with aconitine in alternation, or together with it. If the pulse is weak, digitalin and strychnine arsenate may be given with aconitine, or as combined in the compound granule, dosimetric trinity, one of which, especially in asthenic conditions, may be given every fifteen minutes, every half-hour, or every hour, as required by the severity of the case. In asthenic cases, the defervescent granule may be given in the same dosage, until the circulation is equalized, and then continued at intervals to keep up effect. This contains aconitine and digitalin, with veratrine.

This, with some protective covering to the chest-wall, and for this purpose absorbent cotton is as good as any, especially if the chest be first rubbed with hot oil, is all that is needed in the majority of cases. Sometimes our smaller patients and some of the larger ones derive great benefit from heat to the chest-wall. When the pain is acute, a mustard poultice helps as a counter-irritant. Poultices as usually applied, are an abomination, though the heat does certainly alleviate the discomfort; but not by " jumping spaces "—simply by the dilation of the superficial arterioles by contact of heat, and also through the vasomotor nerves. Heat relaxes spasm, and with congestion and consequent dilatation in the pulmonary vessels, there is a constriction of the capillaries in the skin. Derivate the blood to the skin, and you must necessarily lessen the congestion in the lung.

At this stage, the dry irritative stage, with dry, hard, tickling cough, burning beneath the sternum, fever and thirst, nothing is needed in excess of the above treatment but a thorough emptying of the bowel—most diseases have their origin in bowel derangement—and prevention of draughts.

To empty the bowel, a few fractional doses of calomel followed by a saline laxative are all-sufficient.

If the catarrhal stage is present, with hard cough and the raising after considerable effort of tough viscid sputa, some of the expectorants are necessary. That which acts the pleasantest and liquefies the secretion most readily, is emetine—given in doses of 1-67 grain to children, 1-6 grain to adults and older children, every fifteen minutes or every half-hour till secretion is raised more freely or slight nausea is produced. Then the dose is given at increasing intervals as needed. Scillitin, 1-67 grain, may be given if a stimulant expectorant is required.

If the expectoration is free and purulent, calcium sulphide is indicated, giving grain 1-6 every hour until the breath smells of the drug. Cubebin, ammonium benzoate, stimulants to mucous membranes, may be given.

If the spasmodic element is pronounced, camphor monobromate, grain 1-6, or atropine sulphate, 1-250 grain, may be given to relieve.

In children, aconitine amorphous, 1-134 grain, emetine, grain 1-67, or apomorphine, grain 1-67, or Infant's Anodyne (nickel bromide, codeine, ipecac, etc.), may be given together in sweetened solution—one of each for each year of the child's age, and one additional granule, to twenty-four teaspoonfuls of water —a teaspoonful every fifteen minutes, every half-hour or hour, until the symptoms are relieved. Strychnine hypophosphite or brucine should be given daily.

This treatment will relieve rapidly, pleasantly, and safely. Given early, it will " jugulate " every case.

In diathetic cases the foregoing treatment may need some extension, by giving colchicine, grain 1-250, arbutin, grain 1-6, lithium benzoate, grain 1-6, one of each every hour or two, to increase elimination.

In asthenic or tuberculous subjects, a tonic form of treatment is indicated. Iodoform or calcium iodized (Calcidin), for the alterative effect of iodine, is very helpful. Give also iron phos-phate, grain 1-6, strychnine arsenate, grain 1-134, or the triple arsenates of iron, quinine and strychnine, with nuclein, three tablets every three hours, to increase metabolism and nutrition, and to " take up the slack."

The diet at first should be restricted, and later very nutritious and easily assimilated. Alcohol in any form is unnecessary and positively injurious. The coal-tar derivatives are not indicated or particularly useful. The usual cough mixtures do more harm than good, very often containing antagonistic drugs, and upsetting the stomach digestion by the syrup they contain.

The indications should be met by single remedies, directed against the underlying conditions present. In this regard, the use of active, reliable preparations given dosimetrically, that is, in " small dosage mathematically divided," is essential to rapid, definite, uniform results. With the active principles given in this manner, there is no possibility of uncertain results, provided that the indications for the chosen remedy are present, and the remedy given in sufficient dosage to produce results, stopping short of overaction.

Chicago, Illinois.

Public Health and Hygiene.

... IN CHARGE OF ...

J. J. CASSIDY, M.D., AND E. H. ADAMS, M.D.

REPORT NO. 1 OF THE COMMITTEE ON EPIDEMICS TO THE ONTARIO PROVINCIAL BOARD OF HEALTH.

Mr. Chairman and Gentlemen,—Your Committee on Epidemics wish to draw your attention to the fact, which is being more emphasized each month, that there exists an almost entire disregard for those sections of the Public Health Act which require that each and every case of typhoid fever (enteric) should be notified.

The sections of the Act relating to the notification of this disease are as follows:

" 86. Whenever any householder knows that any person within his family or household has the smallpox, diphtheria, scarlet fever, cholera or typhoid fever, he shall (subject in case of refusal or neglect to the penalties provided by subsection 2 of section 115), within twenty-four hours, give notice thereof to the local Board of Health, or the medical health officer, or by a communication addressed to him and duly mailed within the above time specified, and in case there is no M. H. O., then to the Secretary of the local Board of Health, either at his office or by communication as aforesaid. R.S.O. 1887, c. 205, s. 77."

" 89. Whenever any physician knows that any person whom he is called on to visit is infected with smallpox, scarlet fever, diphtheria, typhoid or cholera, such physician shall (subject in case of refusal or neglect to the penalties provided by sub-section 2 of section 115) within twenty-four hours give notice thereof to the local Board of Health or medical health officer of the municipality in which such diseased person is and in such manner as is directed by rules 2 and 3 of section 17 of schedule B, R.S.O. 1887, c. 205, s. 80."

It is, therefore, quite evident that the Public Health Act requires both the householder and physician in charge of a case of typhoid fever, to notify the local health authorities of each case within twenty-four hours, and for this purpose it is the duty of each local Board of Health, either through its health officer or secretary, to provide each medical practitioner in its municipality with blank forms, upon which to report any case. (Rule 1, sec. 17, schedule B, R.S.O.)

To remove misapprehension respecting the outcome of the notification of typhoid fever, should any such exist in the minds of members of local boards of health or medical practitioners, your Committee deem it advisable to state that while the Ontario Health Act requires the householder and attending physician to report a case of typhoid fever, the local Board of Health is not required to placard the house in which a person sick with this disease is lying. According to rule 4, section 17, schedule B, R.S.O., placarding is required for scarlet fever, diphtheria, smallpox, cholera, or whooping cough, but is not considered necessary for typhoid fever. Primary notification of typhoid fever by the householder and attending physician to the local Board of Health, and secondary notification by the latter to the Provincial Board of Health are required for the following reasons:

First. That inquiries may be instituted at an early date to discover the cause of the disease, such inquiries relating chiefly to the character of the water and milk supplies used by the infected person.

Second. That preventive measures may be adopted.

Third. That trustworthy statistical facts giving information as to the prevalence of the disease, its type, mortality, etc., may be recorded.

In the Bulletin of the Provincial Board of Health of Ontario for February, 1904, the following question is asked: Are typhoid fever cases reported? Replying to this question the Bulletin states that the returns of typhoid fever by householders and physicians received during 1903 by the Provincial Board of Health amounted to only 1,012 cases. An extract is also taken from the statistics of typhoid fever given in the Annual Report of Dr. Chamberlain upon the hospitals of Ontario, for 1903, which shows that 1,231 males and 687 females were treated for typhoid fever in the Ontario hospitals during the year.

Do the hospitals notify their cases of typhoid fever?

The figures just quoted show conclusively that they do not notify them. Now admitting that an hospital is an excellent place in which to treat typhoid fever, a place which will not easily become a centre for the diffusion of that disease, the following facts also remain to be considered:

From the standpoint of hygiene, the medical health officer of a municipality should learn the nature of the local conditions which occasioned an attack of typhoid fever in a person living in his municipality, in order to exercise his preventive powers as promptly as possible.

A patient with typhoid fever is treated in some private house or in an hospital, either of which may be situated in the municipality in which the patient contracted the disease, or in another municipality of this Province. Should the patient be treated in a private house of the municipality in which the disease was contracted a report from the householder and one from the attending physician will answer. If in an hospital of the municipality, one from the medical superintendent would answer. If the patient is being treated in another municipality, similar reports would be called for; and in addition the medical health officer of the municipality in which the patient is domiciled, who should be advised in the notification that the patient was not residing in his municipality at the time when he contracted typhoid fever, would also report to the medical health officer of the municipality in which the patient was residing when he contracted typhoid fever. Notification of this nature would draw expert attention to the local conditions or circumstances which had occasioned the disease in question, and the medical health officer of the municipality where the disease had occurred being informed of the possible source of the trouble would be placed in a position to exercise proper measures of prevention. There can be little doubt, therefore, that public health would benefit very much if such a system of notification were made obligatory, as the majority, if not all, of the cases of typhoid fever which occur in Ontario would be known, not only to the physicians or hospital superintendents who may have medical charge of them, but also to the medical health officers of the municipalities to which they respectively belong.

It is reasonable to think that if superintendents of hospitals who have charge every year of a large number, perhaps the majority, of the typhoid fever cases in Ontario, were bound by law to notify these cases, in the way mentioned above, private medical practitioners would not be so likely to neglect their duty in this particular, but would learn to imitate so excellent an example.

Such a system of notification would inevitably lead to the extinguishment of unsuspected local conditions which regularly produce typhoid fever, and the irrelevancies which now exist between morbidity and mortality statistics of typhoid fever in Ontario would soon disappear.

Your Committee would therefore advise that the facts and figures embodied in this report should receive your careful consideration, and that any conclusions you may form relating to this matter should be drafted in the form of a circular and mailed as soon as possible to the Medical Health Officers, Local Boards of Health, Medical Superintendents of Hospitals, Asylums, etc., and to all the medical practitioners of this Province.

Your Committee would also advise that in the circular here referred to attention should be drawn to the fact that samples of drinking water are examined free at the Provincial Laboratory, and that persons desirous of having such examinations made should apply to Dr. J. A. Amyot, bacteriologist of the Board, for properly sterilized bottles, in which the samples of water should be placed. Emphasis might also be given to the fact that physicians may forward samples of suspected blood to the laboratory in order to have the Widal test made.

It may be feared that the reporting of cases by medical superintendents of hospitals may cause re-duplication, it being possible that physicians, who have seen cases before they were admitted to the hospitals, may already have reported. The attention of medical health officers would need to be drawn to this possibility, with the request that they look over the names and addresses of the persons reported to them to avoid re-duplication.

Your Committee also desire to draw your attention to a leaflet prepared by them and containing personal and general precautions suitable to prevent the spread of consumption. Your Committee ask your endorsation of this leaflet, and if it is satisfactory, request your permission to print copies for distribution throughout this Province. The following is the text of the leaflet:

Personal Precautions Against Consumption.

1. Consumption is contracted by taking into the system, chiefly through inhalation, the germ or microbe of the disease.

2. This germ is contained in the sputum or spit of the consumptive, and the minute droplets which he sprays into the air in coughing or sneezing. The germ may be inhaled directly through the air. When the sputum and droplets become dry they mingle with the dust, and being inhaled with it, introduce the germ into the body; or the germ may be inhaled directly through the air.

3. The consumptive person, therefore, must not expectorate about the house or on the floor of any public building, cab, street car, railway carriage, or other conveyance, nor on the street or other public place.

4. The consumptive must not expectorate anywhere except in a spittoon kept for the purpose, which spittoon should contain water to which a disinfectant has been added—preferably a 5 per cent. solution of carbolic acid, which is prepared by dissolving one ounce of carbolic acid in one imperial pint of hot water.

5. When absent from his own room the consumptive should use a small wide-mouthed bottle with a carefully fitting cap (pocket spittoon), the contents of which when emptied should be

destroyed, and the receptacle carefully cleansed, being kept in boiling water for at least ten minutes.

6. A consumptive should not spit into a handkerchief but, if not provided with a spittoon, should use a piece of cloth or paper, which should be burned at the first opportunity.

7. Handkerchiefs which may have been used should be boiled one half-hour before being washed.

8. Consumptives should not swallow their phlegm, as by so doing the disease may be conveyed to parts of the body not already affected.

9. Kissing by consumptives should be prohibited. When coughing a consumptive patient should always hold a handkerchief in front of the mouth, and should avoid coughing in the direction of another person.

10. The greatest care should be taken to prevent the smearing of hands, face, clothing and bed clothes with the sputa. Should any accident of the kind happen, the parts should be immediately cleansed, and for this reason the clothing and wearing apparel of consumptives should be thoroughly disinfected before being used by others.

11. A consumptive should not hold a situation in which he is required to handle the food or wearing apparel of others.

12. A room occupied by a consumptive should not be swept or dusted. Such few floor rugs as are used should be frequently taken up and exposed to the sunlight and also disinfected at intervals. They should on no account be shaken, beaten or swept. In cleaning such rooms wet cloths must be used to wipe the floor, woodwork, windows, furniture, etc., and these cloths should be frequently boiled. These rooms should be thoroughly cleansed at least once a month, in addition to the daily cleaning.

13. On a room being vacated by a consumptive, it should be thoroughly and completely disinfected. The wall paper (if any) should be removed, and the walls, ceiling and floor well washed with a disinfectant solution and well aired.

14. Special sets of spoons, forks, knives, plates, cups, etc., should be kept for the exclusive use of each person affected, and these articles should be placed for a few minutes in boiling water, before being washed.

15. Milk and other articles of diet should not be permitted to stand in the bedroom of a consumptive; they should be brought to him in only such quantities as are required for immediate use.

General Precautions Against Consumption.

1. The special measures required for producing conditions destructive to the virulence of tubercle bacilli which may have

found lodgment in a house are fortunately those best calculated to preserve and improve the health of the inmates.

2. These are air, light, sunshine and dryness, which, while they aid in rendering individuals able to resist the establishment of the germ of disease, at the same time are most destructive to its vitality.

3. Ventilation by means of fresh air is most important for the preservation of the health of children, as well as adults, fresh air preventing the development and spread of consumption. Ventilation is essential in factories, workshops, offices and houses, particularly when the air of such places is associated with gaseous fumes and fine dust.

4. The breath from the lungs contains foul organic matter, which becomes poisonous if rebreathed. Hence the air of living and sleeping rooms, work-rooms, schools, churches and public vehicles should be quickly changed, otherwise persons breathing it become weakened, and thus may become pre-disposed to consumption.

5. Overcrowding is both dangerous and injurious to health, and should be avoided.

6. Windows should be made to open to the external air; they should be kept open day and night sufficiently to provide for a continuous supply of fresh air, but injurious draughts should be avoided.

7. Open spaces around buildings are necessary for the access of fresh air.

8. Rooms, staircases and passages should be frequently flushed with fresh air by opening windows and doors. This rule applies equally to churches, schoolrooms, factories, hotels, public halls, as well as to the homes of consumptives.

9. All rooms should be kept clean, otherwise the air can never be pure. Cleanliness and good sanitary surroundings are essential for the prevention as well as the cure of consumption.

10. To protect against the germs of tuberculosis, as found in both meat and milk, these articles of diet should be subjected to a temperature of at least 140 F. (60 C.) Meat should be well cooked through, and milk should be heated to at least 140 deg. F.

11. All bed linen and body linen should be disinfected before being sent to the wash.

12. The clothing, wearing apparel and other effects of a consumptive should either be destroyed or disinfected by superheated steam, before being used by another.

13. Never put coins, articles of the toilet, or other small objects in your mouth. Do not use a pipe, wind instrument or implement which goes to the mouth, that has been in use by any other person.

14. The extent to which outdoor exercise and fresh air should be indulged in should be regulated by the physician in charge, as also the character of clothing to be worn, and the daily dietary.

All of which is respectfully submitted.

J. J. CASSIDY.

W. OLDRIGHT.

CHAS. A. HODGETTS.

Toronto, May 4th, 1904.

THE DEGENERATION OF THE NATIONAL PHYSIQUE.

THIS subject is at present occupying a great share of public attention in Great Britain. Questions are asked about it even in the House of Lords. The *Philadelphia Press* comes to the rescue as follows:

"*Physical Decline in England.*—From statistics presented to the House of Commons by the Home Secretary there has been a steady annual increase in the last ten years in the police court cases of drunkenness in England and Wales. Between 1892 and 1896 the cases numbered 583.47 per 100,000 population; between 1897 and 1901, 642.87; in 1901, 644.84; and in 1902, 666.16. The actual number of cases has grown from 175,627 in 1892 to 219,-908 in 1902. This is a very unfortunate showing, and is all the more significant when taken in connection with the returns of recruiting officers. An army officer quoted in the London *Express* says: ' In the last twenty years stature and chest have so dwindled that if we attempted to enlist on the standard of the 80's we should reject 70 per cent. of the men offering.' Since April, 1899, the number of men rejected as unfit was 113,000 out of 365,000 candidates, and in addition 10,000 recruits were invalided within two years of enlistment. Every third man is thus a ' defective.' This is a bad showing for the United Kingdom, and a royal commission is at work to investigate the cause of this condition of the national physique."

Still, we must not get too much excited. We seem to have heard this before, and yet we live. But we like the way some people talk about it better, *e.g.,* Professor William Wright, of the University of Birmingham, who, in a popular lecture recently, on " The Degeneration of the National Physique," advocated the formation of boys' brigades and cadet corps, and suggested that the German plan of allowing ten minutes' or a quarter of an hour's play to every hour's work in school was a good one.

AN ORATION DELIVERED BY DR. W. P. C. BARTON IN 1821.
WITH EXPLANATORY NOTE.

BY WILLIAM PEPPER, M.D.,

Instructor in Medicine in the University of Pennsylvania.

In an old volume of bound manuscript lectures, addresses, etc., by Dr. William Paul Crillon Barton, at one time Professor of Botany in the University of Pennsylvania, I found the following oration, which he had delivered before the Philadelphia Medical Society as their annual orator for the year 1821. This I believe was never published, probably on account of the rather personal, and at times derogatory, remarks it contains, in reference to his fellow-professors, although it was usually the custom for the speakers, at the request of the society, to publish their addresses. The oration, however, contains such vivid descriptions of the appearances, dress, manners, and speech of such University of Pennsylvania worthies as Rush, Physick, Woodhouse, Barton, and Wistar, that I have thought it well worth publication. The manuscript is in Dr. Barton's own handwriting, and on the last page is a note which reads:

" This dream was entirely composed and written between the hours of 7 o'clock a.m. and 3 p.m. of Sunday, the 18th of Feb., 1821, and delivered as an oration before the Phila. Medical Society, without any material revision, on Tuesday afternoon, the 20th Feb., following.   W. P. C. B."

It will perhaps be best to give here a short account of the author of this strange conceit, called by him a dream, written and composed in such a very short space of time.

William Paul Crillon Barton was born in Philadelphia in 1786. While a student at Princeton he assumed the name of Count Paul Crillon, and retained the name for the rest of his life, unlike the rest of his classmates, who merely used the names of the celebrated men they had chosen during their undergraduate days. He graduated in 1805, and then entered the University of Pennsylvania, and studied medicine under the direction of his uncle, Dr. Benjamin Smith Barton, of whom he speaks in the dream. He received the degree of M.D. in 1808. He was resident physician to the Pennsylvania Hospital in 1809, serving for four months, and was not on the surgical staff, as has been stated in some biographies. Shortly afterward he became a surgeon in the U. S. Navy. In 1816 he was elected Professor of Botany in the then newly established Faculty of Natural Science in the University of Pennsylvania. The fact that this chair which he held was not part of the medical faculty seems to have preyed on his mind a great deal. He even printed a memorial to the trustees requesting them to transfer the professorship of botany to the medical faculty. Finally he resigned, probably disgruntled, in 1828; but having previously become, in 1826, Professor of Materia Medica and Botany in Jefferson Medical College. He was a Fellow of the College of Physicians, a member of the American Philosophical Society, and President of the Linnæan Society. He wrote a number of books on medical and botanical subjects. He died in Philadelphia, in 1856, at the age of sixty years.

A Dream.

Alas! the age of chivalry is gone—that of sophisters and self-aggrandizing calculators has succeeded, and the glory of Europe is extinguished forever!

Such as this was the pithy ejaculation of the prince of philosophic politicians, after presenting a rapid sketch of the crimes and enormities of the French revolution. It was midnight when I lately read it—a midnight of restless excitement which caused me to leave my couch, and court, in the prosing periods of some author, that sleep, or disposition to it, which intense study had driven from my pillow. I chanced to light on a book marked at the passage containing the expression of these sentiments; and, seduced by the strain of melancholy regret from a high-minded philosopher, at detailing scenes of anarchy and vice which they breathe, I rapidly ran my eye over the humiliating picture of irrational licentiousness, dissoluteness and perfidy, that the author has so ably portrayed.

The mind, in nocturnal excitement, is prone to revery, and however willing or desirous we may be to shun the fatigue it causes, we indulge, in despite of the faint degree of reason which a semi-consciousness leaves at our disposal, its fantasies and its freaks. The sentiments of the author struck me as strangely applicable to the disturbances, irrationalities and follies, which a history of medicine, and some of the institutions by which its doctrines are extended in the United States, is, at this epoch, unhappily characterized and racked. I know not at this time whether a full degree of consciousness or reflection attended the forcible associations in my mind, of the ruinous effect following the causes to which the author attributed the downfall of Gallic greatness, and those rapidly undermining the dignity and usefulness of the empire of medicine; but this I know, that a train of revery calculated to strengthen the idea of their identity seized irresistibly upon my mind. It was painful. I strove to shake it off. Still the idea haunted me; and gained still stronger and stronger force; till at length, wearied by excitement, and unaided by my book, in courting sleep, I threw myself into bed. Tired nature claimed her boon. Sleep soon overcame my corporeal functions, but not sufficiently profound to allay or subdue the mental excitement. Visions quickly flitted before me, each partaking of the nature of the remarkable words which had been indelibly imprinted on my memory. And, after repeated wandering of the fancy through unconnected flights, it finally presented to my weakened mind a *long connected dream.*

As allegory has always been profitably enlisted in the cause of reason and virtue and harmony, both in society and in science, it occurred to me, as soon as I awoke, to record my dream, believing that the thoughts which it occasioned were worth noticing, and under the impression, too, that there existed ample room for the animadversion they convey, in the feuds and jealousies of our profession. I further believed these causes were rapidly exhibiting such ravages as would end in the disjointed skeleton of medicine there is just reason to fear will take the place of the full and comely system of physic which the unbiased genius and the well-directed talents of our country have taught us a right to look for.

Permit me, then, gentlemen of the medical society, the privilege of a novel, but, I trust, not an uninstructive mode of addressing you on this our yearly meeting for the purpose of receiving from one of your members whom you have honored with the appointment, an annual oration. And if aught in the relation which I shall give you of my dream shall appear incongruous or censorious or sarcastic, pray recollect that it is *but a dream;* and attribute these faults, if such they appear, to a disturbed fancy, rather than a deliberate intention of being too keenly satirical or indulging in wanton sarcasm or animadversion. But if, on the contrary, you should incline to the opinion that, though only a dream, it yet bespeaks the truth—as sometimes dreams come true—unite, I beseech you, with me, heart and soul, to prevent or retard so dangerous, so ruinous a reality.

Methought I had been shipwrecked on wild and rugged shores.* My mess and ship-mates, together with the bilged vessel which had carried us, had been swallowed up in the vasty deep. Though I alone of all the crew had reached the shore, the ocean seemed thirsting for me too; for billow chased billow at my trembling feet, until I was forced to run with speed to avoid

---

*Barton graduated in 1808, and it is the account of medical affairs in that year that he is now about to discuss. The Faculty at that time consisted of Physick, B. S. Barton, Woodhouse, Rush, and Wistar. Morgan had died in 1789; Kuhn had left the Faculty in 1797; Shippen died in 1808; Hutchinson had died in 1793.

being submerged by their greedy haste. This caused me to become so faint and weary that when once assured I was beyond their foaming reach nature began to yield, and, my strength by this time completely exhausted, I tumbled over a ledge of rocks and fell, wounded and bleeding, insensible among them.

Recovered reason discovered me to be in a new but lovely country, and at that moment attended by a surgeon who had kindly dressed my wounds and informed me I had been brought to him by some fishermen who had found me, apparently dead, among the rocks. The language of this disciple of Aesculapius* was soothing and full of wisdom, brief and pithy. His stature was of the graceful height, his carriage erect, his nose rather straight than aquiline; his eyes steady, thoughtful, but not sad, and, when synchronously acting with the pleasant smile into which his lips, by some transitions from the straight of meeting, changed, it was peculiarly expressive, and lightened up his pale and interesting visage to serene cheerfulness. He was apparently on the shady side of fifty years,† with a general physiognomy strongly indicative of invincible probity, and a behavior expressive of close and retired application to business. He interrogated me respecting my country, the cause of my shipwreck, and my profession. On hearing that I had been the surgeon of the ill-fated ship, he seemed to take a new interest in conversing with me; spoke of the improvements of the art which in his country had been made; their benefit and importance, and the reasons which induced them, the chief of which was to alleviate pain and lessen the necessity of frequent operations. In a word, his whole heart and soul seemed engrossed with the principles, practice and improvements of his profession. He had mixed much in the world, in a professional way, which gave him a self-possessed and easy carriage, rendered interesting by the zest of agreeable manners; but he was still a recluse, ignorant of the deceitfulness, the duplicities and artifices of men. Innocent himself of such vices, his honesty did not appear to have put him sufficiently on his guard against the turpitude of others. On expressing my surprise at meeting with such a man as himself in a rude and desolate land, he modestly bowed and informed me that I was mistaken in supposing the country I had entered was wild, uncultivated, or destitute of physical and moral resources. He said there were institutions of a literary nature and rising character, springing up in different parts of it, and ended by telling me that one for medical instruction was in existence in the city in which he dwelt, and that he was himself

---

* Philip Syng Physick, Professor of Surgery in 1808, was born in 1768. The so-called "Father of American Surgery."

† Physick was but forty in 1808.

connected with it.* At this information I was all astonishment, and my happiness was without bound, to find that instead of being thrown on a desolate land of savages, I had been cast on the shores of a country blessed by a lovely and fertile soil, and nhabited by a race of people of native and original intellect, who were imitating all the polish and refinement of older countries, divested of the pollution which their age imparts to the general population, and of the vicious taint which superannuated political, moral and religious establishments inevitably imbibe. Eager to view this school, in one of the teachers of which I had seen so much to admire, I craved an introduction to its walls and the benefits of its instruction. " Come, young man," said this professional mentor, " accompany me. It is but a pleasant walk down yonder slope, and we are there—but mark the termination of that vista. It was an expanded lawn bordered with shrubbery and interspersed with coppices of flowering forest trees, for which this new country seemed remarkable. Thither let us hie, and there let me call your attention to him who courts its charms." Arrived at the spot, my guide pointed to a tall and plain-looking man† breaking branches from the clumps of dogwood which decorated the edge of the vista. He was loaded with twigs of the tulip tree, which appeared also an abundant production of this luxuriant spot, and a little tin box which was slung from his side was filled with gorgeous and fragrant flowers. When we approached the spot where he stood he turned suddenly towards us, and with a cordial but somewhat awkward address, accosted us by a general salutation and a particular inquiry as to who I was. He had a full, keen and brilliant black eye, which beamed intelligence and intellect in every movement. He was habited in a plain and becoming suit of drab-colored clothes, with a large white hat. His visage was small, chiefly characterized by a fine, expressive forehead, and the remarkable eyes just noticed; and his nose was, what Lavater would have pronounced, that of a sage's face. His voice was peculiar, attenuated, delicate, yet penetrating; his enunciation clear, distinct, emphatic. He was communicative, and seemed pleased with the interest I took in the objects of his pursuit. In fine, he was evidently an enthusiast in nature's charms; and became eloquent and animated when he informed me of the names of the plants and twigs of trees with which he was loaded, and dilated on their properties and uses.

A rustling among the leaves of a deep thicket near us attracted his attention from us, and with quickness and vivacity he cried out to know what new plant had been found. To whom this ques-

---

* The University of Pennsylvania.

† Benjamin Smith Barton. Professor of Materia Medica and Botany in 1808, was born in 1766. Uncle of Dr. W. P. C. Barton.

tion was addressed I could not at first understand, but anon a crowd of youths burst from behind the cornice which had screened them from our view, leaped the rill which bordered it, and crowded around him with eager and enthusiastic curiosity, each presenting some plant and interrogating him as to its name, its class and uses. I took this opportunity, while all but myself and guide were thus enwrapped, of inquiring into the meaning of this concourse of youths, loaded, like the older gentleman,. with roots and flowers, and carrying books and pencils in their hands. " That plain and intelligent-looking man," said he, " is a botanist. He is also a teacher in the school to which I belong, and to which I am conducting you. Those are his pupils in whom he inspires the enthusiasm so conspicuous in himself. But he is more. He is an acute, penetrating, and reflecting physician,. and by exploring these lovely lawns and searching those fragrant woods encircling them, he has presented us with medicinal plants of such peculiar power and merited reputation, thus rendering us no longer dependent for our materia medica on foreign countries, but actually makes them tributary to us for the products of our abundant medicinable resources. To him our school is indebted for a large share of its high and still increasing reputation; and to the fascinating and useful science of botany his invaluable medical lectures owe much of their force and utility. He has taught those pupils to depend on the produce of their native soil for active medicines; and so valuable have their preceptors (many of whom have also been his pupils) found this lesson that the class now following his perambulatory instruction contains many members actively and usefully employed in investigating the obscure and detecting the hidden properties of other plants, as the subjects of their inaugural theses. Thus,. he has been instrumental in elevating the character and genius of our country, by commanding respect for its resources, and praise of its native talents, industry and learning."*

At this moment the sky lowered, and a sudden squall of wind, accompanied by a shower, caused the group to disperse and seek shelter where it might be found. The fields were soon enveloped in a mist from the torrents of rain which sheeted the air. My guide and myself sought refuge from the storm in the excavated recess of a vicinal rock, where we had no sooner arrived before

---

* During B. S. Barton's occupancy of the Chair of Materia Medica and Botany the interest he stimulated in these subjects was truly remarkable. To quote from Carson's History of the Medical Department of the University of Pennsylvania: "If the subjects of the theses enumerated in the Catalogue of Graduates during the connection of Dr. Barton with the Medical School be examined, one cannot but be forcibly impressed with the number which treat of the Vegetable Materia Medica of the United States. It was a department which he fostered, writing not only upon it himself, but instigating his pupils to its cultivation. Nor are these essays jejune, for under the conducting hand of the master they took the form of experimental and practical utility, and the present generation is under obligation for valuable researches, in the field of home productions, to many aspirants for medical honors."

claps of loud and alarming thunder rent the heavens. The firma-
ment was overcast with deep-blue, angry-looking clouds, loaded
with rain and fraught with thunder, and finally the scene was
cloaked by dismal darkness, rendered visible by vehement momentary shafts of lightning. The most vivid of these was followed by a sudden and tremendous clap of thunder, which shook
the rock above our heads and rent asunder the shelving barricade
it formed behind us. The fragments separated, and in the breach
appeared a portly man, apparently in the prime of life and the
zenith of good cheer.* He bore a retort in his left hand, from the
mouth of which issued a flame of ignited gas, and his right was
extended toward my guide. He was dressed in full black, and inclined to corpulency. He was bald, and had his hair, of which,
indeed, little was visible, whitened by art. His carriage was bold,
frank, and courteous. He immediately invited us into his subterranean abode, not as to a place of pleasurable sojourn, but as a
safe asylum at least, as he termed it, from the terrific storm.
His conversation was sententious, his manners abrupt and eccentric; but his physiognomy, together with the deep intonations
of his manly voice, bespoke a probity of character, a generosity of
heart, and a cordial welcome, that softened those fears at entering his lonely cavern, which the gloomy aspect of its entrance inspired. My guide had on his first appearance shook him by the
hand, with marks of recognition, a circumstance in which, though
I could not help pondering, added strength to my feelings of safety,
and I no longer hesitated to grope my way, over pots, pans, cruci-
bles, retorts, and all the paraphernalia of an alchemist's abode,
toward the spot whither he led and invited us to be seated. I
now found myself, by the aid of the sudden glare of light which
was produced by a removal of the tin covers from the lantern, in
a chemist's laboratory, and, after some hours' tarry, during
which I learned more of this elegant but eccentric teacher's character, was startled by an ingress of great numbers of young men
to the laboratory, and making their way to the numerous vacant
seats in front of the teacher. Among these persons I recognized
some of those I had seen before the storm in the fields. They
had the same roots with them, and, with a confidence, evidently
inspired by the proprietor of the laboratory himself, advanced

---

* James Woodhouse was professor of Chemistry in 1808. He filled with great distinction
that Chair from 1795 until his death in 1809. In 1808 he was thirty-eight years old. To
again quote Carson's History: " Dr. Caldwell, who was an attendant upon his [Wood-
house's] lectures, informs us that he became in a short time so expert and successful an experimenter as to receive from Dr. Priestly, who had just arrived in the United States, and
had declined the appointment, very flattering compliments upon his dexterity and skill.
That distinguished gentleman, on seeing him engaged in the business of his laboratory,
did not hesitate to pronounce him equal, as an experimenter, to any one he had seen either
in England or France. His enthusiasm was unbounded, and his style of speaking of his
subject sentimentally impressive. He introduced to his juvenile auditors the science by
the term ' Miss Chemistry,' and strenuously urged fidelity and devotion to her as a chaste
and eminently attractive mistress."

toward him, and inquired into the means of making a chemical analysis and investigation of their various medical and economical properties.   A frank, encouraging, and didactic courtesy was paid to each pupil, and by an original, but abrupt, and peculiarly forcible and impressive kind of instruction each, in his turn, was furnished with the information he asked.

As I was informed this was the hour of lecture, I took a proffered seat, and determined to avail myself of the opportunity of ascertaining whether this professor (for such I now ascertained he was) of the medical school was as eminent in his branch of knowledge as the other two decidedly were in their province.   I was not long kept in suspense, for he commenced punctually at his hour, in a clear, concise, and lucid manner, a discourse on the method of making some of the mineral preparations of physic, and, by a strain of didactic precision, sustained and enforced by adroit experiments, arrested the attention of his hearers to a lecture on medical chemistry.   He seemed particularly to feel the necessity of, and ably insisted on, the medical application of the subject, enforcing it with so much energy that I could at once realize the importance of chemistry to a physician.   I was pleased to learn that he succeeded in rendering his numerous classes enamored of his charming science; and many of them, I was told by my guide, became adepts in it.   He finished his discourse by a few interesting experiments on fulminating mercury; but so tremendous was the crash succeeding one of the explosions of this substance that we were stunned with its effects and the clamor of the terrified students, and the whole laboratory being by this time enveloped in the smoke and vapor of the various experiments, everything was concealed from our view but the passage of exit through which we endeavored to force our way.   The scene suddenly changed, and I found myself at the entrance of an extended pile of buildings of striking appearance, though mixed and faulty architecture.*   A colossal statue of bronzed lead was conspicuously planted in its front, which represented, I understood from my guide, the great founder of the province in which the medical institution existed.   Rows of lofty sycamore trees surrounded the walls and reared their stately heads even as high as the spires of the building; and when once we had passed the portal a showy and enticing garden, separated by a low portcullis on either side from smaller and less decorated enclosures, invited my attention. The balustrades were entwined with odorous vines and relieved by hedges of terebinthinate shrubs, rather too formally planted, but adding, nevertheless, to the beauty of the spot.   Choirs of

---

* The Pennsylvania Hospital.   The statue, of course, is the one, still standing, of William Penn, presented in 1804 to the hospital by John Penn.

feathered songsters carolled their peals of grateful music from
the highest branches of the sycamores, and the flowers, with
foliage, threw around a fragrant and salubrious exhalation.
Groups of young men habited in various costumes, indicating their
congregation from different and distant lands, or sections of the
same extended territory, were strolling in careless watchfulness
of the portal; crowds thronged the vestibule of the great hall,
through which a large garden in the rear of the building was
discovered in perspective. All were busily sauntering to and fro
with careless attention to the charms around them, and in evident
expectation of some approaching event of importance.

I could no longer restrain my curiosity, and though I much
feared my importuning interrogatories had fatigued my dignified
and taciturn companion, I ventured to be again inquisitive as
to the use and appropriation of this huge structure, and the cause
of such a concourse of youths, among whom I could not help
noticing many of those I had seen in the fields and the laboratory.
" Can they be students ?" said I; " and is this a place of recreation, a theatre, in which some favorite comedy is to be acted ? or
is it a lounging athenæum which allures, by the richness and
variety of its light reading, these youths to its rooms ?" " You
are right in your conjecture as to the young men," rejoined my
pioneer, " but this is not, as you suppose, a place of amusement or
diversion. It is a hospital, the receptacle of every kind of
disease interesting to students of medicine and surgery. But to
them it is quite as alluring as any place of amusement, owing to
the felicity they enjoy of hearing clinical lectures from the most
learned and eloquent physician of our new country. I also perform a part in this scene; for in this building all my capital operations are executed, in a splendid theatre, constructed to accommodate many hundreds of these diligent and inquiring youths.
Thus they learn practical surgery, without an opportunity of seeing which all didactic closet instruction loses half its weight. But
be patient; anon I will conduct you thither, for this very day I
have two operations of great importance to perform, and those
pupils whom you there see (for we had now entered the hall) will
attend." Some were loading themselves with books from the
library of this fine institution, others examining surgical instruments and dressings, and a few scrutinizing the aspect of medicines arranged in the druggery of the establishment. " They are
all," said he, " the common pupils of the great clinical teacher I
have mentioned, the botanist, the chemist, and myself. But mark
the movement of the students who throng the lobbies of the hall
leading to the wards! This indicates that our Sydenham has
arrived at the seat of his willing and instructive labors; and they

are impatiently crowding around the sick bedside to insure a hearing of his sage and invaluable practical remarks."*

At this moment my attention was arrested by a tall and very slender but venerable old gentleman, habited in drab-colored clothes, who walked toward the sick wards with a quick step, his hands folded before him, among flocks of pupils eager to catch his words. A slight passing introduction to him by my guide gave me an opportunity of seeing in his physiognomy the wise, the watchful, the thoughtful physician; and his conversation evinced the same degree of earnestness or even enthusiasm which had been so remarkable in the other professors in their respective departments. His aquiline, large, and rounded nose, insensibly gliding into his upper lip, gave a peculiar degree of penetrating expression to his face. His silvered locks indicated that his words of instruction had been the product of experience; indeed, I learned that he had for more than thirty years gratuitously served that establishment by his counsel, his attendance, and his skill. His eye was small, quickly moving, and full of genius; his voice full-toned, flexible, and soothing, and his manners possessed an irresistible charm equally felt by his patients, his companions, his pupils, and his friends. I followed for an hour the train which hung on his practical remarks, and could easily discern how *all-important* a branch was this clinical instruction, when I found him at one moment jesting with the hypochrondriac, soothing the melancholy, and recurving the morbid apprehensions and associations of the crazed with equal ability and success, and practically applying his principles to the cure of their diseases. Courteous as a cavalier, after waiting until the operations of my guide were completed, which, owing to his adroitness and skill, was indeed but a few minutes, he placed me in his carriage and drove us both to the same building in which I had heard the chemical lecture. It was, he said, his day of clinical remarks, for by such modest title did he call a long, connected, lucid lecture on the causes, seats and cure of the different cases I had just witnessed in the hospital. He enlarged upon his treatment of those cases, explaining by them his peculiar principles; and such was the enthusiasm of this teacher, and his love of medical science, that when his hour was elapsed by a few minutes he craved, with his watch in his hand, the *favor* of "*only one minute more*"—a boon with how much cheerfulness granted was evidenced by the silence and decorum, the fixed attention of his hearers. When at length he had completed his subject he took leave with these remarkable words

---

* Benjamin Rush, who in 1808 was Professor of the Theory and Practice of Medicine and of the Institutes of Medicine and Clinical Medicine. Born in 1745, he was therefore in 1808 sixty-three years old. He was on the staff of the Pennsylvania Hospital from May 26, 1783, until his death on April 19, 1813. He was celebrated for his punctuality, and it is said that during the whole of this period he never missed his daily visit, and was never more than ten minutes late. As everyone of course knows, he was called the American Sydenham

addressed to his pupils: " Think, young men, read, reflect and judge for yourself!"*—a lesson which might safely and profitably be given to minds disciplined, like those of his pupils, in the legitimate school of practice, nature and observation.

In the rush of students which came from this sage's room I lost my guide, and became entangled in a labyrinth of corridors and lobbies, each of which seemed to lead me still farther from the object of my search, and each becoming more obscure until I was finally lost in utter darkness. Faint and weary and overcome with disappointment and fear, together with the pain produced by too much exertion after the wound I had received on the shelving rocks when I was shipwrecked, I sank insensible on the floor, and when I awakened to a sense of my situation, so dismal and painful was it that I called peevishly on Death to come and carry me from a world of misery. Too readily did he obey; for, before the words had well escaped me, his skeleton figure, hideously grinning in my face, stood before me. Seeing the panic his presence produced, " Wretch," he cried, " why hast thou called me?" Terrified as I was, in vain did I urge that an hallucination of the fancy had caused me to pronounce his name and invoke his relief. In fact it was, I assured him, his desperate enemy I sought, having lost him in a crowd of young men, among whom I had taken a seat to listen to the precepts of an Aesculapian chief, who had strenuously instilled the lesson of resisting and contending with him whenever unhappily he should seem to be near, and never yield to him so long as medicinable arms and ammunition remained unexhausted. "Leave me, therefore," continued I, "for you must be convinced that, as I never could have learned respect for your power, nor been taught to call in your aid to procure relief in such company, a distempered imagination alone caused me to call on you." "Hypocrite," rejoined Death, seizing me, " hie thee with me to the haunts of these my cruel and implacable enemies, and I will show you by what means they contend against my power. It is by midnight robberies of my plunder that they fill their charnel houses; and, by examining with their wily arts the devastations I have made on the mortal frame, learn and teach their pupils—in whom they instil the same degree of hatred which they themselves possess—how to oppose efficient force to my work, and to contend against my power. Among the deadliest of my foes is that guide of yours; and so implacable is he, and so interminable the warfare he has waged against me, that in my contest with him he will sever limbs asunder, and pluck the eyes from their orbits, ere he will surrender the body to my power. You will find him at his work; and as you are not ready for me, and as I know he is at hand to aid you, I must relinquish all claims to your

---

* An oft-quoted remark of Rush.

body for the present. I will conduct you to your guide, and a coadjutor of his whom you have not yet seen; but, as I cannot remain an inhabitant of the same spot with either of those things, and do not like even to peep where they are, for fear of a blow on my poor, emaciated body, I shall leave you." So saying, he thrust me, terrified, into a dissecting-room and clapped the door upon my back.

As promised by Death, here I was greeted by my lost guide, who was instructing his pupils in the mode of removing limbs from the living body, by severing them from the dead. He immediately introduced me to a fat, florid, powdered, gay-looking gentleman of low stature and clumsy form,* who appeared busy in directing other pupils in the arts of injecting the blood-vessels and in guiding their hands into the adroit method of examination of the body *post-mortem.*

(To be continued.)

LOCAL ANESTHESIA.

BY HORATIO C. WOOD, M.D., LL.D.

UNDER any circumstances the use of an anesthetic is accompanied by a very small but distinctly appreciable danger to life; a danger which, in the happenings of practical medicine and surgery, is often increased until it becomes very positive. A perfect anesthetic would be a substance which should act upon the peripheral sensory nerves and have no other influence upon the human organism. Such a substance has not as yet been discovered and it may be, does not exist in nature. The subject of local anesthesia is therefore one of great practical importance.

According to our present knowledge all attempts at the production of local anesthesia may be divided into two sets: those in which the loss of sensation is produced by paralysis of conducting nerve-fibres at a greater or less distance from the seat of pain, or proposed surgical operation; those in which the seat of pain is attacked immediately. For brevity's sake, we shall speak of the first of these subdivisions as neuritic anesthesia, the second as local anesthesia.

Neuritic anesthesia may be produced by injections of the local anesthetic into the vertebral column in such position as shall

---

* Caspar Wistar was elected Professor of Anatomy after Dr. William Shippen's death, which occurred July 11, 1808. The exact date of Wistar's election was December 6, 1808; previous to that time he had been Adjunct Professor of Anatomy since 1792. He was a distinguished citizen of Philadelphia, best known to us now from his having been the founder of the museum that bears his name. He succeeded Thomas Jefferson as President of the Philosophical Society, and was also President of the Society for the Abolition of Slavery. The genial, hospitable character of Dr. Wistar is evidenced by the custom of still holding the so-called "Wistar Parties."

paralyze the cauda equina and lower sensory nerve-roots, as they emerge from the cord. It is not proposed to discuss here this method of producing anesthesia in any detail. Introduced and exploited by Bier, Seldowitsch, and Tuffier, followed by other surgeons, it has been practiced in a large number of major operations upon the legs and even upon the lower trunk. The loss of sensation usually sets in about ten minutes after the injection and begins to pass off in about an hour. In most cases the anesthesia has been complete, but occasionally has been more or less imperfect.

Intra-spinal anesthesia has been practiced sufficiently to warrant judgment as to its usefulness, and this judgment must be that the dangers which surround its employment are greater than those of ether or even chloroform anesthesia. One surgeon reported five deaths in one hundred intra-spinal injections of cocaine, and according to H. Mohr-Bielefeld, all available statistics taken together show that one death is to be expected in every two hundred intra-spinal anesthesias. Moreover, the cases must be rare in which spinal anesthesia is available and can not be advantageously replaced by that form of neuritic anesthesia to which the form of neural anesthesia may be given.

As long ago as 1884, Hall and Halsted suggested the injection of cocaine into the nerve-trunk for the purpose of destroying sensation in the region supplied by the nerve, and this method has in the last few years been somewhat freely employed with general satisfaction, and when properly carried out is free from danger to life. When the nerve to be attacked is a small one, the drug selected may be injected simply in contact with the nerve within the sheath, but if the sciatic or other large nerve is to be paralyzed the local anesthetic should be thrown into the nerve itself. So injected, cocaine, and probably eucaine, produces a complete break in the afferent conducting power of the nerve; not only the fibres which are connected with the pain centres but all afferent fibres have been cut off, so that when the incision is made into the peripheral distribution of the nerve not only is there no pain, but little or no surgical shock, the nerve centre not being, as it were, cognizant of the happening in the affected regions.

Cocaine has usually been injected by surgeons and as the dose used does not have to be large, it is entirely safe, although it is probable that beta-eucaine might be satisfactorily employed. When the nerve is small and easily reached, a two per cent. solution of cocaine may be injected into its sheath without previous incision, but when an amputation or other large operation is to be performed it is essential to expose, under infiltration anesthesia, the one or more nerves involved and inject two to five minims of a solution of cocaine, which should not be stronger than one per cent., directly into the nerve. Of course absolute antiseptic precautions must always be taken, and although, *a priori*, it might be expected that the process would involve the danger of the production of neuritis so far the clinical reports do not indicate that such danger exists.

In the production of local anesthesia by a direct action upon the part, several substances are in use, so that the general discussion may well be preceded by a few words concerning them. The oldest of these local anesthetics is cocaine, a substance whose action is so well known that it is only necessary to point out that its employment in over-dose is not unattended with danger, and that half a grain of the ordinary cocaine salt is as much as the surgeon is justified in using at one time.

Nirvanin (Di-Ethyl-Glycocyl-Para-Amido-Ortho-Oxy-Benzoic-Acid-Methyl-Ester-Hydrochloride) which has been very recently introduced into practical medicine by Einhorn and Heinz, is a pronounced local anesthetic, which seems not to be quite equal in activity to cocaine, but which according to the results reached in the experimental research of Luxenberger is so little poisonous that its two per cent. solution may be freely used for the production of infiltration anesthesia up to a maximum amount of eight grains. At present writing there is not sufficient experience to make it possible to assign the exact value of this substance.

Anesthesin, the *ethyl-ester of P-amido-benzoic acid,* is according to the experiments of Binz almost free from general physiological action, he having found that when given in colossal doses to rabbits it produced only a transient methaemoglobinemia, with renal irritation or methaemoglobinuria.

Subcutin, a compound of anesthesin and paraphenol-sulphuric acid, introduced by Ritsert, has been recommended for the production of infiltration anesthesia. Concerning it, also, practical judgment must as yet be suspended.

The one substance which at present seems to share popular favor with cocaine, is beta-eucaine. The eucaine of the present markets is not the eucaine of the market five or six years ago; originally the manufacturing chemists brought forward as the result of the scientific work of Vinci, two allied chemical substances, alpha-eucaine and beta-eucaine. At first it was believed that alpha-eucaine was the better of the two for use in practical surgery, and so it was sold under the simple name of eucaine. Experience, however, demonstrated that this alpha-eucaine was irritating, producing local soreness, hardness, and even sloughing; whilst beta-eucaine was from a local point of view not objectionable; so the manufacturers, retaining the name of eucaine, simply substituted beta-eucaine for alpha-eucaine, and thereby retained the results of their early advertising. As a poison our present

6

beta-eucaine is very feeble,, though it is not without physiological action; it is a paralyzant of both motor and sensory nerve-fibres, appears to have a direct action upon the heart muscles, and also to be a paralyzant of the vasomotor centres; before, however, its exact general influence can be considered settled further research is necessary.

PRODUCTION OF LOCAL ANESTHESIA.

If, as is the case with an ordinary felon, the part to be oper-ated upon can be tightly surrounded by a constricting bandage so as to almost entirely shut off circulation, it is very easy to pro-duce a sufficiently lasting anesthesia by injecting cocaine or eucaine directly into the part. Ordinarily, however, in surgery this cannot be done, hence the importance of the so-called infil-tration anesthesia. In this process,, as originally devised by Schleich, the point of the hypodermic needle is thrust first into the papillary layer of the skin and a small mass of fluid injected. Then the hypodermic needle is thrust forward, another small injection made and so on until the whole region is filled up, or in cases of tumor the base is completely encompassed with a zone of artificial edema. The fluid used by Schleich contained about one-fourth as much morphia as it did of cocaine. There is no reason for believing that morphine has a distinct local anesthetic power and, therefore, no reason for believing that the addition of mor-phia to the fluid, as suggested by Schleich, was a useful procedure. On the other hand it is very clear that the results obtained by his so-called infiltration anesthesia were entirely out of proportion to the amount of cocaine employed, and also were much more lasting than when the ordinary solutions of cocaine were used. Their results were undoubtedly due to the extreme dilution of the solu-tion which required large quantities of water to be injected into the tissue that was to be operated upon; the water under these cir-cumstances acts in several ways. In the first place by pressure and dilution, it lessened the sensibility of the peripheral nerve filaments and endings, and in the second place by pressure and dilution it interfered greatly with the circulation in the part, this interference having a distinct tendency to lessen the sensibility of the nervous apparatus and especially delaying the absorption of the cocaine. Schleich's method was undoubtedly a great advance on the previous processes,, but it has been greatly improved by Braun. This investigator, in experiments made upon the lower animals, found that if by local cooling the vitality and circula-tion of a part were interfered with, absorption of the injected cocaine was so long delayed that the symptoms of poisoning were put off almost indefinitely, or perchance, failed to develop at all; in the latter case, elimination went on as rapidly as absorption, so that at no time was a toxic amount of cocaine in the general circulation. These facts suggested to Prof. Braun the conjoint use of adrenalin and cocaine. He found that the adrenalin produced so much contraction of the blood vessels as to not only very sensibly increase the benumbing action of the local anesthetic by shutting off blood supply, but also greatly to increase the duration of its local activity by lessening the rate of absorption of the drug. By employing from 1 to 5 per cent. solution of cocaine to which had been added from 1 in 10,000 to 1 in 100,000 of adrenalin, Braun was enabled to do trunkal operations without causing suffering. Braun's method has been reported upon by a number of surgeons with high commendation. The further suggestion of Barker that eucaine should be substituted for cocaine seems to have brought infiltration anesthesia almost to the high water mark and has been followed out in Philadelphia by various surgeons with great satisfaction. The plan is readily carried out as follows: Powders are kept in stock in the operating room containing 0.02 grm. (3 grains) of B-eucaine or the eucaine of the shops and 0.8 grm. (12 grains) of pure sodium chloride. At the time of the operation one such powder is dissolved in 100 cc. of boiling distilled water, and when it is cooled sufficiently 1 cc. of adrenalin chloride solution (1 to 1,000) is added; 100 cc. of the resulting liquid containing 12 grs. of B-eucaine and 0.015 grs. of adrenalin chloride. The whole 100 cc. may be used at one infiltration anesthesia, but according to Barker from 50 to 60 cc. usually suffices, even in such considerable operations as for the cure of hernia, castration. It is of course essential that the syringe used be aseptic and the surgeon should always employ the platinum needle with an iridium point which can, without injury, be disinfected in the flame of an alcohol lamp immediately before use.

If the surgeon should wish to try anesthesin for infiltration anesthesia the formula of Dunbar may be employed. The original solution of Dunbar was:

Anesthesin hydrochloride......................0.25 grm.
Sodium chloride............................0.15 grm.
Morphine hydrochloride..............0.005 to 0.015 grm.
Water. ....100 cc.

The solution should be sterilized by heat. It should also be modified by omitting the morphine solution and adding 1 cc. adrenalin solution (1-1000).

As previously stated, much of the effect of infiltration anesthesia is due to the water injected. Schleich recognized this, and stated also that by the employment of unmedicated water a transitory anesthesia could be produced. Very recently, January 23rd, 1904 (*N.Y.M.J.*), Dr. Samuel G. Gant has asserted as the result of much experience, that for very many surgical purposes it is sufficient to distend the tissues with pure sterilized water. Most of his experience has been in rectal surgery, but he affirms that he. has used the method in explanatory laparotomy.   He describes the technique as follows:

" A fold of the skin at one extremity of the line of incision is caught up between the thumb and forefinger and compressed for a few seconds, which diminishes, and often prevents, the momentary pain caused by the first injections.   The needle is then quickly introduced between the layers of the skin, and a few drops of water are slowly injected.   They should produce a small, localized distention not unlike a blister, and as soon as it appears, anesthesia of the skin should instantly occur at this point.   The needle is then inserted slowly further and further along the line of the cut to be made, and the water is gradually injected as before, care being taken not to go entirely through the skin. When the syringe is emptied it is refilled, the needle is introduced within the anesthetized area, and the injections are repeated as before, until the distention extends the entire length of the line of incision.   The needle is then plunged through this distended line and subcutaneous injections are rapidly made until a firm, whitish, ridge-like swelling, about as wide and thick as the index finger is produced.   These deep injections may cause a temporary discomfort due to the rapid distention of the subcutaneous tissues. If the procedure has been properly carried out, the skin and underlying tissues can now be incised without pain in almost every instance."

In cases of extreme thrombotic hemorrhoids, Dr. Gant injects the sterile water only between the layers of the skin overlying the clot to be removed; when the hemorrhoid is cutaneous, both the skin and the tumor should be distended tightly; when the hemorrhoid is internal, sufficient water should be injected directly into the centre of the tumor to distend it tightly and cause it to turn white, when it will be found absolutely insensitive.   In various surgical diseases about the anus, the skin, subcutaneous structure up to the anal margin, the mucosa and sub-mucosa, the external and the internal muscle must be successively distended until the pressure is sufficient to overcome sensation.   The injections should be given slowly.   In opening abscesses the layers of the skin immediately over the abscesses must be distended, but in deep rectal abscesses requiring extensive cutting and curetting, Dr. Gant does commend the method.

Apparently water, used in the way suggested by Dr. Gant, is a sufficient anesthetizing agent when the lesion is superficial, or when it is so situated that the fluid will be confined in a limited space for the time being.

A NEW CHLOROFORM INHALER.

THE Vernon Harcourt Chloroform Regulator was first introduced to a special chloroform committee appointed by the British Medical Association to investigate the subject of anesthesia in certain directions. One of the committee, Dr. Dudley Buxton, at the instance of the other members of the committee, tested the Inhaler clinically and reported in favorable terms of it. (*Supplement to the British Medical Journal,* July 18, 1903.) Mr. Walter Tyrrell also employed the Inhaler, and his cases, which further demonstrated its value, appeared as an appendix to the committee's report. Since this pronouncement the Regulator has been in con-

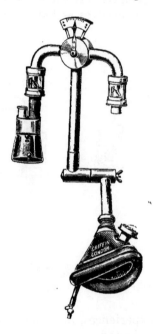

stant use at University College Hospital, and in the hands of several anesthetists, and has earned for itself the warmest approval.

From a clinical standpoint it is not too much to say that Mr. Vernon Harcourt's patient and truly scientific endeavor to produce an exact apparatus has been successful. It was somewhat doubtful, until extended use proved such to be the fact, whether a 2 per cent. vapor of chloroform was adequate for all cases. The common objection urged is that such a low tension vapor could only be applicable to subjects who were easily anesthetised; but when the apparatus is intelligently used it is found to be capable of the widest employment.

The features most noticeable about the narcosis are that as the patient at first inspires a 2 per cent. vapor he is soothed and not excited; if the increase in vapor strength be graduated with precision, the onset of narcosis is gradual, and what is more important, is even. There is no sudden variation. The onset travels as it were along an inclined plane; there are no irregular elevations and depressions, and as a result struggling, whether voluntary or the result of overstrong vapor, seldom occurs. The nerve storms and convulsive respiratory phenomena, at times met with among the alcoholic or muscular during the inhalation of chloroform, seldom if ever occur when the low tension vapor is used, and hence the risks of the period of induction are lessened, if not wholly removed.

After effects are certainly less when the Regulator is used, and most patients express themselves as having found the method less

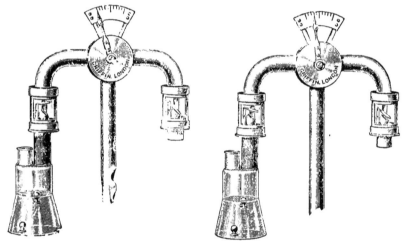

Pointer adjusted to give 2 per cent.   Pointer adjusted to give 1.4 per cent.

painful than former experiences, in which other methods of giving chloroform had been adopted.

There can, we think, be no doubt that Mr. Vernon Harcourt's Inhaler is the best apparatus we possess, and marks an enormous advance in our available methods. It would be premature to say more, but we confidently await the criticism of the next few years; we believe it will more than justify what has been said, and will show that a low percentage vapor of chloroform from an accurate scientific apparatus such as Mr. Vernon Harcourt's, administered by an experienced anesthetist, will give most satisfactory results.

When this method is universally adopted chloroform will once again take the premier place as the anesthetic among anesthetics, and its accidents will, if they arise at all, result from an unwise departure from known physiological principles.

Description of the Apparatus.

Mr. Harcourt's Inhaler provides, in sufficient quantity for full and free respiration, a mixture of air and chloroform, which is automatically limited to a maximum strength of 2 per cent., and can be diluted at will with additional air down to any smaller proportion.

The two-necked bottle is filled with chloroform to near the top of the conical part, and two colored glass beads are dropped into the liquid to indicate when the temperature is within the range, 13 to 15 deg. C. If the temperature of the chloroform is below 13 deg. both the colored beads will float; if it is above 15 deg., both will sink; in the former case the proportion of chloroform inhaled will be less than the pointer of the stopcock indicates; in the latter case it will be greater. During inhalation the chloroform is cooled by evaporation; its temperature may be kept between 13 and 15 deg. by now and then holding the bottle in the hand till the red bead has floated up and the blue bead is beginning to rise.

The stopcock is so made that when the pointer is at the end of the arc nearest the bottle of chloroform the maximum quantity is being administered—namely, 2 per cent. When the pointer is at the opposite end only air will be inhaled; and when it is midway dilution of the 2 per cent. mixture with an equal volume of air will make the proportion 1 per cent. The shorter lines on either side indicate intermediate quantities—namely, 0.8, 0.6, 0.4, 0.2; and towards the chloroform bottle, 1.2, 1.4, 1.6, 1.8.

The valves on the two branches prevent the entrance into the apparatus of expired air, and also serve to show whether the stopcock is working rightly. Only one valve opens when the pointer is at either end of the scale, both equally when the pointer is midway, and for all other positions one valve opens more and the other less, in the degree indicated by the position of the pointer on the scale. The movement of these valves shows also how full and regular the breathing is, and the slight click which they make conveys this information to the ears when the eyes are otherwise occupied.

It is generally found that beginning with the pointer at 0.2 and moving it on towards the chloroform bottle at the rate of one division about every half-minute up to 1.6 or 1.8 produces narcosis as quickly as is desirable.

For the maintenance of narcosis it is believed that 1 per cent. or even less will be found sufficient. The stopcock can be moved by a touch of the finger so as at once to increase or diminish the dose.

The face-piece, which is provided with an expiratory valve and can be fixed in any position, is either attached directly to the inhaler, which in this case is held in the hand, and should be kept as nearly vertical and as steady as possible, or can be connected by about 20 inches of half-inch rubber tubing; the inhaler in this case being supported on a stand or hung on to the back of the bed.

The mask is made of solid toughened rubber, fitted with a rubber air-cushion. It can be washed, or boiled, and as it becomes plastic in hot water the shape can easily be modified, if required, so as better to fit the patient's face.

No chloroform evaporates excepting that which is inhaled by the patient; and only that which is exhaled passes into the air of the room. A great economy of chloroform is thus effected, which should in a short time repay the cost of the apparatus to institutions or medical men in large practice by whom it may be used.

On the use of the Vernon Harcourt Inhaler.

The apparatus must be carefully examined to see the parts are adjusted, and the administrator should inhale to see that the valves are working properly. About 1 1-2 oz. of chloroform should be poured into the conical bottle and the beads seen to be floating. The face mask should then be carefully applied. This is best done when the head is turned to one side. Breathing taking place freely and the air inlet valve and expiry valve flapping properly, the inhaler should be grasped at the horizontal cross-piece with the right-hand, while the lower jaw is pressed forward by the left hand placed behind the angle of the mandible. Firm pressure is necessary, as absolute co-adaptation of the mask to the patient's face is essential. If the pressure used is equal over the whole area of the face the patient will not complain. It is a common fault to allow air to enter by the sides of the bridge of the nose. Absolute fitting of the face-piece having been secured, the strength of the vapor may be gradually increased by turning the pointer. This is done slowly, but unless the patient is restless and struggles, not too slowly. Struggling is an indication for the lessening of the strength of the vapor but not for removal of the face-piece unless duskiness supervenes. When narcosis is attained, the usual signs being relied upon, in most cases the maintaining of anesthesia can be effected with 1.5 or even .5 per cent. according to the physique of the patient and the requirements of the operation. After prolonged administration slight duskiness may appear, and in this case the apparatus may be lifted for a few breaths and then replaced.

The Canadian
Journal of Medicine and Surgery

J. J. CASSIDY, M.D.,
EDITOR,
43 BLOOR STREET EAST, TORONTO.

W. A. YOUNG, M.D., L.R.C.P.LOND.,
MANAGING EDITOR,
145 COLLEGE STREET, TORONTO.

Surgery—BRUCE L. RIORDAN, M D ,C M., McGill University; M D University of Toronto; Surgeon Toronto General Hospital; Surgeon Grand Trunk R R ; Consulting Surgeon Toronto Home for Incurables , Pension Examiner United States Government ; and F. N. G. STARR. M B., Toronto, Associate Professor of Clinical Surgery, Toronto University , Surgeon to the Out-Door Department Toronto General Hospital and Hospital for Sick Children

Clinical Surgery—ALEX PRIMROSE, M B , C.M. Edinburgh University , Professor of Anatomy and Director of the Anatomical Department, Toronto University ; Associate Professor of Clinical Surgery, Toronto University, Secretary Medical Faculty, Toronto University.

Orthopedic Surgery—B. E MCKENZIE, B.A., M D., Toronto, Surgeon to the Toronto Orthopedic Hospital , Surgeon to the Out-Patient Department, Toronto General Hospital , Assistant Professor of Clinical Surgery, Ontario Medical College for Women : Member of the American Orthopedic Association; and H. P. H. GALLOWAY, M.D , Toronto, Surgeon to the Toronto Orthopedic Hospital , Orthopedic Surgeon, Toronto Western Hospital ; Member of the American Orthopedic Association.

Oral Surgery—E H. ADAMS, M.D , D.D.S., Toronto.

Surgical Pathology—T. H MANLEY. M D., New York, Visiting Surgeon to Harlem Hospital, Professor of Surgery, New York School of Clinical Medicine, New York, etc , etc

Gynecology and Obstetrics—GEO. T. MCKEOUGH, M D , M R C S Eng., Chatham, Ont ; and J. H. LOWE, M.D , Newmarket, Ont

Medical Jurisprudence and Toxicology—ARTHUR JUKES JOHNSON, M B., M R C S. Eng ; Coroner for the City of Toronto ; Surgeon Toronto Railway Co., Toronto ; W. A. YOUNG, M D., L.R.C.P. Lond ; Associate Coroner, City of Toronto.

Pharmacology and Therapeutics—A. J. HARRINGTON M D , M R.C.S Eng., Toronto

Medicine—J J CASSIDY, M D., Toronto, Member Ontario Provincial Board of Health , Consulting Surgeon, Toronto General Hospital ; and W. J, WILSON, M D. Toronto, Physician Toronto Western Hospital

Clinical Medicine—ALEXANDER MCPHEDRAN, M D , Professor of Medicine and Clinical Medicine Toronto University ; Physician Toronto General Hospital, St Michael's Hospital, and Victoria Hospital for Sick Children

Mental and Nervous Diseases—N H. BEEMER, M D , Mimico Insane Asylum; CAMPBELL MEYERS, M D., M.R C S., L R.C P (London, Eng); Private Hospital, Deer Park, Toronto ; and EZRA H. STAFFORD, M D

Public Health and Hygiene—J. J CASSIDY, M D., Toronto, Member Ontario Provincial Board of Health ; Consulting Surgeon Toronto General Hospital ; and E. H. ADAMS, M D , Toronto.

Physiology—A. B EADIE, M.D., Toronto, Professor of Physiology Woman s Medical College, Toronto.

Pediatrics—AUGUSTA STOWE GULLEN, M D , Toronto, Professor of Diseases of Children Woman's Medical College, Toronto , A R GORDON, M.D , Toronto

Pathology—W H PEPLER, M D., C.M , Trinity University ; Pathologist Hospital for Sick Children, Toronto; Associate Demonstrator of Pathology Toronto University; Physician to Outdoor Department Toronto General Hospital ; Surgeon Canadian Pacific R.R , Toronto ; and J. J MACKENZIE, B A., M B , Professor of Pathology and Bacteriology T ronto University Medical Faculty.

Ophthalmology and Otology—J. M MACCALLUM, M.D., Toronto, Professor of Materia Medica Toronto University ; Assistant Physician Toronto General Hospital ; Oculist and Aurist Victoria Hospital for Sick Children, Toronto

Laryngology and Rhinology—J. D THORBURN, M D., Toronto, Laryngologist and Rhinologist, Toronto General Hospital.

Address all Communications, Correspondence, Books, Matter Regarding Advertising, and make all Cheques, Drafts and Post-office Orders payable to "The Canadian Journal of Medicine and Surgery," 145 College St., Toronto, Canada.

Doctors will confer a favor by sending news. reports and papers of interest from any section of the country. Individual experience and theories are also solicited Contributors must kindly remember that all papers, reports, correspondence, etc., *must be* in our hands by the fifteenth of the month previous to publication.

Advertisements. to insure insertion in the issue of any month should be sent not later than the tenth of the preceding month. London, Eng Representative, W. Hamilton Miln, 8 Bouverie Street, E. C. Agents for Germany Saarbach s News Exchange, Mainz, Germany.

VOL. XVI. TORONTO, JULY, 1904. NO. 1.

Editorials.

OUR REPORT OF THE ONTARIO MEDICAL ASSOCIATION.

WE have decided, rather than hold our *July* issue too late, to publish our special report of the proceedings of the Ontario Medical Association, which closed the other day, in the August number, and feel that, in doing so, we have acted wisely, our readers preferring, we think, to receive the JOURNAL promptly on the first of each month.

A GLANCE AT THE ATLANTIC CITY MEETING OF THE AMERICAN MEDICAL ASSOCIATION.

WHERE duty called, pleasure abounded, the magic of the sea entranced, the song of its waves lulled to rest, and over all the Queen of Day shone, and pleasant faces reflected her light as they smiled a welcome and uttered the greeting, " Doctor, I am so glad to meet you again." On the great board walk, in the numerous hotels, in every nook and corner the physicians were to be found; but perhaps a glimpse of them as a unit was best obtained at the opening ceremonies in the auditorium on the pier, where standing room even was at a premium. The hall was destitute of floral or other decorations, so that the faces of the vast crowd of men and women stood out clearly, and many a well-known Luminary was easily recognized among the attentive audience as they composed their features and said " prunes and prism " as the camera fiend took the inevitable snap-shot. If we had been fortunate enough to have had a lightning artist with us, and had allotted to him the task of sketching a composite face of the physician representing the leading features of the three thousand followers of Esculapius there assembled, we think the sketch would have shown a young face, firm in expression, with settled convictions, bright eyes looking at life cheerfully and steadily; in a word, the face of a man not laboriously studious, perhaps, but strong in purpose and masterful enough to say to that greedy old reaper, Death himself, " Not yet." From a glance at the audience we instinctively turned " eyes front " to the platform, or rather stage, on which, forming a background, some garish scenery was arranged, which contrasted strangely with the dignified appearance of those seated solemnly in front of it, among whom were the retiring President, Dr. Billings, of Chicago; the President-elect, Dr. Musser; the Secretary; the clergyman who read the invocation; the Mayor of Atlantic City, and as many past and ex-presidents as George Washington has " former residences " in America! Dr. Musser's address was very interesting, especially dealing with that burning question, the proper equipment of the medical student and the high standard of preparatory university education that should be required to fit the young man to become an intelligent student ere he knocks at the door of the medical college for admission. We heartily congratulate the President upon his finished and interesting paper, and only regret that many of the vast audience, owing to the imperfect acoustic properties of the auditorium, were unable to hear it all, and the doctor's voice seemed to strike a musical cadence and dwell continuously upon the one note, till between the lines we seemed to hear the key of an old Gregorian chant as the sound crept out through the bars of a monastery chapel off in New Orleans. With all due respect to Dr. Musser, his splendid " song " deserved a " singer " with a better range.

The appeal made to the audience by a number of leading physicians for funds to erect the Reed Memorial met with a magnificent response, we understand, of over seven thousand dollars, a tribute to the memory of the man who courted death by his investigation of and success in dealing with that awful scourge, yellow fever. Though he sacrificed his life, he left the legacy of an honored name to his profession and a record in the great book of science.

The large body of the Association, after the opening ceremonies, split up into sections, meeting in the various hotels, thereby combining convenience, comfort, and focusing interest, and then each day when " meetin' was out," perhaps the gravest debater or most skilled clinician was just the very funniest thing on the beach, for Dr. Jack knows full well the value of play after work.

Night at Atlantic City is a revelation. Everything in earth and air flashes forth an electric light, and

> " A spirit of delight, scatters roses in her flight,
> " And there's magic in the night
> When the heart is young."

Sufficient to say, a young heart of ninety-two years rushed away from a smoker at eleven o'clock to take " a look in at the dance on the pier," and in our hearts we all said, " Bless the dear old Spartan, who in his professional career has caused so many hearts to dance for joy as he attuned their faltering footsteps, almost slipping o'er the brink, and set them to keep time to the quickstep of perfect health."

To begin to thank the Entertainment Committee for their kind hospitality would occupy a volume, a sequel, and a post script. Musicales, dances, dinners, yachts to sail in, and the three large

receptions—one at the Marlborough Hotel to the ladies, given by
Mrs. Musser; another given by the ladies of Atlantic City in the
ball-room on the pier, and the last by Dr. Musser, also in the ball-
room at the end of the long pier. All were very largely attended
and greatly enjoyed. Unfortunately, Old Ocean was in a strange
mood the night of the President's reception. A storm was
raging—

> " A strange spirit moved the waters ;
>   The wild spirit of the Air
>   It lashed, and shook, and tore them
>   Till they thundered, groaned and boomed "—

and nearly blew the frolicsome doctors off the pier into the sea
as they were making their way, freighted by their " femininity,"
to the entertainment. Several were merrily advocating the bare-
headed treatment as healthful and delightful, as the ocean said to
them imperatively, " Gentlemen, hats off !" The mermaids now
are surely wondering, as they try them on, if they are becoming,
and Neptune, sly old fellow, is perhaps claiming the kisses !

Many of the physicians accepted the cordial welcome extended
to them to visit the new Laboratories at the University of Pennsylvania upon their opening day, and a charming afternoon and
evening were enjoyed by all. Many went on next day also to
Washington, to be present at the unveiling of the Rush Monu-
ment, but Old Ocean called insistently, so we lingered, watching
the unending procession of holiday makers, as restless as the sea
itself, as they strutted by all glistening with jewels, and somehow
Pope seemed ever to whisper—

> " Worth makes the man, and want of it, the fellow ;
>   The rest is all but leather or prunella."
>
> W. A. Y.

MEDICAL EDITORS AT ATLANTIC CITY.

PARTICIPATING again in the proceedings of the annual meeting of
the American Medical Editors' Association in Hotel Dennis,
Atlantic City, and looking at the hale, hearty and alert men
assembled to talk together with voice instead of pen, we felt that
no one could say, these are they who have come up out of the great
tribulations of an editorial sanctum—they all looked as if their
chosen vocation agreed with them. After enjoying the privilege

of attending the yearly sessions of this Association, one always returns strengthened and impressed more than ever by the place the medical journal has made for itself in the library of the universal physician, and at the high standard of journalism demanded by the profession. The pace set by the foremost magazines that are in the hands of the public makes the task to supply every month an up-to-date and strictly ethical and scientific medical journal an increasingly difficult one.

The 1904 meeting was quite a success, and we had the privilege of again shaking hands with Dr. Sajous, the retiring President; Dr. Harold N. Moyer, the incoming President; Dr. W. C. Abbott, Dr. T. D. Crothers, Dr. Macdonald, Jr., the energetic Secretary ; the Drs. Taylor, of Philadelphia, and many of the foremost medical editors of the United States, and from them received many useful pointers as to how to conduct a successful, and yet scientific, medical journal. The papers read were of a high order, the discussions quite lively, and the number of new members proposed greater than any year since the inception of the Association. The banquet held the same night was most enjoyable, the speeches showing the added quality of the ready tongue of the ready speaker to the powerful pen of the forceful writer. Ere many moons may we have the pleasure of again meeting with so pleasant a company, who, as the years roll by, become the "auld acquaintance"—who add the flavor to the annual cup of kindness. W. A. Y.

DISEASES AFFECTING WOMEN ON THE FARM IN ONTARIO.

Acting on the suggestion of the National Council of Women circulars were recently sent to a number of farmers' wives and daughters throughout Ontario containing questions concerning the life of women on the farm. These circulars were distributed through the officers of the women's institutes, and the answers are now being received. The circulars were sent to twenty women in each district. Catarrh and rheumatism are given as the chief complaints from which the women suffer. One woman, however, characterizes the prevailing trouble as "that tired feeling."

Chronic pharyngitis is not a rare disease in Canada. It is commonly known as "the catarrh." It is generally a subacute affection at the beginning, and is developed imperceptibly, so that in most cases, when patients first come under observation, it has existed for a considerable period. The mucous membrance of the pharynx is more or less reddened and thickened; the surface in some cases is smooth, but often presents a granulated appearance, especially marked on the posterior wall of the pharynx. This inflammation often extends to the posterior nares. It may extend around the top of the larynx, but it has no tendency to pass into the larynx. The mucous membrane around the openings of the Eustachian tubes may be swollen and the inflammation, in certain cases, extends into these tubes. As a consequence, deafness is not uncommon from obstruction of the Eustachian tubes, requiring their catheterization.

Writing of the causation of chronic pharyngitis Dr. Price-Brown states ("Diseases of the Nose and Throat") that, "Persons whose occupations keep them exposed to constant respiration of foul or irritating gases are subject to it. Exposure to cold and wet has been thought to have an influence in the causation of chronic pharyngitis." It has also been thought to be rheumatic in its origin.

As the women on the farm are not remarkable for leading lazy lives, and as most of them must, of necessity, spend some portion of their time in pure country air, the breathing of such impure air as they suffer from would arise from a residence in small, unventilated dwellings. Their lives are passed in a sort of workshop, and the work is continued for many years, giving little or no time for recreation. It would be interesting to learn if the men on the farm suffer as much from " the catarrh " as the women. We do not think they do. "It (catarrh) seldom occurs among the so-called laboring classes, and it is much more frequent in cities than in the country. It is accompanied by symptoms denoting impairment of the general health. Patients complain of debility and a want of their accustomed energy; they are generally depressed in spirits and have forebodings of loss of health, they are very apt to fancy the existence of some serious disease, especially pulmonary consumption, and it is sometimes difficult to convince them that the latter disease does not exist. Dyspeptic ailments frequently coexist. Palpitation of the heart is not uncommon." (Flint's "Practice of Medicine.")

Of follicular pharyngitis Dr. Price-Brown says: "In adult life it frequently occurs as a result or complication of previously existing nasal disease. It is said to occur more frequently among women than men, probably owing to the more sedentary occupations of the former, and the consequent greater tendency to disease of the mucous membranes. We should remember, also, how much the pharyngeal mucosa is influenced by the gynecological condition of the sex."

The remedy for "the catarrh," to be effective, must have reference to the system. Alteration of the habits of life is of the first importance. Relaxation and recreation in the open air should be sought for, and exercises, especially those which call into action the muscles of the arms, shoulders and neck should be regularly taken in the open air. Topical applications are useful and tonic remedies may often be advantageously conjoined with proper hygienic management. The diet should be nutritious. The main object of treatment is to restore the general health.

By rheumatism is probably meant chronic articular rheumatism in some cases, and in others, muscular rheumatism. The former usually begins as a chronic affection. Heredity, advanced years, and habitual exposure to cold and wet are the predisposing factors. It rarely results from an acute attack. In the treatment attention to hygiene, especially as regards diet, bathing, clothing, exercise and occupation, should be thought of. The site on which the farmer's dwelling is built is often damp and undrained. There is a close connection between dampness of the soil upon which we live and rheumatism. Most rheumatics are also benefited by a change of residence to a dry, warm and equable climate. The tone of the system is often reduced, hence tonics like iron, quinine, strychnine and arsenic are of considerable value. The special remedies are iodide of potassium, guaiacum, salicylic acid and alkalies like the salts of potassium and lithium.

In muscular rheumatism, an affection of the voluntary muscles characterized by pain, tenderness and rigidity, presenting types such as lumbago and pleurodynia, the gouty or rheumatic diathesis is a predisposing cause, and exposure to cold and wet or muscular strain usually excites it. It may also be remembered that pharyngitis, tonsillitis, laryngitis and bronchitis are sometimes dependent on the rheumatic diathesis. Purpura, erythema nodosum and urticaria are also associated with it.

Some of the women on the farm work hard, perhaps too hard, and this may account for "the tired feeling" mentioned by one of those who replied to the circular. There is much monotony of scene, environment and occupation in their lives, with but little physical or mental recreation. The older women give no time to relaxation, and spend too much time indoors. They should ventilate their small dwellings more frequently and fully, and should partake less freely than they do of fried pork, and hot bread, washed down with libations of very strong tea. They should imitate, also, the example of their American cousins, who go forth in search of recreation, and "visit" regularly.

The habit of building a farm dwelling on undrained soil should be reprobated. A sufferer from chronic rheumatism will have better health by living in a house on a dry, well-drained site. Neither should she forget to keep the alvine secretions in an active condition.   J. J. C.

SOMETHING ABOUT MATERNAL MILK IN ENGLAND AND FRANCE.

STATEMENTS about the milk-giving habits of the English mother are appearing in the English medical journals, which would have astonished our mothers and grandmothers. Thus, in *The British Medical Journal,* April 9th, 1904, Mr. William Hall, whose experience has been principally obtained in the London slums, makes comparison between Jewish and Christian mothers in the matter of suckling children, and gives the preference to the former. He says, "Jewish mothers suckle their children for twelve months, and feed them on fresh and suitable food when they are weaned. Most English mothers are unwilling or unable to suckle their children, or they cease to do so, before they are many weeks old."

To show the outcome of this evil habit he writes: "I have weighed, measured and examined upwards of 4,000 school children, most of them living in the slum district of our city. Not only are the majority of British slum children rickety, but they are also tainted with scurvy. They are stale, they live on stale food;

chiefly garbage." Of the Jewish children he writes: " During the same period I have weighed, measured and examined upwards of 1,000 Jewish children born and bred in the same slum district. They are free from the taint of scurvy, and are superior in physical development."

Another correspondent, " W. H. C. S.," writes to *The British Medical Journal,* April 16th, 1904: " Well-to-do women, when asked why they have not suckled their children, even for a time, answer, ' I really don't know. Nobody told me that I ought to, and I thought they did just as well on the bottle. My husband did not wish me to.' ' The monthly nurse advised me not to.' " He goes on to say that many of these women are perfectly willing to nurse in future, when they know the reasons why they ought to. He thinks that a medical man should give the question of abandoning suckling as much consideration as he does the question of inducing premature labor, seeing that the risk to the child's future welfare is about equal in the two cases.

Neglect or refusal to suckle her baby may not depend on the whim or ignorance of a mother, but on her physical incapacity for the function of giving good breast-milk. At the French National Congress of Obstetrics, Gynecology and Pediatrics, held at Rouen, last April (*La Presse Medicale,* April 13th, 1904), the good or evil done by the Gouttes de lait was very warmly debated. Dr. Pinard said: " The Gouttes de lait gave nursing women the chance of weaning their babies, and giving them artificial milk instead of breast milk. The managers of the Gouttes de lait pretend that they save the lives of sick babies. I want to see babies prevented from being sick, and to accomplish that end nothing is better than nursing at the breast. I think the Gouttes de lait are dangerous, as they offer mothers too many facilities for procuring milk and weaning their babies." Other physicians, Drs. Ausset and Peyron, took the same ground, contending that the Gouttes de lait were an encouragement to artificial nursing, and that wherever a Gouttes de lait was established nursing at the breast was less and less practiced by mothers.

Evidence on the opposite side was given by Dr. Variot, who said that when the babies were brought to the Gouttes de lait their mothers had long before ceased to suckle them, because they had no breast milk to give. Dr. Brunon, director of the Rouen School of Medicine, said: " We are not trying to find out if two per

7

cent. of mothers are unable to nurse their babies. Such a low percentage would not surprise me at all. We are trying to find out, however, how many women of the poorer class get enough to eat to enable them to have breast milk. That is the important question. The question of suckling children is a social one. Stop women from working at trades, from taking situations in post-offices, telegraph offices, and especially in telephone offices; suppress female slavery in school teaching; let woman do the work she is fit for; pay her for her work; protect her from the ferocious selfishness of man. When that much has been done women will suckle their children, and we shall close the Gouttes de lait. But, as nothing of the kind will be done, we shall keep the Gouttes de lait open, because they fill a long-felt social want. We are told that we encourage the artificial nursing of infants and discourage suckling by mothers. When a child, which has tried breast-milk, concentrated milk, farina, etc., and is so wasted as to be at the point of death, is brought to the Gouttes de lait, do you think I " should make a speech to its mother on the immortal principle of a mother suckling her child?"

Very graphically put indeed. All the same, we agree with Drs. Pinard and Ausset that too great facilities should not be extended to women who are quite willing to renounce the natural duty of nursing a baby at the breast for the chance of earning a little money at a trade, or in some situation. That instances do occur in which an infant, whose mother cannot suckle it, is happily raised on the bottle all will admit. That the work of dispensing bottled milk is admirably done at the French Gouttes de lait is equally true. When these facts are admitted the truth remains— the old way of raising babies by suckling them at the breast is the proper one. It speaks well, indeed, for the influences of creed and family life, that the Jewish mothers, living in the slums of London, could and would suckle their babies, and they and their husbands deserve credit for their labor and care, in striving to raise healthy children under deplorable conditions, instead of seeing them turned over to the undertaker, or growing up the victims of scurvy and rickets. It is to be hoped that the influence of Christian charity, co-operating with and assisting the natural feeling of Christian mothers, will assist them to vie with the Hebrew mothers in this respect.   J. J. C.

EDITORIAL NOTES.

Adulterations Discovered in Cider and Ground Spices.— The chief analyst of the Inland Revenue Department states, February 6th, 1904, that of forty-one specimens of Canadian cider examined by him fifteen (36.58 per cent.) were found to contain small quantities of salicylic acid, the addition of which to alcoholic, fermented, or other potable liquors renders them, according to the Adulteration Act, liable to be considered as adulterated in a manner injurious to health. Of ground spices 188 specimens collected in various districts of Canada during the months of August and September, 1903, were examined. Based on the opinions of the analysts, the following recapitulation shows the extent to which adulteration prevailed among these 188 samples:

	Genuine	Doubtful	Adulterated	Total
Black pepper	33	1	42	76
White pepper	23	1	30	54
Red pepper	0	1	2	3
Allspice	13	2	1	16
Mixed spices	3	0	2	5
Cassia or Cinnamon	1	0	10	11
Cloves	9	2	2	13
Ginger	6	0	4	10
	88	7	93	188

Microscopical examination showed in different samples of adulterated black pepper: (1) Wheat flour and charcoal or roasted shells; (2) wheat and rice starch, cayenne pepper, many stone cells, probably cocoanut shell; (3) some buckwheat and wheat starch; (4) little pepper, but much fibrous tissue, hairs, dirt, etc., also rice, starch, mustard, husk and turmeric. Microscopic examination of adulterated white pepper showed: (1) Corn starch and much foreign tissue—fermenting matter; (2) wheat flour and buckwheat; (3) some wheat starch, and turmeric; (4) wheat starch and a little charcoal. The inspection of cassia and ground cinnamon showed that cassia is chiefly used instead of cinnamon. The analyst, A. McGill, says in a note: "Since cassia and cinnamon are the barks of allied species of cinnamomi, they necessarily have many features in common. Cinnamon is distinguished by having been more carefully freed from valueless portions of cortex and wood; and is characterized by a greater preponderance of bast cells and other structural peculiarities. Hence the microscope is the chief and only reliable means of differentiating these species, and even its indications must be accepted with caution, since some samples of each species closely approximate to those of the other." Referring to the inspection of ground cloves, A. McGill says: " The adulteration in some of the samples consists in the addition of foreign matter of a more starchy character, containing stone cells and other vegetable tissues not largely present in genuine cloves. Part of this tissue may come from admixture of clove stems, but this cannot be certainly determined. The effect of this adulteration is shown in the considerable lowering of the total volatile matter, and the very marked lowering of the volatile oil. Of course these features might come from addition of exhausted cloves." In ground ginger microscopic examination showed: (1) Adulteration with foreign starchy matter; (2) exhausted ginger, or is of lower than average quality.

The Genesis of Epilepsy.—In the genesis of epilepsy Dr. Rabinovitch, of Paris, attaches great importance to alcoholism in the parents: " Alcoholism in the parent causes epileptiform attacks, and the descendant of such a parent is apt to be epileptic in a vast number of cases. It is of interest to note in this connection, and the fact has already been referred to, that alcoholic parents who have given birth to epileptic, idiotic or imbecile children, with or without other pathological stigma, can give birth to normal children if the parents abstain from alcoholic drink during a long period of time before conception takes place. The reverse side of this biological phenomenon is also true, as every physician knows perfectly normal parents, with no pathological family record, have been known to give birth to epileptic and other degenerate offspring, if one or both parents have indulged in drink at the period synchronous with the conception of the child." Writing on the same subject, Bevan Lewis (" Text-Book on Mental Diseases," chapter on the pathology of epilepsy) brings to light the important fact that the microscopic appearances of the brains of epileptics are similar to those found in subjects suffering from chronic alcoholism. He says that the change in the cell of the epileptic is not peculiar to epilepsy: "It is found in other diseases and especially alcoholic brain disease. The nucleus of the cell is the earliest portion affected. The cell protoplasm being apparently secondarily involved (p. 522). With the atrophy and disappearance of the nucleus, we find associated declining functional activity and ultimate degeneration of the cell itself. Displacements, distortion, degeneration, enfeebled vitality, and the absence of the nucleus are constant accompaniments of cerebral disturbances characterized by loss of inhibitory control. This idea is not in contradiction to the fact observed in acute anemia, where the suddenly induced absence of nutrition causes—on the mental side loss of consciousness and on the physical side general convulsions (p. 526). A nutritive irritability underlies the morbid activity. Where mental disturbance predominates and actual insanity coexists with epilepsy, there is a notable affection of a special series of cells, not exclusively seen, however, in this disease, for it likewise prevails in other convulsive affections, such as chronic alcoholism, wherein spasmodic discharges of nerve energy are frequent (p. 525). With epilepsy is associated ancestral intemperance. Is it probable that the nuclear and cellular changes bear the imprints of ancestral vice (p. 527)? Disparity between nucleus and protoplasm and the displacement or degeneration of the former seem to bespeak a convulsive constitution" (p. 528).

Duty of Sanitarians Regarding Venereal Diseases.—At the eighteenth annual meeting of the Conference of State and Provincial Boards of Health an excellent paper, entitled "The Duty of Sanitarians Regarding Venereal Diseases," was read by Dr. Holton. A good deal of discussion followed, and the following resolution was put and carried: Moved by Dr. Probst, seconded by Dr. Wingate: "Whereas, the great prevalence of venereal diseases, which is indirectly the cause of many deaths, is a matter of much concern to the public health, and Whereas, the communication of these diseases to innocent persons must be largely due to ignorance, Be it resolved, That a committee of three be appointed by the President to prepare a leaflet that would be acceptable to physicians to give to their patients, setting forth the precautions to be taken by one suffering from a venereal disease to prevent its communication to others, and to make such other suggestions as it may deem proper, such instructions, when

adopted by this conference, to be recommended to State and Provincial Boards of Health for dissemination among the medical
profession, and said committee shall report at the next meeting."
The proposition which Dr. Probst has advanced is in line with
what was done at the Congress on venereal diseases, held at
Frankfort this year. It was there determined to send to every
physician a leaflet or slip in reference to this matter. Dr.
Probst's resolution is likely to start the ball rolling in America,
and it is not a bit too soon. The matter is not tabooed as it used
to be among laymen and laywomen. We think that women,
who are the principal sufferers from venereal diseases, should
agitate this reform, so as to hearten the sanitarians in any preventive measures which they may wish to introduce.   J. J. C.

The More Extensive Use of Diphtheria Antitoxin.—The
opinion is growing in Ontario that the time has arrived when to
neglect to give antitoxin in each and every case of diphtheria is
gross neglect. Several physicians who have obstinately held
out against the general conviction have capitulated at last. That
the free administration of diphtheria antitoxin is the correct
thing was exemplified by the local Board of Health of Brockville
(Ont.) during 1903. When a Brockville physician is called to
see a case of diphtheria he uses antitoxin, and the bill for the
same is sent to the municipality. Not only is this done in the
case of the necessitous person, but in all cases, rich and poor alike.
This free dispensing of diphtheria antitoxin commends itself as
an excellent method of employing municipal funds; the attending
physician in a case of diphtheria being left free to follow the best
instincts of his profession without being obliged to consider in any
degree the financial status of the patient. Another important
consideration is that the free use of diphtheria antitoxin exercises
a great influence in shortening the period of quarantine on those
who have contracted diphtheria. Besides, its immunizing power
protects those who have been exposed to the infection of diphtheria, thus preventing, in a timely and efficient way, the formation of fresh centres of the disease. Antitoxin lessens the expense of treating a case of diphtheria. In fact, if a competent
nurse be placed in charge of a case of diphtheria, the membranous
exudation, which is the source of the disease, being local and con-

trollable, there is no reason why the patient cannot be treated in an isolated room in a private house instead of being compelled to go to an isolation hospital.

Exposure to Flame Does not Disinfect Surgical Instruments. —A report recently presented to the Société de Chirurgie de Lyon (*La Presse Médicale,* April 2nd, 1904) shows that the exposure of surgical instruments to burning alcohol, a much-vaunted method of obtaining the antisepsis of cutting instruments, is a failure. The experimenters placed in an enamelled basin virulent cultures (staphylococci, bacteria of charbon, bacilli of tetanus), and covered them with alcohol. The alcohol was lighted, and the microbes exposed to the flame, but they were not destroyed, because when they were afterwards sown, fine cultures were obtained. A similar result was obtained by Drs. Berard and Lumiere, who, instead of exposing the cultures to burning alcohol, placed them in direct contact with a Bunsen burner. Another circumstance, which particularly shows the inefficaciousness of sterilization by flame, is that the micro-organisms resist the action of fire, not only when they are protected by a layer of dried blood or pus, but also in cases in which they are directly exposed to flame without being protected by an organic coagulum. Hence, one can readily understand that in exposing to burning alcohol a hypodermic needle, which may contain saline or organic concretions, the resulting asepsis may be of a very imperfect character.

Notification of Tuberculosis.—A statute has been passed by the Legislature of the Province of Quebec, providing for notification in municipalities of all cases of consumption that have reached the stages of suppuration or expectoration. The principle of notification of tuberculosis is favored by the Provincial Board of Health of Ontario. As we said in April, the notification of pulmonary consumption is excellent in principle, and, if carried out, would aid the health department of a city in securing the destruction of tubercular sputa in dwellings, places in which by long odds, sputa are likely to do more injury to the well than when ejected on sidewalks, streets and public places.

PERSONALS.

Dr. Lelia Davis has removed from 189 College Street to the Alexandra Apartments, University Avenue.

Dr. Lester Keller, of Ironton, Ohio, has completely recovered from his very severe illness, and, with Mrs. Keller, was present at Atlantic City.

Dr. Ingersoll Olmsted, 16 Bay Street South, Hamilton, announces to the profession that in future he will confine his practice to surgery and consultations.

Dr. and Mrs. Price-Brown sailed from Montreal, on the *Tunisian*, on the 1st inst. They expect to be away for a couple of months in England and on the Continent.

Dr. B. F. Turner, of Memphis, Tenn., was an interested participant at the Atlantic City meeting. He was accompanied by Mrs. Turner, who has the distinction of being the president of the largest woman's club in the South.

Dr. George Wilkins, professor of medical jurisprudence at McGill University, at the termination of his course of lectures for the 1903-1904 session, was presented by his class students with a handsome illuminated address, inscribed in Chinese characters.

Dr. L. Harwood, Montreal, has been appointed Professor of Gynecology in Laval University and chief of the Gynecologic Department of Notre Dame Hospital of that city, succeeding the late Dr. Brennan. He has also been chosen president of the section of gynecology of the Medical Congress of French-speaking Physicians of North America, which is to meet in Montreal this year.—*Jour. Am. Med. Association.*

Among the Canadians who attended the American Medical Association Convention, held at Atlantic City, N.J., last month, were: Dr. Alex. McPhedran, Dr. N. A. Powell, Dr. B. E. McKenzie, Dr. H. P. H. Galloway, Dr. C. J. O. Hastings, of Toronto; Dr. J. H. Elliott, of Gravenhurst; Dr Bruce Smith, Mrs. Smith, and Miss Smith, of Brockville; and Dr. W. A. Young and Mrs. Young, of Toronto.

THE well-known firm, Wm. R. Warner & Co., Philadelphia, Pa., have a most complete exhibit of pharmaceuticals in the Palace of L beral Arts, World's Fair, St. Louis, and all visiting medical men will be made heartily welcome there.

DR. J. H. WILSON, St. Thomas, who for many years sat in the Canadian House of Commons, has been appointed a Senator by the Dominion Government, succeeding Dr. Geo. Landerkin, deceased. The medical profession of the County of Elgin, Ontario, tendered Dr. Wilson a banquet, April 11.

FOUR out of the nine buildings belonging to The Norwich Pharmacal Co., Norwich, N.Y., were destroyed by fire a few weeks ago. Th s has not necessitated any stoppag in business, as the Company's new building, containing 24,000 feet of floor space, had stored in it the bulk of their manufactured products, which, of course, remained unharmed. Business goes on as usual.

THE Ontario Medical Association elected the following officers for the ensuing year: President, Dr. Wm. Burt, Paris; 1st Vice-President, Dr. J. L. Davison, Toronto; 2nd Vice-President, Dr. George Hodge, London; 3rd Vice-President, Dr. Edward Ryan, Kingston; 4th Vice-President, Dr. F. H. Middleboro', Owen Sound; General Secretary, Dr. C. P. Lusk, Toronto; Assistant Secretary, Dr. Samuel Johnston, Toronto; Treasurer, Dr. Frederick Fenton, Toronto.

DR. CHARLES A. OLIVER, of Philadelphia, Pa., has been chosen by the British Medical Association as its official guest from the United States for its seventy-second annual meeting, which is to take place in Oxford, England, in July. With him are associated Prof. Hirschberg, of Berlin, representing Germany, and Dr. Javal, of Paris, representing France. During his stay Dr. Oliver will reside at Keble College as the personal guest of Mr. Robert Walter Doyne, the President of the Ophthalmological Section of the Association and Lecturer on Ophthalmology at Oxford University.

❧ News of the Month. ❧

THE ROYAL AND IMPERIAL STATE INFIRMARY, VIENNA.

A HOSPITAL with 2,000 beds, with a death-rate of thirty a day and a birth-rate of 10,000 a year is what Vienna boasts in its great Royal and Imperial State Krankenhaus, or infirmary.

Dr. A. A. Dame, of Brunswick Avenue, who recently returned from Europe, thinks that the opportunities afforded by this immense institution, which is combined with the university, accounts for the eminence of Austrian medical men. "The great secret, the success of Austrian pathology, is the unlimited material they have there to work on."

Lorenz is known the world over, but Vienna has many other great specialists, such as Fuchs, the eye expert, and Politzer, who must retire in two years at the age of 70, according to the laws of the hospital, and whose superannuation will be a serious loss to the place, though every man there is a specialist.

Teaching in Vienna in very thorough, the anatomical laws being much less strict than in England. Dr. Dame found very few Canadians in Vienna and but fifteen or sixteen Americans in the classes he attended, and in the Anglo-American Society which the medical men maintain there.

Vienna had comparatively no winter this season. Six weeks ago the flowers and foliage in the parks were fully expanded, and Germany had a similar season. "The cold weather seemed to be confined to Canada this year," said the doctor.

"Except in education, Vienna is a century behind us. They are very crude," he continued. "A peculiar thing there is the hearses. They all gather about the hospital, and I have seen as many as thirty at a time. They are not all black, as with us, but some pink and some green and blue and all sorts of colors. Another thing that strikes one in Vienna is the dogs. They are a cross between a boar-hound and a mastiff, and are used very largely for draught animals. They draw most astonishing loads, and with very small wheels on the wagons which makes it all the harder work."

Dr. Dame was also in Berlin, Heidelberg, Leipsic, Prague, Halle and London. While the pathological work in Vienna is the greatest in the world, London holds her own in most lines. Moorefield is the finest equipped special hospital in the world. It is devoted to the eye; and Golden Square, where the ear, nose and throat are treated, is another great institution.

"Colonials seem to get positions as house-surgeons in these hospitals. There were two Australians and one Canadian in Moorehouse, and a Toronto boy in Golden Square, and there will be another Canadian there shortly."

THE M. J. BREITENBACH COMPANY vs. SIEGEL, COOPER COMPANY AND THOMAS H. McINNERNEY.

THE following decision of the Supreme Court of New York State will be of interest to the medical profession: This action having been begun by the service of the summons and complaint on each of the defendants on December 22nd, 1903, and the defendants having duly appeared on January 8th, 1904, by Rose & Putzel, Esqs., their attorneys, and it appearing that no answer or other pleading has been interposed on behalf of said defendants, and that they are in default in pleading, and due notice of application for final judgment having been given to said defendants, and on reading and filing the summons and complaint and the notice of appearance for said defendants, and the affidavit of Harry Eckhard, verified April 20th, 1904, and the copies of affidavits of Max J. Breitenbach and Edward G. Wells, verified December 17th, Henry P. Loomis, Charles O. Weisz, Mortimer Bartlett and Frank P. Ufford, verified December 22nd, all 1903, and after hearing proof on behalf of the plaintiff in support of the allegations of the complaint, and it appearing that the plaintiff's rights in the name "Pepto-Mangan" have been infringed by the defendants, now on motion of Philip Carpenter, attorney for the plaintiff, it is

Ordered, adjudged and decreed as follows:

1. That the plaintiff, The M. J. Breitenbach Company, is the owner of the sole and exclusive right to the use of the words "Pepto-Mangan" as a trade mark and trade name, as applied to medical preparations, throughout the United States and Canada, and has the sole and exclusive right in the same countries, of putting up and selling the preparation known as Gude's "Pepto-Mangan," according to the secret process and formula discovered by Dr. A. Gude, of Leipsic.

2. That the said defendants, the Siegel, Cooper Company and Thomas H. McInnerney, their agents, servants, employees and attorneys, be and they hereby are forever enjoined and restrained from making use of the words "Pepto-Manganate" in any man-

ner whatsoever, either alone or in combination with other words, or from using the words " Pepto-Mangan," or any word or words similar to the words " Pepto-Mangan " in sound or appearance, in connection with the advertisement or sale or otherwise, of any medical or other preparation—excepting only that of the plaintiff.

3. That the said defendants, the Siegel, Cooper Company and Thomas H. McInnerney forthwith deliver to the plaintiff, or its attorney, to be destroyed, all bottles, packages, wrappers, circulars, or other things in their possession or under their control, or that of either of them, bearing the words " Pepto-Manganate " or any similar words.

4. That the said plaintiff, the M. J. Breitenbach Company, recover of the said defendants, the Siegel, Cooper Company and Thomas H. McInnerney, the damages, to be assessed by the court, resulting from the use by said defendants of the name. of " Pepto-Manganate," which is hereby adjudged to be a violation of the plaintiff's rights in the name " Pepto-Mangan."

5. That the plaintiff recover of the said defendants the costs of this action.

Enter,

THOS. L. HAMILTON,   HENRY BISCHOFF,
  No. 136.   Clerk.   *Justice of the Supreme Court of*
STATE OF NEW YORK,   *State of New York.*
COUNTY OF NEW YORK

I, Thomas L. Hamilton, Clerk of the said County and Clerk of the Supreme Court of said State for said County, do certify, that I have compared the preceding with the original decree on file in my office, and that the same is a correct transcript therefrom, and of the whole of such original.

Indorsed filed, May 6th, 1904.

In witness whereof, I have hereunto subscribed my name and affixed my official seal, this 6th day of May, 1904.

(L. S.)   THOS. L. HAMILTON,
                               Clerk.

ITEMS OF INTEREST.

King Edward VII. Hospital in Grosvenor Garden, London, has been opened for the treatment of sick officers of the British army. Thirty London practitioners of eminence are on the staff.

Queen's Recognized.—Dr. J. C. Connell, dean of the faculty of medicine of Queen's University, has received word that Cambridge University, England, has granted recognition to Queen's medical course. This means that Queen's medical students, after spending a session or two here, will have the privilege, if they desire, of going to Cambridge and completing their course, full allowance being made for their attendance at Queen's.

Historical Medical Museum.—The formal opening of the department of medical history in the Germanic National Museum at Nuremberg occurred recently. All over Germany and Austria families have been delving among their heirlooms from medical ancestors and have found many articles of surpassing historical interest, which have been presented to the museum. The collection of books and MSS., instruments, and medals is being rapidly catalogued. Those in charge regard the work as a memorial to Dr. R. Landau, who gave the first impetus to the project.—*American Medical Journal.*

Exhibit of Mosquitoes at the St. Louis Fair.—Dr. Frederico Torralbas, a member of the Havana Supreme Board of Health, will exhibit a large number of mosquitoes, which he has brought from Cuba, for the purpose of illustrating the theory of the transmission of the yellow fever germs. Dr. Torralbas will also erect a series of tents at St. Louis, provided with wire screens, the same as were used when the American and Cuban surgeons made a series of experiments, to show that yellow fever germs can only be propagated by mosquitoes biting human beings. Men will be employed for a practical demonstration.—*Medical Record.*

A Protest.—The medical students of the Province of Quebec are protesting against the proposed action of the Legislature, which would throw open the doors of the profession in that Province to those who have not fulfilled the condition imposed by the present law. The bill now before the Legislature proposes to admit all who had begun the study of medicine before September last, thus avoiding their matriculation examinations. The profession in Montreal is aroused against the measure and is sending a deputation to Quebec to protest before the Legislature. The passage of the measure would benefit nearly 260 students in Quebec and Montreal.

M.D.C.M's. of Trinity.—The following are the results of the final M.D., C.M., examination at Trinity University: Certificates of honor—R. J. Manion, gold medal; J. A. Brown, silver medal; S. M. Lyon, J. A. Durnin, A. J. Fraleigh, R. A. McLurg, W. J. Chapman, H. A. Bray. Class I.—F. J. Rundle, W. A. Atkinson and W. E. McLaughlin (equal), H. E. Knoke, F. H. Hughes, S. J. Hillis, J. F. Adamson. Class II.—W. H. Brown, W. J. Backus, G. R. Luton, D. G. Cameron, J. H. Dickett, W. A. Scanlon, N. G. Allin, B. C. M. Whyte, W. J. Barber, L W.

Lynn, F. C. S. Wilson,, Miss L. Morden, A. V. Brown, G. H.
Boyce, J. Fettes, A. A. J. Simpson, L. Clarke, G. H. Richards,
Miss Allyn. Class III.—B. M. Lancaster, J. H. Cascaden, R. J.
Reade, J. H. C. Henderson. R. H. Taylor, D. Livingstone, H. A.
S. Treadgold. Conditioned in pathology—E. A. Hammond, Miss
D. J. Bower. Conditioned in gynecology—E. R. Frankish.

Dynamite for Butchers.—"A new use has been found for
dynamite," said a butcher, "and perhaps before long we shall be
eating dynamite-killed beef. At the weekly meeting of my
society a member told of some experiments with dynamite that
he had seen in a slaughter-house. These experiments had been
successful, and had proved that a thimbleful of dynamite, ex-
ploded on a steer's or cow's forehead, would kill it more quickly
than the usual 'knocking-in-the-head' method. It was said that
three steers had been placed side by side and about two feet apart.
On the forehead of each a charge of dynamite with an electric
fuse had been fastened, and these charges had all been connected
with a common battery. A touch of a stud on the battery had
set off the dynamite, and the three steers, without a struggle, without a groan, without a violent movement, had fallen back, stone
dead! It was a very impressive sight," the speaker said, "and he
hoped to see the day when all the meat in the world would be
dynamite-killed."

An Ambulance Service for London.—The committee of the
Metropolitan Street Ambulance Association has made the following suggestions for supplying London with an efficient street ambulance service—a long-felt want: 1. A controlling authority
responsible for a uniform well-organized ambulance service under
the government of the London County Council. 2. The division
of London into districts, or "accident areas," with a properly
organized ambulance service in each, consisting of horse or motor
as well as hand ambulances. 3. The conjoint carrying out of the
fire brigade and the ambulance services. 4. The stationing of
ambulances at or in connection with the principal hospitals. 5.
Keeping the police efficient in first-aid training and making them
available in rendering aid, summoning an ambulance, and taking
charge of the patient until the ambulance and attendant arrive.
6. The 800 fire-alarm telephone posts now existing, and all other
telephones to be made available for calling ambulances. 7. The
experience gained in New York,, Chicago, Paris and other cities
is more than sufficient to justify work on a scale large enough to
provide for the removal of 13,000 to 15,000 casualties yearly.—
London Letter, American Medical Journal.

The German Medical Exhibit at the World's Fair.—The committee in charge of the exhibit decided to devote the comparatively small space allotted to Germany to a presentation of the German methods of instruction in medicine. Anatomy, surgery, internal medicine and bacteriology are thus presented in systematic order, as taught in Germany. One-fourth of the entire space is given up to bacteriology and experimental therapy, outlining a complete course, with each of the most important human and veterinary diseases treated separately. The etiology is shown by cultures and pictures of the germs, their pathogenic properties by mounted specimens and plates, and differentiation by production of agglutination and the specific chemical changes in the micro-organisms. The various procedures in bacteriologic examination are also presented, and a complete outfit of one of the " flying laboratories " organized to fight typhoid and other epidemics on the spot. The principle is to fight the disease in the individual and destroy all infection breeders on the spot. There will be ample evidence, pamphlets, statistics, etc., to testify to the value of this mode of prophylaxis of epidemics. The exhibit of serums, their standardization and their practical results is the co-operative display of the Imperial Board of Health, the Institutes for Infectious Diseases at Berlin, and for Experimental Therapy at Frankfurt, the institutes at Halle and Breslau and Dunbar's Institute at Hamburg besides the private firms that manufacture serums. The exhibit for internal medicine portrays a clinical lecture on the subject of tuberculosis, etiology, examination of patient, pathologic findings, prophylaxis and treatment. The surgery exhibit is planned on much the same lines, but comprises two separate displays, one arranged by von Bergmann, the other by Mikulicz, each exhibiting the instruments, etc., preferred. Bergmann presents a portable Rontgen apparatus which allows reduction and fixation of fractures, etc., under constant control of the eye. Nitze's first, original cystoscope is seen in this display. Great efforts have been made to make the exhibit of pathologic anatomy truly representative of German achievements in this line with actual specimens preserved in the Kayserling fluid, casts, photographs, atlases, etc., contributed by many institutions and clinicians.—*American Medical Journal.*

New Medical Building for London, Eng.—Reference has been made in previous letters to the proposal to centralize the teaching of anatomy, physiology, and the other sciences which form the foundations of medicine which at present are taught more or less efficiently in the twelve independent medical schools in which this metropolis rejoices. The scheme is taking practical shape, and already negotiations for the purchase of a suitable site are in progress. Unfortunately it seems to be considered necessary that the site of the proposed Institute of Medical Sciences should be in the near neighborhood of the existing local habitation of the University of London. This means that it will have to be found in South Kensington, one of the most expensive quarters in London. Not only will land be of great price there, but it will be difficult for students, who are not as a rule richly endowed with worldly goods, to find suitable lodgings within reasonable distance of the Institute. It is proposed that premises and equipment adequate for the instruction of 500 students in anatomy, physiology (including pharmacology), biology (zoology and botany), chemistry and physics should be provided. The total cost of the buildings is put at $800,000, while it is estimated that an annual expenditure of $102,500 for teaching will be necessary. Toward all this little or nothing has so far been subscribed by the public, to whom a strong appeal was made not long ago by Lord Rosebery, Chancellor of the University, and the other principal officials of the University. It is almost hopeless to ask a British Government for substantial help in furtherance of such a scheme, and for some reason or another millionaires do not appear to find a stimulus to generosity—or self-advertisement—in the University of London. Yet there are here the makings of a university—particularly in the department of medicine—such as the world has hardly yet seen. The fact is, I believe that there has been so much squabbling about trivialities and so much jealousy and narrowmindedness among those who undertook the reconstitution of the University of London that people are disgusted with the whole thing. The struggle has been going on for nearly a score of years, and is not yet finished. But it really seems as if the obstructives were about to be beaten all along the line, and London at last to have a living teaching university instead of a system of examining boards.—Extract from "London Letter" to *Medical News.*

Trachoma.—In late years the trachoma question has assumed a much greater importance in this country, and especially in New York City, where for about a year a real epidemic of this disease has prevailed. Until now it has shown little sign of subsidence, and new cases are constantly coming under observation. The children in our public schools have been particularly attacked by the disease, and it has been stated that in certain parts of this city twenty-five per cent. of the scholars have been found to be affected. In the special hospital for trachoma cases, established by the Board of Health, over 1,100 patients were treated from December, 1902, to May, 1903. The health commissioner considered the matter of sufficient importance to hold a conference in reference to the best way of suppressing the epidemic. . A trouble until they were refused admission to the schools by the medical examiners with the statement to consult an ophthalmologist.—This was the case even in children in whom the trachoma had developed to such an extent that upon drawing aside the lids the conjunctival folds were found to project as thick, stiff, gelatinous protuberances. The results obtained from instillations of a 2 per cent. protargol solution in the milder cases of trachoma as well as those which had not too far advanced, were perceptibly good; the secretion rapidly diminished; the hypertrophy of the conjunctiva soon subsided, and in most instances, the children, after four to six weeks' treatment, were so much improved that they were permitted to return to school. The energy displayed by the New York Board of Health in the suppression of trachoma is worthy of general adoption in our other large cities. After the disease is diagnosed in a certain case, most stringent precautions should be taken to avoid its communication to others. Especial attention should be given to cleanliness of the patients, and particularly the hands. All rags and cotton that have come in contact with the eyes should be burned at once, and towels, bed-clothing, etc., should be thoroughly boiled, and the patient warned against rubbing the eyes. Children should be excluded from school until the disease is no longer in the infectious stage, and perhaps it might be well to suggest that the books, pencils, and slates be also disinfected. A thorough examination of the eyes of all immigrants and strict precautions in the case of those who have been attacked will reduce the cases of trachoma to a very trivial number, and thus prevent its serious complications. —A. A. Ripperger, M.D., in *American Medicine*.

"By the way," said the gentlemanly-looking person in the black broadcloth suit, " if you mention my name in connection with the accident, you may say that ' Dr. Swankem was called, and the fractured arm was suitably bandaged,' or something to that effect. Please spell the name correctly. Here's my card." " Thanks," said the reporter, looking at the card. " You are next door to Dr. Rybold, I believe. Are you acquainted with him?" " No, sir," replied Dr. Swankem, stiffly. " We do not recognize Dr. Rybold as a member of the profession. He advertises."—*Maryland Medical Journal*.

Obituary

DEATH OF DR. C. W. CHAFFEE.

THE death occurred on May 26th, at 614 Spadina Avenue, of Dr. Charles Walton Chafee, son of the late Dr. T. M. Chafee. The deceased, who was connected with the I.O.F., and not engaged in regular practice, was a promising young man, and had only been ill for a few days. Pneumonia was the cause of death. The funeral took place on Friday afternoon, the 28th, to St. James' Cemetery.

DEATH OF DR. REGINALD HENWOOD.

DR. REGINALD HENWOOD, one of the most successful physicians and surgeons in the Province, died of general decline at his home in Brantford, on May 22nd. Born in England seventy-six years ago, he came to Canada when a mere youth, locating at Toronto, where he secured a Provincial license to practise medicine in 1847. Shortly afterwards he removed to Brantford, where for fifty years he carried on a very large practice. During 1882-1883 he served as Mayor of Brantford. In religion he was an Anglican, a Conservative in politics, and a most prominent member in Masonic circles. Three sons survive—Dr. A. J. and Edward, of Brantford, and George Henwood, of Victoria, B.C. The funeral took place in Wednesday, May 25th.

BOOK REVIEWS.

Manual of Materia Medica and Pharmacy. Specially designed for the use of Practitioners and Medical, Pharmaceutical, Dental, and Veterinary Students. By E. STANTON MUIR, Ph.G., V.M.D.; Instructor in Comparative Materia Medica and Pharmacy in the University of Pennsylvania. Third edition, revised and enlarged. Crown octavo, 192 pages, interleaved throughout. Bound in extra cloth, $2.00 net. Philadelphia: F. A. Davis Company, publishers, 1914-16 Cherry Street.

" This work, originally published eight years ago, and a second edition four or five years later, is intended to give to practitioners and students of medicine, in as concise and clear a manner as possible, those points which are of value, without the lengthy detail usually found in text-books." This announcement the author makes in his preface, and, judging from our perusal of the books, he has carried out his original idea throughout. One good point in the arrangement of the work is that the drugs are arranged in alphabetical order. Dr. Muir has wisely eliminated a lot of matter that is entirely superfluous, a point many authors pay too little attention to. He has divided the book into three parts, Part I. being devoted to Botany; Part II. to Individual Drugs, and Part III. to Pharmacy.   W. A. Y.

Diseases of the Gall-Bladder and Bile-Ducts, including Gall-Stone. By A. W. MAYO ROBSON, F.R.C.S. Hunterian Professor of Surgery and Pathology, 1897, 1899 and 1903; and Vice-President, Royal College of Surgeons of England, 1902; assisted by *J.* F. DOBSON, M.S. (Lond.), F.R.C.S., lately Resident Surgeon to the General Infirmary at Leeds. Third edition. Pp. 485. London: Bailliere, Tindall & Cox, 8 Henrietta Street, Covent Garden. 1904.

Among the many excellent monographs which have appeared of recent years, written on special subjects in surgery, none is more widely or more favorably known than Mr. Mayo Robson's work on "Diseases of the Gall-Bladder and Bile-Ducts." The first edition of this work appeared in 1897, and since that time the author's position as a leading authority on the surgery of diseases caused by gall-stones has been universally recognized. Successive editions became necessary, not only because of the demand for the book, but because such rapid strides had been made by the author and by others in perfecting the technique of operative procedure in this field of surgery. One sentence in the preface of the present edition, which illustrates this fact, reads as follows: " The operation of choledochotomy for the removal of gall-stones from the common duct, which, up to July, 1901, showed a mortality of 16.2 per cent., has since that date, under the more complete exposure which can now be obtained, shown a mortality of only 1.9 per cent.; and I have done a consecutive series of over fifty cases of duodeno-choledochotomy without a death." This remarkable record establishes a claim for recognition of the magnificent work which has been done in the surgical treatment of these diseases. Mr. Mayo Robson has operated on the gall-bladder and bile-ducts 539 times, and, therefore, speaks from the standpoint of an unusually extensive experience. He has also made and recorded some very interesting observations in his book regarding the physiological action of bile. The bearing of these conclusions upon his operative procedure may be appreciated by quoting his statement that " bile is probably chiefly excrementitious, and, like the urine, is constantly being formed and cast out." Again, he concludes that " increase in body weight and good health are quite compatible with the entire absence of bile from the intestines." Under these circumstances he does not hesitate where occasion requires to divert the flow of bile from the small intestine such as he accomplishes in making a permanent artificial opening between the gall-bladder and the colon in cases of occlusion of the common duct. This operation is recommended where, for some reason, the artificial opening cannot be made between the gall-bladder and the duodenum or the jejunum. It is hardly necessary to review this work in detail. Enough has been said to indicate its scope and character. It is undoubtedly the most valuable monograph we have from British surgeons on the subject, and is admirably adapted to serve as a practical guide to the treatment of diseases of the gall-bladder and bile-ducts.   A. P.

The Man Who Pleases and the Woman Who Charms. By JOHN
    A. CONE. New York: Hinds & Noble. Cloth, 75 cents.

For those who would cultivate charm in person and grace in deportment this book has its helpful lesson. It presents the characteristic needs of the present generation and prescribes the means of satisfying them.

The Practical Medicine Series of Year-Books, comprising ten
volumes on the year's progress in Medicine and Surgery.
Issued monthly, under the general editorial charge of Gus-
TAVUS P. HEAD, M.D., Professor of Laryngology and Rhin-
ology, Chicago Post-Graduate Medical School. Volume IV.,
Gynécology. Edited by EMILIUS C. DUDLEY, A.M., M.D.,
Professor of Gynecology, Northwestern University Medical
School; Gynecologist to St. Luke's and Wesley Hospitals,
Chicago; and WILLIAM HEALY, A.B., M.D., Instructor
Gynecology, Northwestern University Medical School.
Chicago: The Year-Book Publishers, 40 Dearborn Street.
1904.

This volume on Gynecology is the March number of the 1904
series, and covers the best of the year's progress in this subject, for
the year prior to its publication. The work is divided into six
parts: Part.I., On General Principles; Part II., Infections and
Allied Disorders; Part III., Tumors, Malformations; Part IV.,
Traumatisms; Part V., Displacements; Part VI., Disorders of
Menstruation and Sterility. While this series is especially prepared for the general practitioner, it is very useful as a reference
for those more interested in gynecology. We are well pleased .
with the volume, and think the whole series not only up to the
high standard of last year, but steadily improving. w. j. w.

Rontgen Ray Diagnosis and Therapy. By CARL BECK, M.D.,
Professor of Surgery in the N. Y. Post-Graduate Medical
School and Hospital; Visiting Surgeon to St. Mark's Hos-
pital and the German Policlinik; with 322 illustrations in
the text. New York and London: D. Appleton & Co. 1904.
Canadian Agents: The Geo. N. Morang Co., Limited,
Toronto.

By way of introduction to his subject, the author has the following words appear on the fly-page of his book:

> "O Light, of all the gifts of heaven
> The dearest, best! From light all beings live—
> Each fair created thing—the very plants
> Turn with a joyful transport to the light."

During the past few years, a good deal of literature has
appeared upon the Rontgen rays, and their application to the
uses of surgery, the only fault with most of the works already published being that they have touched too little upon the clinical
aspect of the subject. This has been a most serious error, and
has detracted considerably from their value up till now. Dr.
Carl Beck has, however, avoided this footfall, and provided the

profession with a volume that is thoroughly practical, as he demonstrates most ably how the rays can be made to aid the surgeon in his work; the book being further added to in value by plenty of illustrations, showing the methods to be employed. Dr. Beck deserves congratulations on the results of his labors, and we bespeak for his volume a hearty reception at the hands of his confreres in the profession.   W. A. Y.

A System of Physiologic Therapeutics, a Practical Exposition of the Methods, other than Drug-Giving, Useful for the Prevention of Disease, and in the Treatment of the Sick. Edited by SOLOMON SOLIS COHEN, A.M., M.D., Senior Assistant Professor of Clinical Medicine in Jefferson Medical College; Physician to the Jefferson Medical College Hospital and to the Philadelphia, Jewish and Rush Hospitals, etc. Vol. VIII.—Rest, Mental Therapeutics, Suggestion—by Francis X. Dercum, M.D., Ph.D., Professor of Nervous and Mental Diseases in the Jefferson Medical College of Philadelphia; Neurologist to the Philadelphia Hospital, Consulting Physician to the Asylum for the Chronic Insane at Wernersville, etc., etc. Philadelphia: P. Blakiston's Son & Co., 1012 Walnut Street. Canadian Agents: Chandler & Massey Limited, Toronto, Montreal and Winnipeg. 1904.

Vol. VIII. of Physiologic Therapeutics is divided into three parts, number one being devoted to Rest, number two to Therapeutics of Mental Diseases, and number three to Suggestion. The book in its first 150 pages will be found to be chiefly exponent of what is frequently spoken of as the Rest Cure, the form of treatment used, chiefly in institutions, for patients of nervous disposition, and whose condition hardly necessitates resorting to any particular form of medication. Part I. goes into Chronic Fatigue (the fatigue neurosis); Rest in Neurasthenia and Allied States, Hysteria and its different Phenomena, Etiologic Factors, Treatment by Rest and Physiologic Methods, Hypochondria, and the Application of Rest in Chorea and Other Functional Nervous Diseases. Part II. consists of less than 100 pages, and deals with the Prevention of Insanity, the General Principles of the Treatment of the Insane and the Treatment of the Special Forms of Mental Disease. Perhaps the most interesting part of the volume is Section III., devoted to Suggestion. The treatment of such conditions as hysteria, hypochondria and neurasthenia by suggestion is dealt with, going to show that in many cases considerable relief can be afforded thereby. The book closes with a chapter devoted to such subjects as Pythonism, Shamanism, Magnetism, Mesmerism, Hypnotism, Metallotherapy, Mind Cure, Faith Cure and Eddyism.

A Practical Treatise on Medical Diagnosis for Students and Physicians. By JOHN H. MUSSER, M.D., Professor of Clinical Medicine in the University of Pennsylvania; Physician to the Philadelphia and the Presbyterian Hospitals; Consulting Physician to the Woman's Hospital of Philadelphia, and to the West Philadelphia Hospital for Women, to the Rush Hospital for Consumptives, and the Jewish Hospital of Philadelphia, etc., etc. Fifth edition, revised and enlarged. Illustrated with 395 wood-cuts and 63 colored plates. Philadelphia and New York: Lea Bros. & Co. 1904.

" The most effective way in which an author can evince his gratitude for favor shown to a book is to keep it a fair exponent of its subject." Such forms the opening sentence to the author's preface to his fifth edition, and it takes but a few minutes for any of his readers to find out that it is Dr. Musser's one desire to keep his now well-known book on Medical Diagnosis to the forefront, by that means sustaining the reputation it has gained for itself in past years. "Musser's Diagnosis " has for some time been considered to be one of the very best works on the subject published, and in its fifth edition it equals any and outstrips several of what might be termed its competitors, *e.g.,* books dealing with the same branch of medicine. The edition is larger than any preceding one, the entire work having been completely revised and many illustrations added. The author lays great stress upon clinical laboratory methods as the only true basis for " precision in diagnosis."

A System of Practical Surgery. By PROF. E. VON BERGMANN, M.D., of Berlin; PROF. P. VON BRUNS, M.D., of Tubingen, and PROF. J. VON MIKULICZ, M.D., of Breslau. Volume II. Surgery of the neck, thorax and spinal column. Translated and Edited by WILLIAM T. BULL, M.D., Professor of Surgery, College of Physicians and Surgeons, Columbia University, New York, and CARLTON P. FLINT, M.D., Instructor in Minor Surgery, College of Physicians and Surgeons, New York. New York and Philadelphia: Lea Brothers & Co. 1904.

The subjects dealt with in this volume are the malformations, injuries and diseases of the neck, thorax and spinal column. The author has the happy faculty of expressing his thoughts concisely; and the translators have done ample justice to the author in the employment of clear, terse, vigorous English. It may fairly be said that in some instances his exposition is too brief. His discussion of wry-neck occupies only twelve pages, and even in this space the subject is well illustrated. The desire for brevity, however, has caused him to dismiss the important feature of diagnosis, while much that is of great importance to the general practitioner remains unsaid. A writer, however, may be excused because of too great brevity when one recalls the fact that the common sin of these large systems is to load themselves up with much that is mere padding. In the treatment of such a subject as goitre it would be confidently expected that the operative treatment would receive full consideration, and it does. His conservatism, however, is manifest in the place which he assigns to the medicinal treatment. One might reasonably look for some reference to the treatment of goitre by electricity; this, however, is not mentioned. In dealing with the subject of spinal bifida the author takes the responsibility of recommending radical operation as being indicated in the great majority of cases. The subject is considered with great clearness and fulness though the account is very concise. His discussion of the diseases and deformities of the spinal column is quite as satisfactory as one may expect outside the pages of a monograph upon that subject. The paper, illustrations and binding do ample credit and justice to the well-known firm who are publishing this work in America.

B. E. M'K.

Commoner Diseases of the Eye; How to Detect and How to Treat Them. By CASEY A. WOOD, C.M., M.D., D.C.L., Professor of Clinical Ophthalmology in the University of Illinois, etc., and THOMAS A. WOODRUFF, M.D., C.M., L.R.C.P., Professor of Ophthalmology in the Chicago Post-Graduate Medical School, Chicago, etc.; 250 illustrations; 7 colored plates; 500 pp. 5 x 8 in. $1.75 net. G. P. Engelhard & Co., Chicago.

One opens this little book with special interest because it is written by two Canadians who have won some reputation in the land of their adoption. It is most satisfying both in its clearness and completeness. Considering Ophthalmology from the standpoint of the physician in general practice it is free from many of the erudite discussions which frighten the general practitioner away from the standard works on the subject.   J. M. M.

Diseases of the Eye. By L. WEBSTER FOX, A.M., M.D., Professor of Ophthalmology in the Medico-Chirurgical College of Philadelphia, Pa., with five colored plates and 296 illustrations in the text. New York and London: D. Appleton & Company. 1904.

The three features which strike the reader in this book are the clearness and good size of the print, the great number of illustrations, and the space devoted to operations. Based upon lectures delivered to students at the Medico-Chirurgical College, it is described by the author as a digested summary of the known facts of Ophthalmology. Facts are very often more or less colored by personal tendencies, and this, in the case of Dr. Fox, seems to be altogether towards operation. This same tendency influences the illustrations, some of which cause one to wonder why they were inserted. " Before and after operation" illustrations may be *de rigueur* in Philadelphia· text-books, but they savor somewhat unduly of a desire to impress upon the reader the operator's skill. The personal element in medical books is all too rare, so that one must not cavil overmuch, for aside from these little flaws the book is no mean addition to one's library.

J. M. M.

A Guide to the Clinical Examination of the Blood for Diagnostic Purposes. By RICHARD C. CABOT, M.D. With colored plates and engravings. Fifth Revised Edition. New York: William Wood & Company. 1904. Canadian agents: Chandler & Massey Limited, Toronto, Montreal, Winnipeg.

In the introduction to this valuable work the author gives his views on the scope and value of blood examination. He says there are probably not more than five or six diseases in which the blood examination gives a certain and positive diagnosis, but there is a very considerable number of conditions in which the blood examination will help in making the diagnosis, and that very often the simple discovery that the blood is normal may be of the greatest value in diagnosis. He also says that improvements in technique have lessened the labor and increased the accuracy of blood examination so much that the most important facts about the blood of nearly every case can be obtained by a practiced observer in fifteen minutes.

These methods for the clinical examination of the blood, as well as its physiology and pathology, are fully described in the first part of the work. The second part of the book is devoted to the special pathology of the blood.

Full descriptions are given of the changes usually found in blood in such diseases as anemia and leukemia, in acute and chronic infectious diseases, in malignant disease, blood parasites and intestinal parasites, and in diseases of special organs.

The Widal reaction in typhoid fever is discussed in a very interesting chapter on examination of serum.

The book contains a very large number of very good illustrations, many of the colored ones being very beautiful. No one who is interested in the subject of blood examination can afford to be without this excellent work by Dr. Cabot. A. E.

Abbott's Alkaloidal Digest, a Brief Therapeutics of Some of the
Principal Alkaloidal Medicaments, with Suggestions for Clinical Application, embodying various articles on important
special agents and certain great phases of Alkaloidal Therapy
that have been developed in my personal practice. By W.
C. ABBOTT, M.D., editor *Alkaloidal Clinic,* etc., etc. Chicago: The Clinic Publishing Co. 1904.

On the title page of this little book appear the following words:
" In therapeutics use the smallest possible quantity of the best
obtainable means to produce a desired therapeutic result." Into
that motto is boiled down the secret of alkaloidal therapy, a new
form of medication, the principles of which are laid down in
Dr. Abbott's book now before us. The Digest will be found to
be a handy vade-mecum, full of suggestions as to the uses of
alkalometry, a system of medication that in many quarters is
rapidly gaining friends.

A Manual of Nursing. By REYNOLD WEBB WILCOX, M.A.,
M.D., LL.D., Professor of Medicine in the New York Post-
Graduate Medical School and Hospital; Consulting Physician
to the Nassau Hospital; Visiting Physician to St. Mark's
Hospital; Fellow of the American Academy of Medicine;
Member of the American Therapeutic Society, etc. Illus-
trated. Philadelphia: P. Blakiston's Son & Co., 1012
Walnut Street. 1904. Canadian Agents: Chandler &
Massey Limited, Toronto and Montreal.

This volume contains the lectures on fever nursing, which
were delivered in substance to the nurses of St. Mark's Hospital during the session of 1903-4. Fevers are first taken up in
a general way; then symptoms, causation and treatment; the
use of the clinical thermometer, pulse and respiration are discussed. After this the various fevers are considered in detail, and
the nurse is given a very clear and practical knowledge of the
subject, and one which, to our mind, is essential for good results.
We have much pleasure in recommending this little work to our
friends in the nursing profession.   W. J. W.

The Bacteriology of Every-Day Practice. By J. ODERY SYMES,
M.D., State Medicine (Lond.), D.P.H., etc.; Assistant
Physician and Bacteriologist, British General Hospital.
Second edition. London: Bailliere, Tindall & Cox, 8 Hen-
rietta Street, Covent Garden. 1904.

This is the second of the Medical Monograph Series, and its
aim is to sketch in brief compass the chief features of given

subjects of every-day interest to students and practitioners. This edition has been largely rewritten, and sections have been added upon the preparation and staining of blood films; upon meningitis, and upon those diseases which science is gradually unfolding to the professional world.   A. J. H.

Medical Laboratory Methods and Tests. By HERBERT FRENCH, M.A., M.D. London: Bailliere, Tindall & Cox, 8 Henrietta Street, Convent Garden. Price, $1.00. Canadian Agent: J. A. Carveth & Co., Toronto.

This little volume aims at giving in detail the commoner methods used in explaining pathological fluids and substances. The conclusions which may be drawn from the various tests are carefully given, while at the same time care is taken to point out the fallacies to which each is liable.

A separate chapter is devoted to each of the following subjects: examination of the urine, blood, sputum, pus, gastric contents, feces, skin, serous exudates, and tests for the commoner poisons.

We have not seen a more useful or more carefully prepared hand-book for the medical laboratory.   A. E.

A Text-Book of Physiology. By ISAAC OTT, A.M., M.D., Professor of Physiology in the Medico-Chirurgical College of Philadelphia. One hundred and thirty-seven illustrations. Philadelphia: F. A. Davis Company. 1904.

This is an elementary work containing the chief facts of physiology, which have a direct bearing on the practice of medicine. The various topics are thoroughly discussed; the whole text is carefully written, and is well adapted to the needs of medical students, for whom it is chiefly intended. The book is well printed, and contains the usual number of satisfactory illustrations.   A. E.

Case Teaching in Surgery. By HERBERT L. BURRELL, M.D., Professor of Clinical Surgery, Harvard University, and JOHN BAPST BLAKE, M.D., Instructor in Surgery, Harvard University. Philadelphia: P. Blakiston's Son & Co., 1012 Walnut Street. 1904. Canadian Agents: Chandler & Massey Limited, Toronto, Montreal and Winnipeg.

A useful list of the history of surgical cases collected by Dr. Blake, at the Harvard Medical School, and Dr. Burrell in his clinical demonstrations. The history of the case is given the student, and he makes his diagnosis and prognosis, and then states what he considers proper treatment for such a case. There are seventy-five cases tabulated, including those most frequently met with day by day. A most useful form for teachers.

A. J. H.

A Guide to Urine Testing for Nurses and Others. By MARK ROBINSON, L.R.C.P., L.R.C.S. (Ed.). Second edition, Bristol: *John* Wright & Co. London: Simpkin, Marshall, Hamilton, Kent & Co. 1904.

The second edition of this booklet on urine testing comes to us in a revised condition. It deals with the first principles of urinary examination in a very clear style, thus making it suitable for those whom the author intended it.   W. H. P.

Aseptic and Antiseptic Preparations, and Treatment of Emergencies after Abdominal Operations. By GEO. WACKERHAGEN, M.D. New York: E. R. Pelton, Publishers.

The first thing that comes to one on looking into this little book is the fact that though it is very small it has many useful hints. To nurses and young practitioners, I suppose, it is most useful.   S.

The Canadian
Journal of Medicine and Surgery

A JOURNAL PUBLISHED MONTHLY IN THE INTEREST OF MEDICINE AND SURGERY

VOL. XVI. TORONTO, AUGUST, 1904. NO. 2.

Original Contributions.

THOUGHTS ON CANCER.*

BY THE HON. SIR WM. HINGSTON, F.R.C.S., MONTREAL.

WHATEVER may be the state of our knowledge in other departments of the healing art, we must admit we know but little of the etiology of tumor formation generally, and especially of those forms we are accustomed to call "malignant." These are still, as Kelynack observes, "shrouded in darkness and mystery." Yet at no time in the history of surgery has cancer occupied a greater share of thought than at the present. France and Germany have long been pursuing diligent investigations to unravel its hiddenness. In Great Britain a Cancer Research Fund has been recently established, and the function of General Superintendent of Cancer Investigation has been created: to supervise workers; to collect statistical, dietetic, topographical, and other information; to organize a system of correspondence with Home, Colonial, Indian, and foreign laboratories; to invite the Colonial Offices to assist in obtaining information as to the relative prevalence of cancer in the various colonies of the British Empire; and to trace, if possible, any connection with the mode of life, food, habits, environment, and so forth, of the inhabitants. How much will be accomplished by organized investigation of this character and how much by the unobtrusive, individual worker in the quiet of the hospital and the laboratory, time alone will determine.

A few months ago the Cancer Research Fund of the Royal College of Physicians and Surgeons made its first report. It consisted of three papers, the first, " The Zoological Distribution of Cancer,"

* Read at meeting of the Ontario Medical Association, Toronto, June, 1904.

4

showing the disease to exist in most of the domesticated animals, in many of the wild, and in several of the fish tribe; the second dealing with the " Transmissibility of Cancer," establishing without a doubt—at least in the case of mice—that carcinoma can be transmitted from animal to animal; the third taking exception to the view that cancer consists of a change from normal tissue to malignant, or, as stated by Campbell, " that cancerous growth is caused by the degenerative reversion of epithelial cells to a germinal type, in association with a local irritant, and in the presence of an abundant blood supply."

In other parts of Great Britain private charity comes to the aid of a local research fund. Thus, in Liverpool, for instance, one person leads off with a subscription of $50,000. The Liverpool Royal Infirmary furnishes a ward for facility of observation and experiment, and its University has placed five large rooms at the disposal of the research fund for the same purpose.

It is quite beyond the scope of this paper to discuss the nature of cancer. That aspect of the question is as yet incomplete. One writer expresses the view that the disease is due to a pathogenetic organism belonging to the numerous yeast family; another, that it is an animal organism; a third, that it is in any case a parasite; a fourth, that it arises from some (not always recognizable) disturbed action of the natural component parts of the body. At the present time the tendency of thought is towards the theory that the origin of cancer is extrinsic—that there is, as Meyer observes, an extrinsic cause, and that it remains only to discover it.

If cancer has a parasitic origin, has it a micro-organism of its own? If it has, so soon as the nature of that organism is understood we may indulge the belief that a specific cure of cancer may ultimately be found. So far, however, there has not been successful cultivation, outside the body, of those micro-organisms which have been supposed to be of malignant growth, and this notwithstanding what the French style " Cancer a deux," an accident so extremely rare as scarcely to deserve mention. But where attempts have been deliberately made, as by Alibert upon himself, his medical friends and students, the result has been invariably negative.

So far, therefore, it may be said, the origin of cancer remains an enigmatic secret. For my part the conviction is forced in upon me from bedside observation, that the cause of cancer is perverted action, possibly inflammatory, without, at first, the usual evidences of inflammation; or, in other words, that it is perverted nutrition. This view I have held for many years.

But while every diligence is being exerted to unravel the causes and nature of cancer, something less problematical, something less doubtful, is forced upon our notice—its increase.

Cancer is greatly on the increase, and reliable statistical information is at hand in support of that opinion. "After all the necessary corrections," says the *British Medical Journal,* "there is an enormous increase in the registered mortality from malignant disease in all civilized countries having a complete register of causes of death."

"In London alone," says Dr. Caldwell Smith, "the cancer death rate has increased from 65 per 100,000 to 95 per 100,000 in five years; in fifty years it more than doubled. Observers have remarked that the increase is chiefly from visceral cancer."

The cancer death rate in England and Wales has increased between four and five times in fifty years.

On this side of the Atlantic the question of the increase of cancer has been carefully gone into by Warren, of Boston, and Roswell Park, of Buffalo—and no men in America, you will admit, are more competent to conduct an investigation of this nature—and the conclusion arrived at by both, independently of each other, is in favor of increase.

The State Board of Health of Massachusetts says: "Every year there is an increase in the reports to the State of the number of deaths from cancer, even when allowance is made for age and greater population." And Professor Roswell Park, speaking of his native State, says: "If for the next ten years the relative death rates are maintained, we shall find that ten years from now there will be more deaths in New York State from cancer than from consumption, smallpox and typhoid fever combined."

Statistics in Canada are as yet too incomplete to be of much value, but the experience of hospital physicians and surgeons is to the effect that cancer in Canada is greatly on the increase. It has been said by those who do not share this view that "a surgeon's personal experience is often misleading, as cases in which he is specially interested are constantly being sent to him by friends and former pupils, and one case brings another from among the public." That view I have taken carefully into consideration, but I am the more impressed as to the greater frequency of cancer than formerly, and as to its steady increase, from observation outside of my own special field of labor.

And while the fell disease is on the increase, medicine has effected little save by co-operating with surgery, to enable the knife, with all the safeguards asepticism can secure, to penetrate parts of the body hitherto regarded as beyond its reach.

The internal specific treatment of cancer, either local or general, has rarely been without claimants to the possession of some special knowledge of a remedy—knowledge claimed to have been acquired, inherited, or revealed. I should not be disposed to treat at all seriously the claims of those who pretend to cure cancer by the internal administration of remedies, for, notwithstanding the certificates of cure which are daily appearing in the public press and elsewhere, it may be safely stated that hitherto, internal remedies have been found to be without any value whatever.

And what can be said of the claims for excellence put forth on behalf of those external applications which are imposed upon a credulous and easily deceived public? *Pari passu* with the admittedly occult nature of the disease, the treatment, it is contended, is not within the usual bounds of ordinary medical knowledge. And thus the cancer curers, by plasters and unguents of mysterious action, have increased in numbers and in presumption. The ordeal to which patients sometimes subject themselves at the hands of ignorant but pretentious quacks, for the removal of supposed cancer, and the suffering and disfigurement which sometimes result, are conditions we occasionally witness, from the use of plasters long since discarded by the profession as unsafe, unscientific, unsurgical and uncertain. I once saw a woman who had had a wart on the back of her hand. It was a harmless excrescence on the skin, but a cancer-curer assured her it was malignant. Contrary to the advice of her family physician, she permitted a plaster to be bound upon the part. On her arrival at the hospital a few weeks later not a vestige remained of the dorsal aspect of the hand, neither skin, tendon, ligament, nerve, nor blood vessel; the metacarpals, from carpus to phalanges, were black as charcoal, and dead. The cutaneous palmar surface, however, still retained vitality, and after a while the patient returned home, carrying with her a limp, flexed hand, without the usual bony support, but buoyed up with the assurance that while her hand had been lost, her life had been saved. If the charlatan knew nothing of surgery, he could form some fair estimate of the patient's credulity, and he plied her with a text which suited her case exactly: "If thy right hand offend thee," and so forth; and was it not her right hand which had offended? Verily the text had been written in anticipation of her case.

I turn from esotericism and occultism to something more intelligible, where deduction from certain manifest qualities is the result of experimentation.

Its Treatment.

The treatment of malignant disease by electrical methods has for some time attracted notice. Although success has not generally followed these attempts, yet patience and energy have sometimes been rewarded by marked improvement. "The healing of an ulcerated cancerous surface," says Lewis Jones, "has been observed in a certain proportion of cases; relief of pain in cancerous parts is a fairly common experience, and superficial nodules, undoubtedly cancerous in nature, will sometimes decrease notably in size under electric treatment."

The science of electricity, however, is yet in its infancy, and the technique of its application is imperfectly understood, while the reluctance of the surgeon to counsel treatment involving delay is and will be for some time, a hindrance to the more general use of electricity, save in those cases which cannot be easily reached by the knife. It is yet too early to speculate on the results of the electric treatment; some are of the opinion that they can bring about the painless removal of the slow-growing epitheliomas. I shall content myself with stating that the treatment which is said to be successful in causing diminution of hyperemia, inflammation, infiltration, and serous exudation, may, ultimately, be found to be of permanent value.

A new, a powerful, and as yet not thoroughly understood, and not always easily controlled, therapeutic agent, has been added to our armamentarium in the treatment of cancer and other diseases. By one or other of those wonderful deductions from light and heat, and from certain modifications of the electric waves, or from their analysis and separation, whether as the X- or Roentgen-Ray, the N-Ray, or Cathode Ray, the Rays of Blondlot, or the Alpha, Beta, Gamma Rays, the Finsen Rays, or the Rays of Charpentier, or that mysterious phosphorescent ray, likened to that which is developed during muscular action or mental effort—whatever name they bear and whatever the source of their potency—a power has been created to be utilized to our advantage.

Have these rays, or any of them, the therapeutic value claimed for them? The illustrations we find in medical journals on both sides of the Atlantic would seem to speak encouragingly of this painless form of therapeutics. The latest at hand is from the London Middlesex Hospital Cancer Research, where, after trying various remedies with generally unsatisfactory results, it says: " In rays we have an agent capable of doing more for superficial cancer than any other hitherto known." The work already done in Canada is evidence of intelligent and persevering effort. From personal observation I may state: Dr. Girdwood has effectually cured intractable rodent ulcer and benefited recurring epithelioma, and Dr. Leforest has effected the extensive destruction of hair-follicles in bearded women without producing even an erythematous blush.

With the assumption—and it is so far only an assumption—that cancer is a micro-organism, the therapeutic value of some of those forms of electric force most amenable to control may yet be found capable of bringing a hitherto distressingly frequent and cheerless malady under subjection. But it must not be forgotten that improvement occasionally noticed in the more superficial forms of cancer, as epithelioma, for instance, must not be allowed to lull the sufferer into dangerous security. I have many times, by the application of an escharotic, kept under subjection, for many years, epitheliomata of the eye-lid, face and lip, and have obtained their final disappearance without the use of the knife. But of the deeper form of cancer it may still be said with MacIntyre, of Glasgow, " that the serious deep-seated affections which, in the public mind at least, may be considered synonymous with the word cancer, have so far baffled us. The problem remains to-day as great as ever." Perhaps, in the future, the penetrative ray may be isolated from its surroundings and be sent on its errand of mercy deep through the normal tissues without affecting them, and attack the hidden morbid growth at greater or less depth, as, in our northern lakes and rivers, the sun's rays sometimes pass through the thickest ice without melting its surface, and establish centres of liquefaction in many places in the interior of the frozen mass.

So far the various forms of the X-Ray, whatever names they bear, act as stimulants and excitants, producing, at first, tingling; then as irritants and caustics, producing pigmentation, as in sunburns, erythema and other evidences of dermatitis; then, if continued, vesiculation or desquamation; then deeper congestion and stasis, leading to all the changes we may notice in burns. But these severer effects are begotten, in some measure, of inexperience in adjustment, on the one hand, or of accommodation on the other, and are becoming less frequent as the new power can be more intelligently measured, and the tolerance or power of resistance of the individual better understood.

I can only allude, *en passant,* to artificial fluorescence of living tissue, and wish for it more than has hitherto been vouchsafed· to other methods.

The still more modern treatment by radium, it is claimed, has given promise of success. But reports, so far, as to its value as a therapeutic agent are not encouraging.

Notwithstanding · the advantages sometimes resulting from the employment of the Roentgen or other rays, Symes' dictum of upwards of half a century ago remains as true as it was then, that in the treatment of cancer, when the disease can be wholly removed, reliance must still continue to be on the knife. But why the knife? Is cancer curable by operation? To this I unhesitatingly reply in the affirmative, provided the operation is done sufficiently early, permitting the entire removal of the disease, and that it is removed.

I now proceed, but most hurriedly, to deal with some of those forms of cancer to be met with, and first of the digestive system. As to the tongue. Although sharing the opinion that its partial removal is wrong in principle, there are cases arising from local irritation where partial excision affords excellent, and in some cases, permanent results. In total extirpation it is marvellous. what recuperative power is sometimes met with. I once removed a cancerous tongue down to the hyoid bone, separating it close to the epiglottis, pharynx and soft palate; and, with the tongue, I removed the whole of the lower jaw, as well as the sublingual and submaxillary glands on one side; yet the patient—an old man— made an uninterrupted recovery.

Concerning cancer of the throat. One might read Sir Morell Mackenzie's book on the late Emperor of Germany's fatal illness; and then the comments of the German surgeons, and of the German and British medical press, and decide as to what is and what is not cancer in those regions, and act, or not act, accordingly.

As to operations on the stomach for cancer, it may be said they will be satisfactory or otherwise in direct ratio to the care and prudence with which cases are selected for the knife, and the cases are few. The delay sometimes caused by medical treatment; the difficulty, often, of diagnosis when seen, and of deciding as to the extent of the disease, will always make operations on the stomach anxious, and too often uncertain. It is only when the disease is confined to the stomach itself—where it has not gone beyond that organ nor infiltrated into neighboring glands or organs —that any hope of success need be entertained.

Gastrotomy is yet on its trial, and the time afforded has not been sufficient to enable one to decide whether the operation introduced by Billroth, some years ago, possesses all the advantages claimed for it.

Let me guard you against an error which is too prevalent— the belief that disease of the pyloric end of the stomach from ulcer passes, after a time, into cancer of that organ. Ulceration, often with resultant stenosis, continues as such, and rarely, very rarely, becomes cancerous. Treatment should be based on this assumption, and should not be influenced by a dread lest the painful, but non-malignant gastric ulcer might eventually become the more formidable malignant affection.

I pass over gastro-intestinal operations hurriedly, as each case of malignant disease of the stomach and bowel has a law unto itself. But the cases are comparatively few where surgical interference is warrantable. When malignant disease is limited to the pyloric end of the stomach, and when its constricted condition interferes seriously with the passage onwards of the contents of the stomach, relief is often obtained from the junction of that

viscus with the duodenum or jejunum. But while relief is sometimes marked, it is often unhappily for a time, when, as Maylard
observes, " vague but suggestive symptoms insidiously reappear,"
prompting one to ask: " Is it for the real benefit of our patient to
rescue him after death, simply to die over again ?" I should have
been disposed to answer in the negative, but the recent address
in surgery by that brilliant writer and operator, Mayo Robson,
leads to the conclusion that, not only as a palliative, but as a
curative measure, gastro-enterostomy must take its place among
the regular operations in surgery.

Cancer of the large intestines, whether of the cæcum, ascending or descending colon, or of its hepatic, splenic or sigmoid
flexures, may, in some few cases, demand surgical interference.
But while contemplating operation on the lower bowel, it is well
to bear in mind Jonathan Hutchison's recognition of exaggera-
tion in two directions: " The danger of the operation," he says,
" is put much lower than it really is, while the probable duration
of life without it, and the possible freedom from pain are much
underrated."

Although the diagnosis of cancer of the head of the pancreas
may, with the aid of Courvoisier's law, often be made out—" deep
painless jaundice and enlarged gall bladder "—the recognition of
these conditions is sometimes insufficient as a safe prelude to surgical interference.   In a case mentioned by Stewart of Leeds,
where cancer of the head of the pancreas was found at the autopsy,
" a prolonged search of over half an hour was made for the gall
bladder, but none was present."   ·

A considerable number of cases of cancer of the rectum having
come under my notice, I may, perhaps, be in a position to express
an opinion as to the best means of dealing with them. In general
terms I may say: In the early stages, when the disease can be cir-
cumscribed, and its base well defined with the finger, Langen-
beck's operation, called the low operation, offers many advantages.
When the disease is not so limited, colotomy may, with advantage,
be resorted to, or it may precede proctotomy.   When, however,
the disease is more advanced, Kraske's operation presents itself
as a last—an almost forbidding—alternative. I have performed
the operation with Bardenheuer's modification several times, and I
am not enamoured of it. As the lower excision of the rectum is
practicable in but a small percentage of cases, Kraske's operation
is advisable in a still fewer number. There may be comfort, however, in knowing that cancer of the lower bowel, being usually a
columnar carcinoma, as Rose and Carliss observe, is not so malignant as cancer elsewhere. Most of you will recall, no doubt, cases
where well-marked carcinoma of the bowel existed for years
without producing any great disturbance.

In suspected cancer of the womb, the early diagnosis of malignancy is of the first importance. The diagnosis clearly made—even sometimes by microscopical examination of scrapings of the curette—what operation should be performed?

Some surgeons give preference to the vaginal, others to the abdominal method. We should not be prejudiced adherents of either, although I have practised both. When the disease is clearly limited to the os and cervix, the vaginal method, it appears to me, is preferable, as being less hazardous to life. When disease is in the body of the uterus, with possible involvement of the appendages, the abdominal route, methinks, offers superior advantages. The extent to which the disease has spread when within the uterus should not deter from operating. In other parts of the body the lymphatic system is generally involved at an early period, whereas, in cancer of the womb, the lymphatics are not affected until the disease has advanced, by direct extension, into the adjoining parts. This circumstance seems to have led the editor of the *British Medical Journal* to state: " If cancer of the womb is only recognized early enough, it can be removed with small risk, and with a good prospect of years of freedom from recurrence."

In those inoperable cases where closing the vagina, draining through the rectum, ligaturing through the arteries, etc., have been proposed—methods, I am free to confess, I do not endorse—curetting offers, methinks, a much better result, especially when followed by the application of a proper caustic, or, perhaps, by one of the forms of the X-Rays.

Concerning cancer of the uterus and ovaries, the observations as to surgical interference are almost identical, for the risk of operating upon either is about equal. An early operation in cancer of the appendages, as of the uterus, is, when successful, usually attended by relief of the more distressing symptoms. Moreover, the differential diagnosis is comparatively easy, and the limits of the disease may be somewhat correctly defined.

What has been said of the ovary may be applied to cancer of the Fallopian tube. The difficulty, nay, the impossibility sometimes, of disuniting affections of these two organs, and the unwisdom of attempting, even were it possible of accomplishment, to remove the one and retain the other, renders it usually necessary to excise both or neither.

Perhaps I should notice, *en passant,* the operation of oophorectomy, not for disease of the ovary, but for recurrent or reappearing disease of the breast. It is not easy to explain how the removal of a healthy organ at a distance can destroy cancer germs in the organ involved, however intimate sympathy may be between the two. Besides, oophorectomy is not always the harmless operation it is claimed to be by those who regard it as a cure, or even as a palliative, for cancer of the breast. The operation has been performed many times, and we have yet to learn a result which might be called satisfactory. Williams, of Clifton, goes so far as to say: "Not a single definite cure can be instanced unless one of Herman's cases may be so regarded." But even if a score or so of " cures " could be cited, the sources of fallacy are so numerous that little weight would attach to them in the face of the overwhelming preponderance of negative results. " In fact every new specific for cancer," says Williams, " has had no difficulty in justifying itself by far more convincing crops of ' cures ' than any that has been adduced on behalf of castration."

I should not have alluded at such length to this mischievous meddlesomeness had it not been that the mutilation undergone for that and other purposes has been somewhat too frequently resorted to on this side of the Atlantic, where ovaries bid fair to be considered, ere long, useless and troublesome appendages to be got out of the way.

While I am speaking of cancer in different parts of the body, I am sure the minds of many of you travel, not to those more formidable affections of organs hidden in the interior of the economy which can be visited only by a limited and expert few, but to that more tangible form of the disease which so often afflicts the female breast. As it concerns the well-being of the mothers of our race, I shall deal with it at some length.

And first as to diagnosis. It is at the earliest moment that an examination of the breast is most valuable, and it is then it should be most thorough. As inspection sometimes conveys the earliest, and sometimes the only information, the whole chest should be freely uncovered, so that both breasts may be readily compared. The patient should stand or sit on a stool or chair without a back, so that the examiner may stand behind her, permitting the educated palmar surfaces of the fingers, not their extremities, to impinge upon the parts to be examined. Both hands should be used in the examination, one to support the breast if necessary. But the examination is not complete until the patient is afterwards examined in a recumbent position, the examiner being, at will, at the patient's head or at either side. These are elementary suggestions, but they are too often neglected.

A few words as to the mode of operating, the manner of which, as generally practised, has always appeared to me to be, in many respects, faulty. I am free to confess that for the first twenty years of my professional life, although I followed always the most recent text-book, I was not satisfied with my own way of operating, nor with that of others. Having before my mind the instructions of surgical writers to cut and dissect parallel with the mus-

cular fibres, the knife was used too freely—almost exclusively—
and a doubt often remained with me as to the sufficiency of my
dissection, on the one hand, and as to the needlessly extensive mutilation on the other. Gradually I learned to do less with the knife
and more with the finger in the work of separation, and with
greater satisfaction. Although sanctioned by very eminent
authority, I could not regard the early separation of the skin from
the subjacent mammary gland as a wise procedure. And here let
me observe that an error has long been indulged in as to the form
and attachments of the mammary gland. Anatomical works often
describe the female breast much in this fashion: " Two hemi-
spherical eminences, nearly circular, flattened, or slightly concave,
on the posterior surface, convex on the interior aspects." The
female breast sometimes sends off cusps above, below,
and to the axillary region; sometimes to and across the
sternum; sometimes even to its fellow on the opposite side. The
breast gland, aptly called by Dennis a cutaneous sebaceous gland,
is sometimes connected most closely with the skin, through fatty
tissue of varying thickness.

To ascertain the form and extent of the mammary gland, my
first incision down to and below the gland is usually at the most
dependent part of the breast. I must see, and feel, the outer
margin of the gland and then separate it from the subjacent
pectoral with my finger, not with my knife, and thus throughout.
If the separation takes place easily, I am satisfied the disease has
not extended to the muscle beneath, and I do not remove it.

But when there is the slightest suspicion of adhesion and the
large pectoral is to be removed, how should this be accomplished?
Not by separating it at the wide circumference of its broad, fleshy,
basal attachments to ribs, sternum and clavicle, but at its narrower
tendinous attachment to the humerus. By turning forward the
now liberated muscle, its freedom from or adhesion to the pector-
alis minor may be established, and the preservation or removal of
the latter follow.

When large quantities of skin and muscle are removed with
the breast gland, leaving the ribs to a large extent uncovered, skin
grafting may sometimes be resorted to with advantage, but when?
I share the opinion of Le Dentu that it is better to wait till the
wound has begun to granulate and has contracted somewhat, and
to have recourse to Thiersch's method at a later period than is
often practised.

To resume: is it advisable to go beyond the mammary gland
when there is no evidence of disease outside of it? My practice,
notwithstanding weighty opinion to the contrary, is invariably to
confine myself to the mammary gland, when it alone is diseased,
and to the elliptoid integument to be removed. I am confirmed in

that practice by having noticed that when the disease reappears it is usually in the cicatrix, and rarely in the axilla. The supply of lymphatics leading to the axilla is doubtless abundant, but the lymphatics above and beneath one mammary gland anastomose freely across the sternum with those of the opposite side, yet it does not usually occur to the surgeon to remove both breasts when one only is affected. Besides, removal of the axillary glands adds greatly to the patient's discomfort and to her risks, and is, I contend, in the vast majority of cases of early cancer of the breast, unnecessary.

To my mind there is no more reason to remove the axillary gland, when not diseased, than there is to remove the network of lymphatic glands which encircle the chest in all directions. I ventured to so express myself in Washington several years ago, and I have not since found it necessary to modify the views I then gave utterance to.

But should the disease again show itself, what then? As I am firmly of the opinion that it is a returning, or coming again into view, of what had been removed merely from sight and apprehension, but not thoroughly and entirely, I repeat the excision as completely as possible once, twice, thrice, or oftener, as often, indeed, as any appearance of the disease is visible, or as the anatomical relations of the parts will continue to permit. In this way I have had the satisfaction, sometimes, of being able to obtain final success after many efforts. But this success, it must be admitted, is only occasional; it is sufficient, however, to encourage the surgeon to repeat his efforts, even if frequent failure almost forces him to look at any effort on his part as to that of which there is but little hope.

In conclusion, Mr. President and gentlemen, it may appear to many of you that I have stated nothing which could not have been said by any of my listeners; but when I was honored with the invitation to address you to-day, it occurred to me that it might possibly interest you to view a few features in a disease which is attracting an unprecedently large share of attention, through the optics of one, who, during years not a few, has had exceptional facilities for clinical observation.

NEURASTHENIA IN SOME OF ITS RELATIONS TO INSANITY.*

BY CAMPBELL MEYERS, M.D., M.R.C.S.(Eng.), L.R.C.P.(Lond.)

Neurologist to St. M chael's Hospital, Toronto.

Mr. President and Members,—The disease upon which I purpose making a few remarks to-day, is so wide in its distribution, and, at times, so disastrous in its effects, that any contribution to its study, however slight, may be of some service to those interested in its nosology and treatment. In a paper read at the meeting of the Canadian Medical Association in Quebec in 1898, I pointed out that, contrary to the opinion then generally expressed by authors, neurasthenia in certain of its forms frequently terminated in insanity. Further experience has confirmed the opinion I then expressed, and I may add that certain symptoms, which are usually classed as neurasthenic, are really the incipient stages of mental disorder, and that their early treatment may avert an attack of insanity. To no members of the profession has the study of these conditions a greater interest than to the family physician, since it is under his observation that these cases always come in the early stage, the period when active treatment is of most avail, and when delays are most dangerous. While we have numberless excellent authors on insanity, the result of study of these cases after the boundary line has been passed, we are still much in need of further writings on the early history of these cases. This is due largely to the fact that so little has been taught in our medical colleges and hospitals about neurasthenia, and, as a consequence, medical men must learn by experience the symptoms and treatment of this important disease. That such experience is often costly, there can be no doubt, since the non-recognition of symptoms and the lack of proper treatment often leads to mental disaster. When we consider the large amount of insanity in this country in proportion to its population, the importance of any means which may avert an attack is at once apparent. In using the term "insanity" in this paper, I do so with reference only to the idiopathic insanities or those mental diseases without ascertainable pathological alteration of brain substance (the psychoneuroses of Krafft Ebing). These may be defined as acquired forms of mental disease, arising in individuals who have a sound mental constitution. I refer, of course, to mania and melancholia, but especially to the latter.

Time forbids any lengthened discussion of neurasthenia in

---

*Read bef re the Ontario Medical Association, June, 1904.

general; but the type of this disease to which I would like to-day to direct your attention is that of cerebrasthenia or brain exhaustion, arising also in an individual of sound mental constitution. In order to better study the relations which exist between neurasthenia and the idiopathic insanities, let us first consider the causes of both these troubles. In regard to the etiology of neurasthenia, we find chiefly mental over-work, especially when combined with excitement of a depressing character, such as worry and disappointment, vexation and grief; trauma, especially when combined with much emotional disturbance; psychical shocks, such as an unfortunate love affair or death of a well-known friend or relative; exhausting processes, such as are incident to the various fevers in influenza or to pregnancy and lactation; auto-intoxication from the absorption of toxins from the intestinal tract, as evidenced by the excess of the ethereal sulphates in the urine; all forms of dissipation and excess, such as alcoholism, drug habits, etc.

If we now turn to the etiology of the idiopathic insanities, we find precisely the same causes given for their development by the best authors on mental diseases. Hence we have exactly similar causes acting on the same nervous elements in both these conditions. With this short discussion of the etiology, let us now take up some of the symptoms of cerebrasthenia, and see what relation, if any, they bear to the symptoms of the idiopathic insanities. Among the chief symptoms of cerebrasthenia we find a diminution in the capacity for sustained intellectual effort, and this difficulty of concentrating the attention may be so great as to lead to an habitual state of distraction. The patient's ideas do not present themselves as readily or in as rapid succession as in health. His will power and energy are markedly lessened, and he has no confidence in himself. He is morbidly sensitive, and often feels intensely hurt by fancied neglect of friends. His emotional equilibrium is readily disturbed. The patient becomes introspective, and is habitually on the alert for suspicious symptoms, suffering from nosophobia. Mental depression is another marked symptom in most of these cases, the patient becoming gradually depressed from his inability either to continue his work or to find relief from his symptoms. A distinct loss of the sense of the proprieties is often visible, and these patients, from their introspection and morbid sensitiveness, will discuss their intimate ailments with non-medical persons in a manner that at times is distinctly repulsive. There is at times, too, a distinct lessening of the affection for near relatives, and a patient will say, " I no longer care for my children as I should," etc. The patient often experiences an apparently causeless fear, which, combined as it is with weakness, is only natural. These attacks of fear may arise from visceral disturbances, and the terror of approaching death from heart failure, etc., may be overwhelming. Or fears may arise which are associated with certain definite ideas, such as the fear of open places, etc., due, probably, to the fact that the faculties are so weakened that ordinary surroundings give no sense of security. Another symptom which is most important, and often one of the earliest, is insomnia, which is often accompanied by the most distressing dreams. We have now and then peculiarities in the speech and handwriting, both being slurred and slovenly, especially in writing letters to friends, when syllables or words may be omitted.

With this enumeration of some of the symptoms of cerebrasthenia, let us now turn to the symptoms of the most simple form of the insanity under consideration, viz., simple melancholia. In the study of this affection, I think we find the same symptoms as have been described in cerebrasthenia, except that they are present in an intensified degree. The mental depression, which is the prominent symptom, becomes much more marked, so that a patient may sit all day long in one position. The patient, after repeated attempts to be relieved of his ailment, has gradually been forced to the conclusion that he can no longer be cured, and consequently it is useless to try. The constant introspection of an earlier date has steadily deepened, and he now becomes wrapped in his own misery and overpowered by the feeling of hopelessness and despair. The incapacity for intellectual effort is increased, so that thought is slow, and often a considerable time is taken to reply to a simple question. His fears of various kinds have added to his mental burden. His will power and energy have become more deeply implicated, and he can only be roused with difficulty from his torpor. The preservation of his reasoning faculties makes the mental pain from which he suffers only the more acute. A feeling of aversion to friends and relatives is, he feels, contrary to nature, but he cannot overcome it. With the concentration of his thoughts on himself, all his relations with the outside world gradually become obliterated. With the consideration of his condition, his hopelessness and despair, the conviction that he will never recover and that his life can only be a burden and expense to his friends, is it any wonder that his thoughts now turn to suicide to end his unhappy existence? During all this time his reasoning faculties may be perfectly good, except in regard to his own condition.

If we now take up the other more advanced forms of melancholia, we simply find an intensification of these same symptoms, but along with them the reasoning faculties become impaired. The patient begins to argue with himself as to why this dreadful calamity should come upon him, and the answer takes various forms according to the condition of his mind at the time. He feels that he must have offended God, that he has committed the unpardonable sin, that he has committed some dreadful crime against humanity, etc., etc., and the suppression of his reasoning faculties makes this all the easier to be believed by him. The more profound derangement of the cells in the centres for the special senses leads to hallucinations of various kinds, and a fully developed attack of insanity results, taking either the form of melancholia or mania.

Having thus very shortly discussed the conditions leading to insanity, owing to the very limited time which, of necessity, is allowed for the reading of a paper, let me add by way of illustration two examples as quoted by Berkley in his excellent treatise on mental diseases: " (1) A mother loses her only son. She is naturally depressed, takes hardly any interest in her surroundings, the conscious mental pain is great and energy is lost. She does not, however, go so far as to become inattentive to the needs of her person; she remains capable of performing her most pressing duties, and when called upon in an emergency will cast aside her own woes and look after the welfare of others, finding relief from her own depression in the work of cheering the sufferers and alleviating their misery. This woman has not been insane; the depression has remained within physiological limits. (2) Another mother may, after a similar experience, not only become depressed and lose all interest in her surroundings, but may even neglect her dress and the imperative duties of daily life. It may be impossible to convince her that the death of the child was not due to some fault on her part, and she may sit day by day, brooding over her misfortune. Even when called upon in an emergency to rouse herself and assist others in the direst distress, her sympathies cannot be awakened, but she will remain inactive, enwrapped in her own loss, and overcome by the impellent delusions resulting therefrom. In fact, she is wholly incapable of mental or physical exertion. In this case the physiological limit has been overstepped; the woman is insane, and the danger of suicide may be great.' Here we have a very good illustration of the difference between sanity and insanity; but what about the clinical aspect, which is the vital point? We have been, I think, too satisfied to stop with the terms " sanity " and " insanity," without going further and considering the clinical side of this disease. The two examples above quoted may, to my mind, be considered quite rightly as different phases of the same disease, but we have been too inclined in the past to consider that, having made the diagnosis of insanity, we had done our duty, and all that remained for us to do was to hand the case over to an alienist for asylum treatment. We have been too inclined to consider only the apparent condition of the patient without studying the features of the disease which produced it.

I believe that, clinically, there should be no boundary line, and that this term should be reserved solely for its medico-legal usefulness. We distinguish by a separate title, in the disease of no other organ, a later from an earlier stage, then why do so clinically in an affection of the brain? Had phthisis been studied only after the stage of cavity formation in the lungs, where would our knowledge of tuberculosis have been to-day? Why apply the title insanity to an advanced condition of disease only, and leave the earlier stages of this same disease without a name, or with some designation entirely different? If we are, from a medico-legal point of view, to consider a delusion as the basis of insanity, as advocated by Dr. Wherry in the last *Alienist and Neurologist,* let such be the case from a medico-legal, and not from a clinical, point of view. Rather let us study the symptoms and treatment of brain exhaustion from its earliest symptoms to its final termination as a single clinical entity which has no boundary line. The disease does not begin when we apply the term insanity to it (often from a medico-legal standpoint), and yet this stage alone has constantly been studied as a clinical entity. When the period arises that a patient is described as insane, it simply means that his case has progressed beyond a certain point, and that the original disease has become intensified. A proper designation for this clinical entity would be most useful, although very difficult to discover. The term cerebrasthenia, while open to several objections, might, if the prefix " acute " were added to it, serve to distinguish this disease until a more satisfactory name were found.

That mental disorders rest upon a physical basis is well recognized, and that we may, with reasonable certainty, regard deranged function of the cells of the higher centres as the cause of all the symptoms mentioned in this paper, is assured. The time is past when any of these symptoms can be regarded as imaginary or chimerical, and the results of prolonged clinical study have shown that these symptoms increase *pari passu* with the more profound derangement of function of the above-mentioned nerve cells. The researches of Hodge and the later experiments of Van Gehuchten and Marinesco point to much that is interesting in this regard. Time, however, allows me only to add a few words in regard to treatment. Since the celebrated dictum of the immortal bard, " How minister to a mind diseased," the impression has remained with us that little could be done. In the past few years, however, a decided change has taken place, and we now rightly conclude that the cells of the brain are just as susceptible to treatment, and respond to treat-

5

ment equally as well as, for example, the cells of the liver, in view of the importance and function of these two organs. The first essential in treatment is isolation, without which treatment is often disappointing. The reason is apparent, in that the good which may be accomplished by drugs is more than counterbalanced by the irritation which still continues, while the patient remains in his accustomed surroundings. The question of travel arises, but, except in the very early stages, a much more satisfactory result is obtained by other treatment first and travel later, when he is able to enjoy it. Hydrotherapy is a most important adjunct at all stages of the disease, and massage and electricity also have their period of usefulness. When combined with isolation, the various drugs yield as good results here as in any branch of medicine, while rest and moral suasion play a prominent part in the successful treatment of these cases.

A word in conclusion. In regard once more to the urgent necessity of suitable treatment in the early stage of this disease, and before the development of any delusions, I am convinced, after an experience of more than ten years, devoted exclusively and under exceptionally favorable circumstances, to the study of nervous diseases, and especially of those of a functional nature, that in their early treatment we have a prophylaxis of insanity which, for practical value, can scarcely be overestimated.

Proceedings of Societies.

THE ONTARIO MEDICAL ASSOCIATION CONVENTION.

In the new Medical Building of the University of Toronto, the Ontario Medical Association celebrated its twenty-fourth anniversary on the 14th, 15th and 16th of June. The spacious and comfortable lecture-room was tastefully decorated with palms and flowers, and, as President J. F. W. Ross remarked, it gave one a comfortable feeling to hold a meeting in such pleasant surroundings. There was a goodly sprinkling of members present when the president called the meeting to order, and these increased from time to time until upwards of two hundred were assembled. The secretary, Dr. C. P. Lusk, had all matters of business and papers carefully arranged, and everything went along rapidly and smoothly. The papers read were of a superior order, and subjects of general interest. Under the skilful direction of the chairman the discussions were prompt, brief and pointed. "Altogether," said Dr. Ross, as he was vacating the chair for his successor, Dr. Burt, "we have certainly had the most excellent meeting in the history of the Association."

Dr. C. J. Hastings, Toronto, gave a paper on "Myxomatous Degeneration of the Villi of the Chorion." The various theories advanced by the earliest writers to explain this condition were briefly considered. Early in the sixth century Amidi taught that each vesicle contained a living embryo. Later the echinococcus was blamed for the condition. Velpeau first showed the cysts to be distended villi.

Among the causes given for this condition are diseases of the blood vessels, disease of the lymphatics, and degeneration of the mucus in the villi. The whole chorion is usually diseased; sometimes the placenta alone is involved. Marshand demonstrated that it was the epithelial covering of the villi, more than the stroma, that was affected, and that both the syncitium and Langhan's layers of cells underwent profuse and irregular proliferation. The terminal blood vessels disappeared, the stroma degenerated, and the cells necrosed. (The fluid contents is not mucin, but serum.)

Etiology.—The causes are not known. Maternal causation is at present most favored. Syphilis, tuberculosis, and endometritis are mentioned as predisposing causes.

Symptoms.—Usually manifest before the tenth week; to the

usual signs of pregnancy there is added a sudden bloody discharge and a disproportionately large uterus, with no evidence of symptoms and pain.

Diagnosis.—The enlarged uterus, the irregular flowing, with the absence of fetal signs, is suggestive. Exploration may be necessary. Twins and threatened abortion must be differentiated.

Treatment.—The indication is to empty the uterus at once, using the finger or the long-handled ovum forceps to remove the neoplasm. Firm contraction must be secured subsequently.

Morbid Anatomy.—The vesicles are characteristic; their mode of attachment to the main stem is by a pedicle. The embryo may or may not be found. Dr. Hastings further pointed out the fact that chorion epithelioma is frequently preceded by hydatidiform mole. He presented a series of three cases illustrating the condition.

Discussion.—Mr. Cameron called attention to this condition as illustrating an epithelial growth from the fetus to the mother tissue. He cited a case of a woman pregnant of an hydatid one year after the menopause, followed by abortion and a subsequent deciduoma malignum.

Dr. McIlwraith pointed out that secondary infections in deciduoma malignum frequently disappeared after operation.

Dr. John Sheahan, St. Catharines, presented a most carefully prepared paper on " The Treatment of Appendicitis in Pregnancy." The question as to whether or not the surgeon should interfere in these cases was ably discussed. Until quite recently non-interference has been the practice; now, however, in acute infective cases pregnancy must be considered no bar to immediate and radical operation.

CASE.—Mrs. B., aged 25, primipara, four months pregnant. No history of previous appendicial trouble—seized with sudden severe pain in the hepatic region. The following day temperature and pulse normal, frequent desire to urinate, with pain in the bladder and over the liver. Three days later a chill, followed by a temperature of 104, pulse 140, respiration 30, and some vomiting. Pain in hepatic region and tenderness over McBurney's point, with but slight rigidity. Two days later a thickened and inflamed appendix was removed, an uninterrupted recovery following. At the eighth month premature labor was induced for albuminuria, with the birth of a dead child.

A summary of one hundred cases prior to 1899 showed that abortion most frequently followed operation; when pregnancy went to full term the fetal mortality being fifty per cent.

Etiology.—The same causative factors as exist in uncomplicated cases, pregnancy itself affecting only those cases where the appendix hangs over the pelvic brim, or where the enlarging uterus separates the adhesions of former attacks, or presses on an appendicial enterolith.

Pathology.—The frequent occurrence of abortion, estimated at forty per cent., is referred to the intimate vascular connections existing between the appendix and the uterine adnexa. Cases with abscess involving the uterus are most unfortunate, as the uterine contractions aid in extension of the pus.

Diagnosis.—The uterine tumor prevents palpation. The muscles are stretched and the intestines are pushed up. The following points are important: 1. A history of constipation. 2. The sudden onset of acute abdominal pain in the right iliac fossa. 3. The localization of the pain over McBurney's point. 4. Vomiting. 5. High temperature and rapid pulse. 6. Rigidity of right rectus. 7. Examination per vagina under an anesthetic is advisable. Conditions such as right tubal pregnancy, acute salpyngitis, cholecystitis, gall stone colic and kidney crises must all be carefully differentiated.

Prognosis.—In simple catarrhal forms, good without operation; all cases favorable if operated on early. Abrahams says the prognosis is gloomy. He observed sixteen cases with eight deaths, and an infantile mortality of eighty-six per cent.

Treatment.—An inflamed appendix is a source of extreme danger, and as its removal is attended by few additional dangers to the mother and fetus, Munde's dictum is, " Treat the case early, regardless of pregnancy." W. Meyer, of New York, lays down the following rules: 1. Operate within twelve hours in acute perforating appendicitis. 2. A rapid pulse (116 to 120) is an indication for operation. 3. In case of doubt, operation is better than waiting. 4. A sudden lull for ten or twelve hours is an indication for operation. 5. The recurrence of an old appendicitis during pregnancy also demands surgical interference.

Discussion.—Dr. Webster, Toronto, advised operation by the vaginal route in pelvic peritonitis during pregnancy. It entailed less shock to the patient. He reported a case of suppurating appendicitis with pelvic abscess opened by this route with excellent results.

" Occipito-Posterior Presentations " was the subject of a paper by Dr. A. A. Macdonald, Toronto. Since the advent of antiseptics and anesthetics a new era has arrived in obstetrics as in surgery. They are exceedingly useful in correcting faulty presentations. Occipito-posterior presentations occur in one and one-half per cent. of all labor cases. Formerly the single blade forceps were used to cause the head to rotate. Herman, in his " Difficult Labor," gives three directions for the use of forceps in treatment: (*a*) Pull, (*b*) Flex, (*c*) Rotate. The practice I advocate is briefly as follows: If you are called to a case late, but before the membranes have ruptured, wait until the os is dilated, then introduce the hand and rotate one quarter turn, converting the case into an occipito-anterior. To do this fully, anesthetise the patient, sterilize the parts and your hands, insert the whole hand and grasp the head. The occiput being now anterior, flex the head and hold it in position until the forceps are applied and locked. There is no injury to the child's neck, as the turn is only one-quarter. With the forceps on, delivery is readily effected, and without laceration.

Discussion.—Dr. Barrick, Toronto, said that he endorsed the methods of Dr. Macdonald. In cases where the head is out of proportion to the pelvis, how can we use the forceps? The rotation or quarter turn may be impossible when the pelvis is narrow. My treatment is, where the child is viable, perform version, as it preserves the mother from injury.

Dr. A. F. McKenzie, Bracebridge, noted the importance of the paper, but took issue with Dr. Macdonald's percentage for posterior presentations. In his experience there was about 20 per cent. of such cases, but nature generally rotates them herself. He emphasized the importance of diagnosis; it is not always necessary to insert the hand, external palpation being sufficient, especially if the abdominal walls are thin. In vaginal examinations, if the anterior fontanelle is felt first, the case is generally left occipito-posterior presentation.

Dr. Hastings, Toronto, drew attention to the importance of strict asepsis, and emphasized the usefulness of abdominal palpation as an aid to diagnosis.

Dr. Todd, Toronto, said in his experience the method of introducing the hand and rotating the head was accompanied by a greater mortality to the child.

Dr. Hunter, Parkdale, advised leaving the cases largely alone and not meddling with them. Nature would nearly always correct the position and effect delivery.

Dr. Temple, Toronto, said that early anterior rotation forward is always the treatment for posterior presentations. He could see no reason for an increased mortality, provided surgical asepsis was maintained.

Dr. McIlwraith, Toronto, said that leaving these cases to nature for a time and then applying the forceps was a cause of increased mortality. He advised early anterior rotation.

Dr. Ross, Toronto, explained, on request of Mr. Cameron, his father's method of treatment in these cases. He passed two fingers in front during a pain and the head rotated itself on them.

Dr. Macdonald (reply) could see no reason for an increase of mortality by introduction of the hand. The following points are essential: 1. Choose your time, *i.e.,* before the membranes rupture, the os being dilated. 2. Fully anesthetise the patient. 3. Cleanse the parturient canal and your hands, rotate the head the quarter turn; rotate the shoulders by external manipulation. 4. Keep the occiput down and in position until the forceps are on and locked. Then make traction in the correct direction.

Dr. H. P. H. Galloway, of Toronto, then read his paper.

Discussion.—Dr. B. E. McKenzie, Toronto, said the diagnosis of congenital dislocation is usually easy; to exclude infantile paralysis is sometimes a difficulty. The value of X-rays in diagnosis is well illustrated by the excellent photographs presented by Dr. Galloway. Other reasons of failure in reduction are that sometimes the head of the femur is absent or is very small, or that there may be no acetabulum, or a very small one. The anatomical conditions are such as to render failure inevitable. He reported fifteen cases with three cures.

In the discussion on Sir Wm. Hingston's paper, appearing in this issue, it was moved by Mr. Cameron, Toronto, seconded by Dr. Harrison, Selkirk, that the hearty thanks of this Association be tendered to Sir Wm. Hingston for his most excellent paper. Carried with applause.

Dr. Dickson, Toronto, said that the electrical treatment of epithelioma of the face is accompanied by good cosmetic results. He advocated the establishment of a chair of electrical therapeutics in the University. He referred to the method of electrometallic treatment with the decomposition of mercury and zinc in the tissue forming an oxychloride of mercury and zinc, as being especially useful in epithelioma of the tongue and sarcoma. He advised the ray treatment to follow operation on malignant cases, citing examples to show that the secondaries frequently disappeared under the raying.

Dr. W. Oldright, Toronto, gave an account of a case of amputation of the breast, in which he had not removed the glands in the axilla, with a good result. He believed that the glands should not always be removed.

Dr. A. McPhedran, Toronto, discussed the importance of early diagnosis in gastric carcinoma. The patient should be submitted to careful examination, with special attention to the age, pain and discomfort in the epigastrium, its nature and relation to food, etc. Many cases may be relieved if diagnosed sufficiently early.

Dr. John Hunter, Toronto, emphasized the importance of good hygienic and systematic after-treatment in these cases; it helped to prolong their lives.

Sir Wm. Hingston (reply) supported Dr. Dickson's electrical treatment. In operations he aimed to cut wide of the

growth, and considered it a great misfortune if, during the course
of an operation, he should see the cancer.   Never operate for
purposes of diagnosis.   Take time and exercise patience.   The
less experienced the man, the sooner he will operate.

Dr. McIlwraith, Toronto, then read his paper on " Placenta
Previa." From a careful consideration of the various methods
of treatment, the conclusion was reached that when you decide
to interfere in these cases, *i.e.,* when the fetus is dead, or the
mother in danger from hemorrhage, the best method of procedure
is to do a combined or Braxton-Hicks version, bringing down a
leg and then leaving the delivery to nature.   The leg serves to
check hemorrhage, whilst, by leaving the case to nature, you avoid
post-partum hemorrhage from laceration of the cervix or rupture
of the uterus.   To perform version, dilatation of the os sufficient
to admit of the introduction of two fingers is all that is necessary.
When the os is not dilated, plug the cervix with iodoform gauze
or a Lysol tampon, and repeat if necessary in from four to six
hours.   Champetier de Ribe's bag is not satisfactory.   For rapid
dilatation no instrument is equal to the skilled use of the fingers.

Discussion.—Dr. Holmes, Chatham, has tried and discarded
most methods.   The tampon has given him the best satisfaction
in most cases.   The patient should be in a hospital or under the
constant care of a trained nurse.   No patient should be left alone
in the country with the danger of a hemorrhage coming on suddenly.   The doctor related an instance in which he had spent a
whole week in the country watching one patient.   The tampon
should be sterile, but in introducing it do not draw the uterus
down, as when the tenaculum is taken off the uterus returns to
its position, leaving a space between it and the tampon.   Use a
Sims' speculum, and introduce the cotton tampons one by one
until the canal is packed full.   The pains will come on rapidly,
and the presenting part come down and check the hemorrhage.

Dr. W. J. Wilson, Toronto, would not risk the tampon if the
waters have come away.

Dr. John Hunter, Parkdale, said it is important to resusci-
tate the patient before commencing delivery.

Dr. McIlwraith (reply) expressed his opinion that the tampon kills the child, and is not sufficient in checking severe hemorrhage.

Dr. N. A. Powell, Toronto, gave a very interesting and instructive demonstration of technique of intestinal anastomosis
by elastic ligature and other devices.   He first traced the history
of intestinal anastomosis, making mention of Senn's bone plates,
Murphy's button, and McGraw's elastic ligature.   " The trend
of opinion to-day is to do away with complex devices, the surgeon
endeavoring to become more proficient in manipulation."   The

doctor performed two gastro-jejunal anastomoses, illustrating the method of employing the elastic ligature, and the later improve- ment by means of the triangular stitch introduced by Drs. R. S. Weir and *J.* W. D. Maury, of New York.

Dr. Geo. Hodge, London, in an exhaustive paper, reviewed the causes and diagnosis of pain in the upper abdominal zone. Among the causes noted were pleurisy, pneumonia, gastric crises, caries of the dorsal vertebræ, uremia, appendicitis in the early stage, cardiac cases (*a*) pericarditis, (*b*) angina, (*c*) eneurism, rheumatism, especially in children, subphrenic peritonitis fol- lowing gastric ulcer, hyperacidity of the stomach, hypersecretion with spasmodic vomiting, gastric ulcer, carcinoma of the stomach, chronic gastritis. In the liver, abscess, carcinoma, Hanot's hyper- trophic cirrhosis, cholecystitis, cancer of the gall-bladder, chole- lithiasis. Of the spleen, movable spleen, infarct, abscess, spleno- medullary leukemia. In the pancreas, acute pancreatitis, chronic pancreatitis, cystic disease, and cancer. In the intestines, duodenal ulcer, impacted feces in the transverse colon. In the kidney, enteroptosis, nephrolithiasis, abscess, tuberculosis, and malignant disease.

Discussion.—Dr. H. A. McCallum, London, complimented Dr. Hodge on his masterly paper. He drew attention to the dif- ficulty of diagnosis in cholecystitis, reciting a case with pain over the gall-bladder with rigidity, following typhoid. It proved to be suppurating cholecystitis.

Dr. McPhedran, Toronto, also complimented Dr. Hodge on his excellent treatment of this important subject, in which mistakes in diagnosis are extremely numerous. He drew attention to the fact that many abdominal lesions were accompanied by identical symptoms, the pain in the early stages being practically always referred to the umbilicus. He called especial attention to dia- phragmatic pleurisy complicating central pneumonia, and to a tender area just to the right of the eleventh dorsal vertebra, de- scribed by Boas, and occurring invariably in cholecystitis. In faulty conditions of the gastric secretion, especially accompanied by an excess of hydrochloric acid, the pain is extreme and is not relieved by food or the administration of antacids; this class of patients, moreover, are neurasthenics and bear pain badly. The stomach contents varies greatly; it mav be scanty, or copious if associated with pyloric spasm.

Dr. Oldright, Toronto, said that the pain of appendicitis and perforation of the intestine was frequently referred to the upper abdominal zone.

Sir Wm. Hingston, Montreal, was pleased to note that Dr. Hodge, in his most exhaustive enumeration of causes, had not forgotten to mention that most important condition, uremia. He instanced a case in which he and a confrère had been puzzled by this condition for some days.

Dr. Holmes, Chatham, gave the history of an interesting case. The patient had been sick for three or four years with pain in the right side, extending from the iliac region to the liver. Paroxysms of severe pain, with acute suppression of urine, followed by a copious discharge of pus in the urine, occurred at various intervals. The diagnosis lay between appendicitis, movable kidney, and suppurating cholecystitis. An exploratory incision over the region of the gall-bladder revealed a tongue-like projection of the liver, which in some mysterious way pressed on a suppurating kidney, and under certain conditions prevented the discharge of pus. He was at a loss to satisfactorily explain the mechanism of this action. The patient was immediately turned on his side, a nephrectomy done, perfect cure following.

Dr. Marlow, Toronto, called attention to small hernial protrusions of fat in the linea alba, sometimes producing severe pain. He had seen two cases.

Dr. Webster, Toronto, said that pain may be due to dislocation of the spleen, with rupture of the gastro-splenic omentum. Tumor of the ovary and herpes zoster were other causes of pain.

Dr. C. B. Shuttleworth, Toronto, in an able paper, gave a complete and critical review of the subject, " Lithotomy *versus* Litholapaxy." From statistics of all the large hospitals available, the writer concluded:

(*a*) Litholapaxy is certainly the operation of election in all simple cases of stone in the urinary bladder.

(*b*) When the stone is too hard or too large to be crushed through the urethra or removed by the lateral method without injury, the suprapubic method should be adopted, or, perhaps better, perineal lithotrity.

(*c*) When the stone is encysted or associated with a tumor of the bladder or prostate, choose the suprapubic route and remove both at the same time. The mortality of a large number of cases is about 20 per cent. by the suprapubic method.

(*d*) Where there is a tight, deep, urethral stricture, especially when fistulæ exist, requiring a long operation to overcome, select the suprapubic or median perineal operation.

(*e*) In anchylosis of one or both hip joints, which interferes with the use of urethral instruments, and excludes all perineal operations, do suprapubic lithotomy.

(*f*) In the presence of foreign bodies in the bladder, which may form the nucleus of a calculus and resist the lithotrite, perform one of the perineal methods.

(*g*) Although the litholapaxy applied to children is very successful in the hands of experts, for the present lateral lithotomy is the safer operation for the general surgeon.

(*h*) Litholapaxy should be carried out, whenever possible, when senile degenerations exist, or when there are morbid changes in the genito-urinary apparatus, and the necessary treatment afforded to the complication either before or after litholapaxy.

Discussion.—Dr. Cockburn, Hamilton, said that as a matter of practical importance we do not get a sufficient number of cases to afford the necessary practice to become expert in the operation of litholapaxy. The suprapubic method has undoubtedly a bad record, but is an easy operation to perform, and with no chance of blank lithotomy. The safest method is perineal litholapaxy, but I consider the method of dilating the prostatic urethra with the finger, as advised by Reginald Harrison, a dangerous proceeding. The surgeons should practise the operation on the cadaver.

Dr. Powell, Toronto, drew attention to the importance of litholapaxy as a method of extracting stones from female children. He instanced two cases; one, a girl five years old, from whom he removed a large and a small calculus, weighing 241 grains, by litholapaxy. This was some years ago, and, so far as he knew, was the first instance of the method being employed in female children. At the request of Dr. Bigelow, these cases were published; the first may be found in full in Skene's text-book on the diseases of women. The method has now become the established procedure. " I have never been able to overcome my dread of the suprapubic route, based on the mortality reports of the large hospitals. So far, I have only removed 107 stones by the suprapubic method—it is only fair to say, however, that 106 of these came from one case. On the whole I prefer the lateral section when the case is not suitable for litholapaxy."

Dr. Primrose, Toronto, regretted that he had not heard the whole paper, but considered the suprapubic method quite as difficult as the perineal operation. He told of a case where the surgeon attempted litholapaxy and failed; then anesthetised the patient and attempted the suprapubic method, which was given up after wounding the peritoneum twice; the patient was finally put in the lithotomy position and the stone extracted with the greatest ease by lateral section. He took issue with Dr. Shuttleworth's tables of mortality of the various methods, pointing out that the more difficult cases, those with prostatic complication, were the subjects of suprapubic section. Consequently the mortality compared unfavorably with the simpler cases in which the other methods were employed.

Dr. Ross, Toronto, had recently visited Mr. Freyer in London, and had seen some of his work. Mr. Freyer had become so skilful in litholapaxy that he now practically never cuts for stone.

Dr. Webster, Toronto, wished to know which method would be employed with encysted stone.

Dr. Shuttleworth (reply) thanked the gentlemen for the interest taken in the discussion. His statistics had been gathered from a great number of cases in large hospitals, and embodied the results of operations on all cases.

Dr. Perry Goldsmith, Belleville, was then called upon for his paper, " The Treatment of Ophthalmia Neonatorum."

Discussion.—Dr. Trow, Toronto, did not consider that Dr. Goldsmith should call his treatment unorthodox; in fact, he considered it quite the orthodox method. He emphasized the importance of the careful treatment of the cornea. Argyrol is a god-send in many cases; a 20 per cent. solution may be dropped into the eye, and, if the child is lying down, will reach all parts of the conjunctival sac. No thickening of the conjunctiva results, as with the old painting method in which abrasion of the cornea was so dangerous. Cocaine should be used with caution; it hardens the cornea, and causes some proliferation of the epithelium. Bichloride does this also, and should not be used in eye work. Protargol has not the advantage of being painless, as is argyrol.

Dr. Goldsmith (reply)—Theoretically, the bichloride is of no use, as it precipitates with mucus and forms an insoluble albuminate of mercury.

Dr. Parfitt, Gravenhurst, presented an account of the work done by the Free Hospital for Incipient Tuberculosis, recently opened in Muskoka by the National Sanitarium Association. He appealed to the members of the profession for a fuller recognition of the importance and need of this work, pointing out that the hospital was dependent upon the charity of the public, and that the medical profession could do a great deal towards keeping its doors open to the needy poor by their co-operation. He presented statistics of the hospital, showing that excellent results followed the systematic out-door treatment, and closed his most interesting paper with a hearty invitation to the members of the Association to visit the Free Hospital and see for themselves the out-door treatment in active operation.

Discussion.—Dr. Elliott, Gravenhurst, joined with Dr. Parfitt in inviting more of the profession to visit the sanatorium. He assured them of a hearty welcome, and was quite convinced that the visit would be of profit to themselves.

Dr. Goldsmith. Belleville, had visited the institutions, and could testify to their excellent work, especially in laryngeal cases. The patients were under the constant supervision of the resident physicians, and received treatment, inhalations, applications, etc., once or twice daily, if necessary. He had no hesitation in advising patients to go to the sanatorium.

Dr. Milner, Toronto, said that from his experience in examining for life insurance, he was convinced that the early diagnosis of phthisis, in which stage it was favorable for sanatorium treatment, was often overlooked. He considered it the duty of every family physician to examine carefully at least every six months those of his patients with a phthisical tendency. He should pay special attention to hemic murmurs, and the character of the breath sounds.

Dr. Trow, Toronto, related the experience of a patient, a neurasthenic, phthisical, sallow-faced book-worm, who lived in a tent at Gravenhurst throughout the summer and through most of the severe winter months, coming back to Toronto robust and healthy.

Dr. Parfitt (reply) regretted to say that laryngeal cases usually do badly unless the patient be in otherwise good health. He was sorry that doctors would continue to send to the sanatorium patients in advanced stages of the disease with only a few more months to live. He would much prefer to have patients sent merely on suspicion, as they were prepared to make most delicate tests by means of tuberculin and the injection of sputum into guinea-pigs.

Dr. Wm. Oldright, Toronto, exhibited specimens of tumors removed, in which the diagnosis had been complicated. He related the history of these cases, and gave a *resume* of the differential diagnosis.

Discussion.—Dr. Perfect, Toronto Junction, asked how Dr. Oldright would control vomiting following abdominal section.

Dr. Oldright said that vomiting after operation is often difficult to control. Washing out the stomach is useful, and a hypodermic of morphia over the epigastrium successful in stubborn cases.

On Wednesday morning a very excellent series of papers dealing with the various phases of life insurance as it more especially interests the doctor, was read by the following gentlemen: Dr. H. R. Frank, Brantford; Dr. F. Le M. Grasett, Toronto (Canada Life); Dr. R. J. Dwyer, Toronto; Dr. Edw. Ryan, Kingston (Canadian Order of Foresters); Dr. H. C. Scadding, Toronto (Canada Life); Dr. B. L. Riordan, Toronto; Mr. Percy C. H. Papps, A. I. A., Toronto (Actuary, Manufacturers Life).

A vote of thanks was moved by Drs. Harrison and Davison to Mr. Papps for his interesting and instructive paper.

Discussion.—Dr. J. L. Davison, Toronto (Imperial Life)— While it may be true that adolescence is especially the age of tuberculosis, and old age that of cancer, yet it must be emphatically understood that no period of life is exempt from tuberculosis. Concerning the influence of heredity on cancer, at the present day not much attention is paid to it, the report of the recent German committee of investigation being that cancer is not hereditary. In regard to syphilis, I hold that three years of active treatment, as advised by Jonathan Hutchison, is the only safe method. The patient should not be considered cured until he has remained free from symptoms for a period of ten years, and even then he cannot be certain of complete safety. Examining physicians should be more careful of their reports, and should not hesitate to write confidential letters to the medical director explaining obscure points. As to the examination of the blood vessels, any degree of sclerosis, or visible pulsation in the radials, is of great importance, often of more importance than the existence of a heart murmur.

Dr. Machell, Toronto (Crown Life), suggested that owing to the excellence of the papers and their importance to practitioners in general, they should be published in book form and distributed to members of the Association.

Dr. Ferguson, Toronto (Excelsior Life), held in regard to syphilis that Sir Wm. Gowers was right. "It damages the vitality of the system, and paves the way for the entrance of other diseases, such as tabes, aneurism, and paresis." The descendants of long-lived parents are not necessarily good risks. Alcoholism is an evidence of neurosis—50 to 60 per cent. of neurotics having alcoholic tendencies. In reference to tuberculosis, I hold that without the seed there is no crop. The nature of the soil is also important, some soils being much more favorable to the growth of the germ than others. The following points are important: (a) Family history; (b) Personal condition; (c) Past history; (d) Collateral influence of occupation, habits, etc.

Dr. Hay, Toronto (People's Life), emphasized the importance of completely exposing the chest. In a recent case, a woman objected to exposing the chest, and upon insisting, he discovered that one breast had been removed for malignant disease, and the other one showed infection also. The woman was even at that time under the care of a surgeon who proposed to remove the remaining breast.

Dr. Oldright, Toronto, considered that some cases of mitral regurgitation with good compensation were as deserving of acceptance as were many other cases which were shoved through. Moreover, that a man operated on for appendicitis, with a good, clean, well-healed scar, should be accepted without difficulty.

Dr. Freel, Stouffville—We have heard much good advice from the medical directors, but I would like to speak a word in behalf of the unfortunate examiners. (Applause.) The difficulty of getting correct answers cannot be over-estimated; especially is it almost impossible to get accurate information concerning the habits and history of the applicant.

Dr. Britton, Toronto, considered that the examiner who was on the spot, and frequently personally acquainted with the appli- cant, was in a much better position to judge of the acceptance of the risk than the medical referee. He considered that the referees should pay more attention to the examiner's answer to that question.

Dr. Hunter, Parkdale, considered that the pay was much too small for the trouble to which the examining physician was oftentimes put. Recently he had made three attempts to ex- amine an applicant, and on the occasion of the third visit the man informed him that " he hadn't time to be examined then, as his wife had some friends in to a card party."

Dr. Webster, Toronto, wanted to know if it was true that some physicians in Toronto were examining applicants for life insurance at twenty-five cents apiece.

Dr. Scadding, Toronto, said it was true that the doctor was not sufficiently paid in some cases, but the applicant paid the doctor's fees, and in many cases these were poor patients who could not afford to pay more. Moreover, the fees were cash, with no difficulty in collecting accounts.

Mr. Papps said that if the doctors are not sufficiently paid, it is largely their own fault. There are physicians who are willing to accept the present fee, and as long as the company could get the services of such men, they could not be expected to pay more.

Dr. Sheard, Toronto, read an excellent paper on " The Relative Importance of the Clinical and Bacteriological Evidences in Diphtheria," as follows:

I have not thought it wise to present to you a set paper this evening, but shall submit some ideas with the object of eliciting an expression of opinion from those members of the profession assembled here. Many physicians imagined that the discovery of the Klebs-Loeffler bacillus and the proof by injection into guinea- pigs and cats of the production of diphtheria, settled the question beyond further discussion. But I make bold to state that the physician who imagines we know all about diphtheria is con- fronted with difficulties and troubles at every turn. I am fully convinced we cannot depend exclusively on the findings of bac- teriological examination in these cases. There are many cases which present no physical signs, but in which the bacilli are un- doubtedly present, and the generally accepted opinion that when the Klebs-Loeffler is present we have diphtheria is not always true. Whether the absence of symptoms is due to a personal immunity or not I am not prepared to say.

There are four distinct varieties of the Klebs-Loeffler bacillus: the long forms, the short, the attenuated, and the pseudo-bacilli. They produce soluble toxins, and are sometimes associated in their action with pus organisms—these toxins produce the symptoms which we designate diphtheria.

I have a series of seven cases diagnosed as posterior fibrinous rhinitis, in which not one but a series of bacteriological examinations failed to reveal the presence of the Klebs-Loeffler, but each case was followed by paralysis. We generally admit with paralysis we have diphtheria. The virulence of diphtheria varies much according to the seed, the mortality being sometimes over 90 per cent. I remember a man from Buffalo with diphtheria who stopped at the Brown Hotel; seven new cases developed from exposure, of whom six died. Some time ago a Russian family of nine set out for Toronto; two of them died at sea of diphtheria, two more in Montreal, and two others in Toronto. All this bears out the teaching that diphtheria is due to a particular form of vegetable organism, and as such is subject to the laws which govern the growth of all seed in various soils.

1st. The sequelæ are due entirely to the toxins, the extent of the membrane being of no consequence in this connection. If we have cellulitis, and no adenitis, the condition is most serious, the toxins entering the nerve trunks and destroying their vitality. The sequelæ may be expected at any time from the third week to the third month.

2nd. Many conditions are due to the associated pus organisms, such as the secondary eruptions, which are identical with those of septicemia, and in no way dependent upon the Klebs-Loeffler.

Another form of bacterial diphtheria is the post scarlatinal type, in which during the second week of the fever the patients have the Klebs-Loeffler, but exhibit no symptoms; they invariably get well and are not infective. I have records of sixteen such cases. Again we have the association of scarlet fever and diphtheria, the diphtheria not following the scarlet fever, but both diseases existing simultaneously in the same patient as the result of two separate exposures—the incubation period of scarlet fever being four days, whilst that of diphtheria is about six days. At the Isolation Hospital we have a separate ward for these mixed cases. Again we have those cases of post-diphtheritic scarlet fever where the scarlet fever follows closely on the heels of the diphtheria, and where, in spite of any form of treatment, we have a mortality of over 80 per cent. And as these cases occur as frequently in private houses as in hospitals, they cannot be accounted for by infection from one hospital patient to another. A frequent experience at the Isolation Hospital is to have whole families sent in, half of whom are suffering from diphtheria, the other half from scarlet fever; showing the correctness of Sydenham's contention that there exists a far greater intimacy between these two diseases than the private physician would care to admit.

I can report several cases in which, after weeks of most energetic treatment, the bacilli could not be gotten rid of, and though such cases were discharged, no new cases have been known to result from them. One patient in the scarlet fever ward developed otitis media, in the discharge from which the Klebs-Loeffler bacilli were found. He was discharged, and no cases resulting have been reported. From these experiences I am convinced that when the bacillus of diphtheria exists in pus it is innocuous and non-virulent.

In conclusion, these questions naturally arise: 1st. Is scarlet fever antidotal to diphtheria? The answer appears to be in the affirmative. 2nd. Does not diphtheria aggravate scarlet fever? The answer again is " Yes." 3rd. Is the difference in the two diseases due to the evolvement of a soluble toxin by the Klebs-Loeffler bacillus? Osler once said to me, " If the rash appears, disappears, and re-appears, it is in all probability a septic rash." The scarlet fever rash, we know, does not disappear and re-appear, but there are many septic cases, such as recurring erysipelatous rashes, all closely connected clinically with diphtheria and scarlet fever.

Dr. McMahon followed Dr. Sheard with a masterly paper upon " The Uncertainties of Diagnosis and the Necessity of Early and Vigorous Treatment of Diphtheria." He emphasized the importance of the early injection of adequate doses of antitoxin in all suspected cases, even before the results of a bacteriological examination could be obtained. He called attention to the great reduction in the mortality, especially of laryngeal cases, since the introduction and the general use of antitoxin. In his own practice he was pleased to report that since he had adopted the rule of early and efficient treatment with antitoxin, he had not had a single death. From the reports of the Hospital for Sick Children, he was convinced of the effectiveness of immunizing doses of antitoxin, and advised that members of a family in which a case occurred should each receive adequate immunizing injections.

Discussion.—Dr. A. R. Gordon, Toronto, strongly verified Dr. McMahon's statements, and expressed himself in favor of the early, abundant, and fearless treatment with antitoxin.

Dr. Allan Baines, Toronto—I must congratulate Dr. McMahon upon his happy experience with antitoxin. I wish it to be emphatically understood that I am a believer in antitoxin, but I can report no such good results. . . . In one case I injected 4,000 units, followed in four hours by 2,000 units, in four hours more by 2,000 more units; in all 8,000 units in eight hours, but in spite of this the patient died. Pure cases of diphtheria are undoubtedly benefited by antitoxin, but those cases of

6

mixed infection, with the streptococcus and the staphylococcus, are not cured by antitoxin.   It is just ten years since this question was thoroughly thrashed out in the Pediatric Society at New York, when this same conclusion was reached.

Dr. W. J. Wilson, Toronto—My experience is the same as Dr. McMahon's. My practice is to inject antitoxin early, make swabs in all suspicious cases, and make my own cultures, in which case I have a report in eight hours. I believe calomel fumigation and intubation to be valuable adjuncts in the treatment of laryngeal cases, but my rule is, " When in doubt, use antitoxin." A difficulty we encounter is that when the swabs are sent to the Health Office on Saturday evening, no report can be received until the following Tuesday morning.

Dr. John Ferguson, Toronto—I endorse Dr. McMahon's posi· tion. I use antitoxin freely and early, and in young children rather increase the size of the dose than diminish it, as their tender constitutions have little power in producing self-immunity. Concerning the cases of mixed infection, with the staphylococcus or streptococcus present, I maintain that if you control the Klebs-Loeffler bacillus, you materially aid the child in its struggle. I am pleased to report that I have not had one death since using antitoxin; in all I have had nine intubation cases, three before the period of antitoxin, and all died, and six since the introduction of antitoxin, and all recovered.

Dr. B. Z. Milner, Toronto—I wish to call Dr. McMahon's attention to the fact that there is diphtheria in the Sick Children's Hospital at the present time, and that recently when I wished to operate on several cases, I was informed that they were in the isolation ward with diphtheria.

Dr. Sheard, Toronto —I would like to ask Dr. Machell concerning fifteen cases in the Children's Home. Did these all receive immunizing doses?

Dr. Machell, Toronto—As far as my memory serves me, I believe all did not receive immunizing doses before being ill, and that but one or two cases occurred in those patients where immunizing doses had been given. . . . Diphtheria varies markedly in epidemics. In some epidemics all die, in others all get well.

Dr. F. N. G. Starr, Toronto, pointed out that the cases at the H. S. C., where the present epidemic commenced, were in children from eight to ten years old, and that the ordinary immunizing dose of 500 units for a child of two or three years was not sufficient for these older children.

Dr. John Hunter, Parkdale, expressed the opinion that the mortality was greater with the use of antitoxin than without it.

Dr. Webster, Toronto, has never seen any good result follow the use of antitoxin after the child once has diphtheria. Of four cases in one family, sent to the Isolation Hospital, one only received antitoxin, and she died; the other three received no antitoxin, and all recovered.

Dr. A. A. Macdonald, Toronto, believes in the effect of immunizing doses, but that in most cases the dose is too small. Do the thing early and do it thoroughly. "Is not your experience the same as mine in laryngeal cases; formerly did not practically all our laryngeal cases die, while is it not now your experience that the child suffering from marked dyspnea after the injection of the antitoxin, soon commences to breathe freely and easily?"

Dr. McMahon (reply) reiterated his former statements, and said that if Dr. Webster had used antitoxin immediately, the little girl would not now be under a small mound on the hillside.

Dr. Sheard (reply) wished to be understood that there were other things in the treatment of diphtheria besides antitoxin, such as cleansing sprays and swabs; and moreover that laryngeal cases will die in spite of antitoxin, not from the toxemia, but from laryngismus stridulus. He doubted the immunizing effects of antitoxin.

On Wednesday afternoon the Association held their annual luncheon. The affair was a most enjoyable one, excellent speeches being given by Premier Ross, Hon. Mr. Harcourt, Dr. Harrison, of Selkirk, and Dean Reeve. Immediately after the luncheon, through the kindness of the Automobile Club, the members of the Association were treated to a ride around the city.

"The Treatment of Prostatic Hypertrophy" was the title of a paper by Dr. T. K. Holmes, Chatham.

From a careful consideration of the subject, Dr. Holmes concludes that castration and vasectomy are of little value; that the Bottini operation, while not in general favor, has many good points, and is deserving of a more careful study and a wider employment; that suprapubic prostatectomy is difficult in fat subjects; the perineal method is the one most generally useful. The gland is drawn down into the wound by means of Sims' rubber bag, and carefully enucleated from its capsule. If it is desirable to avoid damage to the ejaculatory ducts, Dr. Young's (Baltimore) device for pulling down the gland and performing the operation visually is recommended. Dr. Holmes gave the history of two successful cases; in one he employed the Bottini operation, in the other median perineal prostatectomy was done. In conclusion he warned the profession against the constant use of the catheter, as it almost invariably resulted in cystitis. "There are one hundred men in this room, and probably twenty of us will have to seek relief for an enlarged prostate. We should advise to others the same treatment that we ourselves would like to receive."

Discussion.—Dr. Bruce, Toronto, preferred the suprapubic operation, although he had not acquired the dexterity of Mr. Freyer, who shelled out the prostate in two minutes. He had never met with any special difficulty in reaching the gland in fat patients. Within the last month he had operated on one very stout gentleman, and by pressing the prostate forward from below had experienced no difficulty in removing it.

Dr. Powell, Toronto, had not intended to take part in the discussion, but was drawn into it by the good-natured raillery of one of the speakers. He was pleased to say that, although he dreaded the suprapubic route, he had as yet no mortality in the operation. Statistics from large centres, however, showed the operation to be attended by a mortality of about 20 per cent. He cited a recent aggravated case, and had just that day received a letter from the patient announcing that " he was able to dispense with his catheter."

President Ross told of a recent visit to Mr. Freyer, in London, and gave short extracts from letters of rejoicing nobility, upon whom Mr. Freyer had operated for enlarged prostate. " Duke —— writes, ' Dear Dr., . . . I can now pump ship like a two-year-old.' " " Earl —— writes, ' Dear Dr., . . . I tell you I can now make the pot hum.' "

Mr. Cameron, Toronto, was pleased to have heard Dr. Holmes' interesting and able paper. He agreed that the older perineal route was the better method. It was not absolutely necessary to damage the urethra in all cases. He took exception to the expression " the anatomical middle lobe," as there is no middle lobe to the prostate. He regretted to report a serious mortality by the suprapubic method. He did so, however, out of the hope that those present might benefit from his misfortunes. Within the last year and a half he had done fifteen suprapubic sections, with five deaths. Two of the fatalities could not be attributed to the operation, one being from facial erysipelas and bronchitis, the other from hemiplegia; but the other three, who were promising and otherwise healthy patients, died suddenly; one acutely insane in twenty-four hours, who was perfectly well twelve hours after the operation; one unaccountably, without either hemorrhage or shock, in about twenty hours, having been in excellent condition twelve hours after the operation; and the last in about forty-eight hours, of albuminous edema of the lungs, the pulse and temperature having been normal and the general condition excellent twelve, twenty-four, and thirty-six hours after the operation. With the old perineal operation he had had no mortality.

Dr. McKinnon, Guelph, operated wholly by the suprapubic method. He considered it much easier, involving less danger of wounding the rectum, and rarely followed by fistulæ. His mor-

tality had not been great. The perineal route is simple, involves
less shock to the patient, but is frequently followed by fistulæ.
He reported a series of cases with successful operation and recovery, in patients from 65 to 83 years old. He had only had
two deaths.

Dr. Olmstead, Hamilton, said that all methods are simple to
those practised and skilled in the method of their choice. On the
continent the perineal method was used almost exclusively and
with great success; in England and Canada the suprapubic route
was the method of election and enjoyed the same success. He
advocated the more frequent use of the cystoscope. Freyer was
able to announce good results, and he was surprised that, with
the immense amount of material at his disposal, he did not
announce more of them, because he was able to carefully select
his cases. We in Canada here could not so pick and choose, but
were forced to do our best to relieve all sufferers. In his mind
the one objection to the suprapubic method was the poor drainage
obtained.

Dr. Hohnes (reply) strongly advised more careful study of
the Bottini operation. No general anesthetic was required, and
he believed it had a great future before it.

Dr. Bingham—The contracted bladder was easily raised by
the hand in the rectum. The bladder should be sutured to the
abdominal wall before opening.

Dr. J. Campbell Meyers, Deer Park, read a splendid paper
on " Neurasthenia in Some of its Relations to Insanity." We
print it in full in this issue.

Discussion.—Dr. McKenzie, Bracebridge, emphasized the
importance of the subject, stating that neurasthenics were frequently met with in country practice. These cases fall easy victims to the quacks. It was a matter of great difficulty to carry
out isolation in many cases.

Dr. Ferguson, Toronto, said that neurasthenia and the earlier
forms of insanity are several links in the same chain; the exact
situation of the boundary line is beyond human judgment. Pronounced cases of neurasthenia or insanity are easy of diagnosis,
but between these there is a series most puzzling to us all. The
question is one of physical disturbance, the great feature being
that the slightest mental effort produces exhaustion. Again, the
nerve system becomes so depleted of all energy that physical
exertion is impossible. The condition is a nutritional change
first, followed later by an anatomical one. The dendrites fail to
absorb sufficient nutriment from the brain matter, and the slightest possible effort exhausts this limited supply. Disorganization
sets in and the sickly, weakly, though normal, cell becomes a
morbid and pathological one, and ultimately disappears. The

conditions producing these effects are: 1. Prolonged worry; 2. Sudden mental shock; 3. Over-work and no rest; 4. Some toxemia which affects the brain, destroying the nerve cell.

Dr. Hunter, Parkdale, would like to know the position hydrotherapy occupied in Dr. Meyers' treatment. A woman under his care, suffering from a pronounced form of neurasthenia, for whom he had prescribed a cold bath every morning (preferably at 5 a.m.), followed by a brisk bicycle ride, was now a perfect picture of ruddy health.

Dr. Bruce Smith emphasized the use of hydrotherapy in treatment, the etiological value of toxemia, and the importance of early recognition of the symptoms in neurasthenia. " Insanity," he concluded, " is the culmination of nervous derangements in the patient, undiscovered and uncorrected."

Dr. Holmes, Chatham, said that women are born with unstable nervous systems, and later in life misfortunes overtake them which lower their vitality and produce the symptoms of neurasthenia. We must search carefully for the cause; it may be a movable kidney, an inflamed gall-bladder, faulty position of the uterus, inflammation of the ovary, laceration of the cervix, or eye-strain. The correction of these conditions, he believed, would, in most cases, result in the entire disappearance of the nervous symptoms. In a case of puerperal insanity recently under his care, he repaired a torn cervix, and the insanity disappeared. Many cases also were due, he believed, to auto-intoxication from the alimentary canal.

Dr. McPhedran, Toronto, said that cases on the borderland between neurasthenia and insanity are difficult of diagnosis. Neurasthenia should include all cases of nerve prostration; *e.g.,* in one patient weakness of digestion may be the prominent feature; another patient cannot sleep or rest; still another may have disturbed cardiac action; but all are neurasthenic. He believed that there should be better provision for more careful attention to the incipient insane. There should be one or more stations for the temporary treatment of such patients, and wherein incurable and curable cases could be separated. This would materially relieve the asylums and save the patient from the stigma attached to the inmate of an insane asylum. There are such institutions in Europe and the United States. An inherited difference in the vitality of tissue is responsible for the easy break-down in neurasthenics. Some have poor vitality of brain, of kidney, or of stomach, with the result that these organs are readily exhausted.

Dr. W. J. Wilson, Toronto, agreed with Dr. Holmes that putting all the organs right and changing the environment of the patient would accomplish many cures. He deprecated the wholesale removal of ovaries for trifling causes, the ultimate result being bad.

President Ross could not agree with Dr. Holmes. Some years ago, through the kindness of Dr. Beemer, of Mimico Asylum, he operated on a number of women patients, repairing lacerations, correcting uterine displacements, etc., with no change in the mental condition of the patients. They were insane before, and they are insane yet, and will probably remain so.

Dr. Meyers (reply)—Any pathological condition should certainly be treated, but improvement in the mental condition could not be expected to follow. He could see no reason why an operation on a woman's uterus should influence the condition of her mind.

Dr. McPhedran discussed some forms of skin disease.

1. *Impetigo Contagiosa.*—The disease is contagious, most commonly occurring on the face or pubic regions, and due to the streptococcus or staphylococcus (or some believe to a specific organism). The disease tends to recur from time to time.

Treatment.—Cleansing, and the application of antiseptic ointments, such as ung. hyd. amm. chlor., or, better, Resorcin, 20 to 30 grains in an ounce of Lanolin. The principle in the treatment of all skin diseases is, cleanse and apply antiseptic, soothing, or stimulating applications.

2. *Erythema Multiforma.*—The trouble commenced in March, four years ago, as a vesicular eruption, occurring on the hands, face, and neck, *i.e.,* the exposed parts only. The eruption lasted all summer, faded in the fall, leaving no mark. It returned in March of the following spring, and went through the same cycle. The lesions are first vesicular, then pustular, and finally coarse crusts, which drop off in a few weeks, leaving faint marks. No inflammation precedes the vesiculation. It is, doubtless, purely a congestion with a serous exudate, followed by an exudate of leucocytes and ultimate crusting.

3. *Acne and eruption on the leg* (syphilitic or tubercular).

Treatment.—Acne, difficult in phlegmatic types. Stimulate until slight desquamation, and then soothe. He prescribed Resorcin, 20 gr.; B. naphthol ½ dr.; sulphur, 2 dr.; green soap and vaselin, aa, 1 oz. To soothe the leg ulcer use Unna's paste: zinc oxide 1, gelatine 2, glycerine 3, aqua 4. Add, if necessary, Ichthyol 2, 3, 4, or 5 per cent.

4. *Tinea Tonsurans.*—Difficult to cure, as the microsporon is deep down in the hair follicles. Two principles to be observed, thoroughness and perseverance, *i.e.,* use any parasiticide and keep it up. He prescribed sulphur, 2 dr.; Lanolin, 1 oz.; or chrysarobin, 1 dr. to the oz.

5. *Cycosis non-parasitica.*

6. *Leucoderma* in a man with pernicious anemia.

Dr. H. B. Anderson, of Toronto, followed Dr. McPhedran.

1. *Urticaria pigmentosa.*—Present since birth. Small wheels, leaving yellowish or brownish pigmentation spots; recur at intervals in the same spot, leaving a deeper stain. Pigmentation due to the escape of red blood corpuscles and deposit of their pigment.

2. *Weeping eczema.*

3. *Psoriasis.*

4. Exhibition of cholene crystals from the blood of a nerve case, prepared by Dr. F. H. Scott, according to the method of Dr. Haliburton.

5. *Molluscum fibrosum.*—A man with many hundreds of small cutaneous tumors.

Dr. H. B. Anderson then read a paper on " Strain in Heart Disease." The influence of severe bodily exertion in inducing rupture of the heart or blood vessels, in patients with arteriosclerosis, or in those unused to physical exertion, was illustrated by the exhibition of a number of specimens, with a short history of each.

1. A patient dropped dead on the street, following rapid walking. The specimen showed rupture of the aorta. Presented by Dr. Powell.

2. A woman, aged 60, died suddenly during the passage of a stomach tube. Specimen reveals rupture of the left ventricle.

3. Captain on a boat attempted to carry a heavy tie, fell unconscious, suffering from tachycardia. Died nine months later, aged 55. Specimen shows rupture of the sinus of Valsalva, with aneurismal dilatation pressing on the right heart.

4. Patient a moderate drinker, good liver, no history of syphilis. After a week of unusual exertion was seized with a sudden pain and sense of weakness, and died the same night. The autopsy showed a dissecting aneurism involving the whole of the descending aorta down to the bifurcation of the iliacs. The blood had burst the middle and inner coats of the aorta, making a false passage for itself under the adventitia.

Dr. J. H. Elliot, Gravenhurst, gave an illustrated paper on the advantages of a pictorial record of chest examinations. By means of lines, circles, dots and crosses, he represents the degree of dullness, adventitious sounds, the nature of the breath sounds, pleuritic rubs, etc. The method commended itself for ease, simplicity and efficiency to all present. Dr. Elliot very kindly offered to explain the details of the system, with illustrations, etc., to anyone who cared to communicate with him.

Dr. R. N. Eraser, of Thamesville, then read his paper, and reported a remarkable group of cases of malignant disease occurring in members of the same family and attendants who waited on them.

Discussion.—Dr. W. J. Wilson, Toronto, recited the case of a gentleman in Germany, who by mistake drank the stomach contents from a patient with gastric carcinoma, and he himself died of cancer some months later. Another case, where a physician by mistake sucked up the stomach contents of a cancer patient from a tube, he himself dying of cancer some fifteen months later, was mentioned.

Dr. Ferguson, Toronto, referred to the excellent record of family cases of malignant disease reported in a recent number of the *British Lancet*.

Dr. Marlow, Toronto, asked if the undescended testicle in No. 5 of Dr. Fraser's series had been found to be cancerous.

Dr. Fraser (reply) did not wish to give the impression that he held cancer to be infectious. It is probably auto-infectious. He could not answer Dr. Marlow's question, as the gland had not been examined.

Dr. A. Primrose, Toronto, then read a paper on " The Surgical Relief of Epilepsy."

Dr. Primrose presented the history of two cases of traumatic epilepsy operated on with good results so far. The first patient was a young lad, about 20, who gave a thrilling history of shipwreck and exposure at sea, after which the fits developed. The seizures always commenced in the first two fingers of the left hand; the wound, however, was on the left side of the head. Was this, then, a case where the pyramidal tracts did not cross, or had there been a lesion on the right side, owing to bursting as a result of the blow on the left side? The left Rolandic area was first trephined, and electrodes applied in the hand area. causing immediate movement of the fingers of the right hand. This proved that the pyramidal tracts did cross. An opening was immediately made on the right side, which revealed a thickened dura mater, and but little other change. Some of this was removed, tension relieved, and the wounds closed up. The patient had two or three fits the night after the operation, but since then (some six months now), has been free from them. The second case was the result of a depressed fracture involving only the inner table of the skull, the result of a pitch-fork wound. The operation revealed an abscess, which was opened and drained. The patient has since been free from seizures.

Discussion.—Dr. Dickson, Toronto, explained the method of localizing motor centres in the cortex by electrodes from a Faradic current. Experimenting should not be done, as it involves great shock to the patient. Fine platinum electrodes are inserted into the cortex and the current turned on gently.

Mr. Cameron, Toronto, said that a lesion giving rise to cortical irritation should be removed. Epilepsy is a discharge of nervous energy from the motor centre in which the cells go off at halfcock. He believed Case 1 of Professor Primrose was a hystero-epileptic, probably a disciple of Captain Marryat's. There is no use operating unless you find some focal symptom. Personally he had not met with much success in the operation; the patients were better for about a year, but the epilepsy almost invariably returned.

Dr. Ferguson, Toronto, said that statistics show that less than 5 per cent. of epileptics are relieved by surgical procedure. Idiopathic cases, with focal symptoms, and especially Jacksonian epilepsy, are most favorable. Cases operated on almost invariably recur, owing to the contraction of cicatricial tissue, and the last condition is worse than the first. He reported a case of depressed fracture, operated on with complete recovery.

Dr. Bruce, Toronto, reported a case of traumatic epilepsy in which he had removed some of the cortex corresponding to the hand centre. At first there was paresis of the hand, but this recovered, and later on the patient developed epilepsy on the opposite side. "So I transferred him from a right-handed to a left-handed epileptic," said the surgeon.

Dr. McConnell, of Las Cruces, Mexico, read a most instructive and interesting paper on "Climatology and its Influence in the Cure of many Cases of, especially, Chest Trouble."

Dr. Oldright, Toronto, complimented Dr. McConnell on his excellent paper. Was always pleased to meet their former students, and learn of their successes. He asked Dr. McConnell to explain the action of the alfalfa in stopping dust.

Dr. Wishart, Toronto, said that we should congratulate ourselves on the information gained from this paper. It will be of great assistance in directing patients to suitable health resorts. He asked the doctor about the winds and the feeding in the arid zone.

Dr. Hunter, Parkdale, had visited the arid regions and could add his testimony to that of Dr. McConnell. The medical men in those districts were prominent physicians from New York and other large cities, forced to live in these health resorts. "Do not load your patients down with directions how to live, but place them in the hands of resident medical men." He would like to know about the disinfection of houses and the removal of patients in Pullman cars.

Mr. Cameron highly complimented the writer; the paper was as full of pabulum as an egg, and might be well taken as a model.

Dr. Webster, Toronto, said that many consumptive people have but limited means, and cannot afford to take long journeys and live in expensive resorts. Lots of them are able to get well right here in Toronto.

Dr. McConnell (reply) said that the alfalfa meadows were effective barriers to the dust. Patients did better to provide themselves with tents, and then they ran no risk of infection from houses. One could live comfortably on $10 a week.

Dr. Burnham, Toronto, then read a paper on " Inflammations of the Lachrymal Apparatus."

Inflammation of the lachrymal sac is the result of struma, violence, or the entrance of irritating fluid, or, most commouly, stricture of the nasal duct. This last condition results in insufficient drainage to the duct, and a chronic blenorrhea is set up. This mucocele is attended by much suffering and constant disturbance, and demands effective treatment. Initial leeching, calomel, etc., usually fail to abort the attack; hot linseed poultices and free incision on fluctuation are necessary in the acute stage. To remove the cause, and consequently relieve the condition, Dr. Burnham operates as follows: Having slit the canaliculus into the sac, he introduces by means of a syringe a 5 per cent. solution of cocaine, and passes probes Nos. 1 and 2 only. He then irrigates freely with adrenalin, followed by potassium permanganate, 1 in 12,000; and last of all he passes a silver style, which is allowed to remain in position. In three or four days the style is removed, the cocaine, adrenalin, and permanganate irrigation repeated, and the style replaced. This method of treatment is much less painful and much more effective than the old method of passing the largest probe possible and using no medication. During the process of healing, little fibrous bands appear along the floor of the divided canaliculus, which act as dams, preventing the free exit of the tears, and which must consequently be divided.

Discussion.—Dr. Wishart asked Dr. Burnham if the inferior turbinate was not frequently enlarged close to the outlet of the nasal duct, and if cauterization was not indicated? Would like Dr. Burnham to explain more fully what he meant by the constriction bands in the canaliculus lachrymalis.

Dr. Burnham (reply)—Where the turbinate was enlarged, it should certainly be treated. By the constrictions he meant little cicatricial bands, 6, 8, or 10 in number, which prevented the free passage of the probe into the lachrymal sac, and had to be divided time and time again until no obstruction was offered.

Dr. D. J. Gibb Wishart then read his report of a case of double otitis media, with mastoid involvement. Operation and termination in fatal purulent leptomeningitis.

Dr. Wishart reported a case of mastoid involvement which presented no symptoms except pus in the middle ear, which seemed to well up through the opening in the drum, and some indefinite headache. The man was under the careful observation of both himself and the family physician, a careful record of temperature having been kept, which showed at no time any marked elevation. The patient did not improve, however; was sent to the General Hospital, the mastoid opened, but fatal leptomeningitis followed. The interesting feature of the case is that at no time did the patient exhibit the usual symptoms of mastoid trouble; at no time was there local pain or tenderness, nor any elevation of temperature nor rigors.

Dr. B. Z. Milner, Toronto, read a paper on "Lympho-sarcoma." The tumor occurred in a young man about nineteen, a strong, athletic fellow. It was situated in the neck, and examination showed it to be a round-celled sarcoma. It was removed by operation, but the glands in the neighborhood were found to be involved, and the growth recurred. The patient was treated with X-rays, with no apparent improvement. Coley's fluid was then used, and after a thorough trial was abandoned, no benefit having resulted. Finsen's rays also proved useless. The patient was seen at various times by Dr. Powell, Toronto, and Dr. Coley, New York. It was now about a year since the first appearance of the trouble, and the patient was in bad condition. As a last resort X-rays combined with quinine-fluorescence (the quinine being given internally before the raying), were tried. Under this the growth made no further progress, and some improvement even was noted. The patient, however, was so exhausted that he succumbed.

"Some of the Newer Methods of Diagnosis in Kidney Cases as applied to Renal Surgery" was the title of a paper by Dr. W. A. Hackett, Professor of Genito-Urinary Diseases, Detroit.

Dr. Hackett briefly reviewed the more important devices and methods introduced since 1885, pointing out the use and advantages of each. Chromocystoscopy is a useful method of determining the activity of the kidneys. The patient is given a dose of methyl blue or indigo carmine, which are normally excreted by the kidneys in fifteen to thirty minutes. By watching the urethral openings with a cystoscope, the exact time of the appearance of colored urine from each kidney can be determined. If one is manifestly slower than the other, it is evidently the diseased kidney.

Urethral catheterization and segregation enable us to collect the urine from the individual kidney. The former method, while becoming more and more popular, is expensive, and demands skill and patience on the part of the operator. Segregation is open to the objection that the bladder may be diseased.

The history of cyroscopy, or the determination of the freezing point of urine, and the application of Dr. Coppet's law, that the lower the freezing point the greater the concentration, was

considered in some detail. The method combined with segregation has been shown to be a most valuable aid in diagnosis, and
has removed the fear of the surgeon after nephrectomy to a large
extent.

Phloridzin Test.—After the hypodermic injection of phloridzin a diseased kidney is found to excrete sugar less rapidly
than a normal one. . . . Electrical conductivity of urine,
X-rays and various bougies were briefly mentioned also. In
concluding, the writer explained that these new methods of diagnosis are gradually replacing the old exploratory operation.

Dr. R. D. Rudolf, Toronto, followed next with a paper on
" Diagnosis of Functional Heart Murmurs."

Functional murmurs, as first described by Laennec, are soft
and blowing in character, occur most commonly in the position
of the pulmonary area, opposite the second left costal cartilage,
and are in no way connected with valvular diseases. They are
due, not to the anemia, as so often taught, but to a condition of
hypotonus of the muscles of the circulatory system; that is, there
is a relaxation of the sphincter muscles guarding the mitral and
tricuspid orifices, and permitting of a leakage. In the pulmonary area, the fibrous band around the orifice permits of no dilatation; but the muscular structure of the pulmonary artery permits
it to dilate, and consequently we have a condition in which the
blood stream flows from one chamber, that is, the right ventricle,
through a relatively constricted orifice, into the dilated pulmonary artery. This is the most favorable arrangement for the production of a murmur. Dr. Rudolf laid down the following rules
to aid in the diagnosis of functional from organic murmurs:

1. They occur in adolescence and young adults.

2. They are more common in males than females.

3. They all occur during ventricular systole.

4. While the pulmonic area is the most common situation
for functional murmurs, it is a rare site for organic murmurs
(congenital stenosis being the only one found).

5. Functional murmurs are heard in the neck; *e.g.,* bruit de
diable.

6. As the general health improves, functional murmurs tend to
disappear; organic murmurs, on the other hand, tend to get
louder with increasing strength.

7. Functional murmurs are soft, and accompany rather than
displace the first sound.

8. They are not so widely propagated as are organic murmurs.

9. They vary under certain conditions; *e.g.,* they are louder
after exertion, and are especially increased on lying down.

10. The pulmonic second sound is accentuated early, even

before the murmur is heard; this is not so in organic pulmonary stenosis.

11. They are accompanied with little signs of dilatation or displacement of the apex.

12. Cardio-respiratory sounds are sometimes mistaken; ask the patient to hold his breath and they will disappear.

13. Signs of failing compensation are rare in functional cases.

14. The patients are not conscious of the existence of the murmur. An analysis of the patients in the surgical wards of the H. S. C. showed that in 60 per cent. functional murmurs were present. An analysis of a number of wards in the Toronto General Hospital and St. Michael's Hospital showed the existence of functional murmurs in 50 per cent. of the patients.

15. Fever gives rise to functional murmurs. They occur in 66 per cent. of scarlet fever cases, and are apt to recur in rheumatic fever. A useful rule in this connection is, " Functional murmurs tend to occur late in fever (*e.g.,* rheumatic fever), while endocardial murmurs appear within the first ten days."

16. Pressure has not much effect as a rule in altering functional murmurs.

Finally, we are all too apt to conclude that there is organic disease when we hear a murmur, and we are too easily soothed into believing the patient organically sound when no murmur can be discovered.

Dr. Chas. Hodgetts, Secretary, Ontario Board of Health, read a capital paper on " The Diagnosis of Modified Smallpox," which will appear in next month's number.

Dr. Hodgetts employs the word " modified " to designate those cases where the course is in any way atypical, not to cases modified by vaccination—the so-called varioloid.

About five years ago the disease appeared in Essex County and Northern Ontario, and was variously diagnosed as chickenpox, impetigo and syphilis. The spread of the affection and the fact that those unvaccinated were its victims, soon, however, established the nature of the epidemic. Since then the disease has continued from year to year, with the maximum number of cases in January and the minimum during the summer months. The virulence of the contagion has been variable, during the early stages (preceding pustulation), but slightly contagious, and in many mild cases the contagion seems slight throughout. The regulation incubation period of twelve days has been the rule, but many cases of fifteen, sixteen and eighteen days have occurred, necessitating the period of quarantine being extended to eighteen days.

The initial symptoms have varied all the way from a passing malaise to severe headache and backache, accompanied by
nausea and vomiting. The initial temperature has been from
100 to 102 F. The mildness or severity of the onset, however,
has been no indication of a mild or severe attack. The fever drops
with the appearance of the characteristic rash in about seventy-
two hours. The rash runs through its regular series of macules,
vesicles, pustules and crusts.

The affection is most frequently mistaken for chicken-pox,
impetigo and pustular syphiloderm, and in the differentiation
the following points are important:

Chicken-pox.—1. A disease of childhood. 2. Runs a rapid
course; lesions are papules, vesicles and scabs, all in twenty-four
hours. All over in a week. 3. Premonitory symptoms slight or
none. 4. Temperature appears with the rash. 5. Vesicles soft
and irregular. 6. Eruption occurs on covered parts. 7. No scar
or pigmentation left.

Impetigo.—1. No elevation of temperature. 2. No initial
stage. 3. Begins as a vesicle or vesicular pustule. 4. Occurs
on the face, hands and exposed parts. 5. Unsymmetrical and
superficial, large blebs. 6. Crust friable, leaves no scar. 7. Fin-
ger-nails carry the infection.

Pustular Syphiloderm.—The large indurated base of the
vesicle, which lacks umbilication, and the history and persist-
ence of the symptoms should prevent mistake.

" Enlargements of the Prostate Gland " was the title of a
paper by Dr. F. W. Marlow, Toronto.

Dr. Marlow gave a very comprehensive account of the anatomy
of the prostate, explaining most carefully the position and variations of the anatomical middle lobe.

Prostatic enlargement, he said, does not necessarily mean
prostatic obstruction; according to Sir Henry Thompson, while
30 per cent. of men beyond the age of 55 have prostatic enlargement, but 5 per cent. have obstruction. The etiology of the condition is still obscure; two theories most in vogue at the present
time are: (*a*) Prostatic enlargement is a local result of a general
arterio-sclerosis (held by Guyon and the French school). This
is opposed by Freyer, Casper, Bruce, Clark, etc., who regard
arterio-sclerosis as conducive to atrophy and not hypertrophy.
(*b*) On account of similarity in the structure of the prostate and
the uterus, Velpeau claims the existence of an analogy between
prostatic enlargement and fibromyoma of the uterus.

The enlargement may be uniform or more frequently asym-
metrical, the enlarged portion raising the vesicle outlet, stretching the urethral walls and forming a pouch in which residual

urine collects.   The symptoms of the trouble are increased frequency of micturition, due first to irritation of the growth, but later to diminution of the bladder capacity.   There is difficulty in starting the stream, which is small, without its normal projection curve, and followed by dribbling.   With proper attention to the history and symptoms, and careful digital examination, the diagnosis should be easy.

Dr. G. A. Bingham, Toronto, read a paper on " Surgical Treatment of Enlargement of the Prostate."

The methods employed will depend entirely upon the individual case.   One man with no symptoms but increased micturition may be carefully and scientifically introduced to catheter life.   While in another case with overflow, cystitis and probably pyelitis, drainage by median perineal cystotomy, done under a local anesthesia, is demanded.   Between these extremes are a number of cases amenable to radical treatment, and for these the following operations have all been done: (*a*) Orchidectomy. The shock is severe and the operation not generally useful, and is now abandoned. (*b*) Vesicotomy.   Slow and uncertain, and applicable to but a limited number of cases. (*c*) Perineal and suprapubic prostatectomy.   Of these the most rational and scientific procedure is the suprapubic.   In this the field is freely exposed, the gland readily reached, and easily shelled out of its attenuated capsule.   The results are usually most satisfactory.

Dr. E. Clouse, Toronto, then read his paper, " Notes of an Uncommon Case of Rectal Surgery."

Dr. Clouse recounted a remarkable instance of a patient's unfortunate adventures with hemorrhoids.   The patient, a prominent clergyman, fell into the hands of a quack, who attempted to do Whitehead's radical operation, but was so unfortunate in the result that the mucous membrane and the skin outside would not unite.   Shortly after, having moved to British Columbia, he came under the care of a friendly jeweller.   This ingenious individual invented for the hapless minister a manner of stem pessary, by means of which the rectum was kept in position.   The clergyman wore this device for six long years, suffering the inconvenience and discomfort of having to remove it once or twice a day.   Dr. Clouse now saw him again, and had in consultation several other prominent surgeons.   They decided that nothing could be done to relieve the situation except a colotomy.   This the patient refused, and again besought Dr. Clouse to do something for him.   Dr. Clouse consented to try what could be done, and, with the patient under an anesthetic, discovered that by snipping the skin just beyond the red border he was able to relieve the tension on the bowel, and a perfect cure was wrought.

Dr. J. H. Peters, Hamilton, prepared a paper on "Anomalies in Fetal Development, with Specimens."

The Secretary read Dr. Peters' paper, which gave an illustrated account of a fetal monstrosity exhibited. The specimen was what Hirst calls a celosoma and of the type agenosoma. The liver and bowels are exposed, with an absence of the genital organs. This is one of the two or three cases of agenosoma reported.

Motions, Resolutions, Etc.

Moved by A. McPhedran, seconded by N. H. Beemer, That in the opinion of this Association there exists an urgent need for the establishment of hospital accommodation for the temporary reception and treatment of suspected and incipient cases of mental alienation. The establishment of such institutions offers the only efficient means for the cure of such cases, and would save many of them from the stigma of having been incarcerated in an asylum for the insane. Carried.

Moved by W. H. Smith, and seconded by F. Fenton, That the thanks of this Association are to be extended to the Automobile Club of Toronto for the kindness exhibited to the members in the very pleasurable ride about the parks of the city. Carried.

Votes of thanks were also passed to the President and Senate of the University of Toronto for the use of the Medical Building; to the retiring President, the Secretary, the Assistant Secretary, and other officers of the Association for their painstaking work in arranging for this excellent meeting.

The motion of Drs. Cameron and Thistle, that the Ontario Medical Association be changed to constitute a branch of the British Medical Association, was, on motion of Drs. Powell and McPhedran, referred to a committee to be named by the incoming President and Mr. Cameron, which committee should report to this Association. In connection with this Mr. Cameron pointed out that the membership fee of one guinea to the British Medical Association included the subscription for the *British Medical Journal.* By constituting this Association a branch of the British Medical Association, we would in no way interfere with our own autonomy. Dr. Bingham pointed out the difficulty already existing in getting men to attend the Ontario Medical Association meetings, and that the matter was one of too much importance to be passed over hurriedly.

The following officers were elected for the ensuing year: President, Dr. W. A. Burt, Paris; 1st Vice-President, Dr. J. L. Davison; 2nd Vice-President, Dr. George Hodge, London; 3rd Vice-President, Dr. Edw. Ryan, Kingston; 4th Vice-

President, Dr. T. H. Middleboro, Owen Sound; General Secretary, Dr. Chas. P. Lusk, Toronto; Assistant Secretary, Dr. Samuel Johnston, Toronto; Treasurer, Dr. Fred T. Fenton.

The following names were elected by the Nomination Committee to serve on committees: Credentials—Dr. Olmstead, Hamilton; Dr. Boyd, Bobcaygeon.   Public Health—Dr. Trimble, Queenston; Dr. Fraser, Thamesville.   Legislation—Dr. H. D. Livingstone, Rockwood; Dr. Chas. Sampson, Windsor.   Publication—Dr. Alex. Taylor, Goderich; Dr. W. J. Charlton, Weston.   Ethics—Dr. H. A. McCallum, London; Dr. T. McKeough, Chatham.

ONTARIO COLLEGE OF PHYSICIANS AND SURGEONS.

THE members of the Council of the College of Physicians and Surgeons of Ontario assembled on the afternoon of June 28th in their board-room in the Medical Council Building, for the first session of their annual five-days' convention.   There was a full attendance of members, and the proceedings of the afternoon were marked by expedition and harmony.   The prosperous year which the College has enjoyed, was indicated by the treasurer's statement, which showed receipts of $36,200.19, and a cash balance, after disbursements had been made, of $5,127.91.

On the meeting being called to order, the resignation of Dr. Thorburn was laid before the members.   Dr. Thorburn said that as Toronto School of Medicine had surrendered its charter, he did not consider that its representative had any longer a right to a place on the Council.   In accepting the resignation, the members of Council expressed regret at losing such a useful and esteemed colleague as Dr. Thorburn.

Dr. J. A. Robertson, of Stratford, the retiring President, in delivering his annual address, welcomed the members of Council to the labors of another session.   He referred feelingly to the death of two valued members, Dr. W. H. Moore, of Brockville, and Dr. Sangster, of Port Perry, and extended a welcome to their successors, Dr. Herald, of Kingston, and Dr. Bascom, of Uxbridge.   He spoke also of the retirement from active life of Dr. W. B. Geikie, Dean of Trinity Medical School, and expressed the hope that he would long continue to enjoy health and prosperity.   He congratulated the members on the satisfactory showing of the treasurer's report, and on the fact that the Council's building had increased in value as an asset.   Dr. Robertson said that he had personally attended the examinations, and he was convinced that the methods in vogue were quite on a par with those of the profession in the Mother Country. In concluding, he thanked the members for their assistance and consideration, and called on them to name his successor.

Hon. Dr. Sullivan, of Kingston, was the only name placed in nomination for the office of President, and his election was, therefore, unanimous. In taking the chair, he thanked the Council for conferring such an honor upon him. He said that he had spent nearly fifty years in the profession, and the longer he remained in it the more impressed he was by the nobility and usefulness of the calling. He feared that doctors did not fully recognize the possibilities for good which their work gave them. He said he was averse to the discussion of the physician's " tariff," as he believed that the doctor's services could never be measured by any money value. The doctor should regard his fee as an honorarium. He expressed the hope that the College would continue to maintain the high standing of the profession, not only by increasing fees, but by keeping up a rigid standard of qualification.

The other officers were elected as follows: Vice-President, Dr. A. A. Macdonald, Toronto; Registrar, Dr. R. A. Pyne, M.P.P., Toronto; Treasurer, Dr. H. Wilberforce Aikins; Solicitor, Christopher Robinson, K.C.; Auditor, Dr. J. C. Patton; Stenographer, Alex. Downey; Prosecutor, Chas. Rose.

The following committees were then appointed: Registration --Drs. Campbell, Lane, Johnson, Stuart, Thornton, Klotz, MacArthur. Rules and Regulations—Drs. Lane, Bascom, Adams, Hillier, Spankie. Finance—Drs. Henderson, King, Griffin, Brock, Bray. Printing—Drs. Temple, Stuart, King, Hardy, Hillier. Education—Drs. Moorhouse, Henry, Luton, Gibson, Spankie, Temple, Robertson, Herald, Britton. Property—Drs. Johnson, Campbell, Glasgow, Britton, Thornton. Complaints—Drs. Griffin, Hardy, Mearns, Glasgow, Johnson.

A communication was received which had been forwarded to Lord Minto by Hon. Alfred Lyttelton, Colonial Secretary, stating that a private members' bill had been introduced in the British House of Commons, providing that when any part of a British possession was under both a central and a local legislature, the King might by Order-in-Council declare any such part under a local legislature to be a separate British possession. The object of this measure was to enable reciprocal arrangements to be entered into under the Medical Act of 1886, with such provinces of Canada as desired to do so. The Colonial Secretary wished to have the views of Canadian Ministers on the measure. The Government had in turn forwarded it to the Provincial Secretary, who had transmitted it to the Council.

After a short, informal discussion, in which the opinion was expressed that Great Britain would be having decidedly the best of the bargain if such a measure became operative, the matter was referred to a special committee composed of the following members: Drs. Bray, Brock, Campbell, Hillier, Johnson, Macdonald and Spankie.

Communications regarding inter-provincial registration from the Nova Scotia and Quebec colleges, and one from Johns Hopkins University, regarding reciprocity in medical degrees, were referred to the same special committee.

A lengthy report on cancer research was received form the Imperial Government. It was forwarded to the Dominion Medical Association.

The following notices of motion were given:

That the Council consider the advisability of disposing of the college property.

That annual examinations be held at London similar to those held at Toronto and Kingston.

That legislation be sought compelling manufacturers of patent medicines to print their formulæ on the packages.

The Council adjourned to resume at 10 o'clock next morning.

SECOND DAY'S SESSION.

The special committee, consisting of Drs. Spankie, A. A. Macdonald and Britton, appointed by the Ontario Medical Council to secure all the information possible in relation to matriculation, presented their report at the session on June 29th. It was the first order of business taken up that morning. According to their recommendations, the requirements for passing the examination will differ little from those at present in vogue. Two changes will be effected. At present a minimum of $33\frac{1}{3}$ per cent. appertains for those candidates who have passed the joint university examinations for junior matriculation in Arts, as conducted by the Ontario Education Department. It is recommended to raise this minimum to 40 per cent. At present this joint matriculation, with honors in two subjects, entitles the candidate to be passed by the Council. The committee advises that one honor subject suffice in future.

The following credentials will in future be accepted, if the committee's report be adopted:

" 1. A certificate of having graduated in Arts in any university in His Majesty's dominions, or any other university approved of by the Council.

" 2. A certificate from the registrar of any chartered university conducting a full Arts course in Canada, that the holder thereof has passed the examination conducted at the end of the first year in Arts by such university.

" 3. A certificate of having passed the joint university senior matriculation examination in Arts as conducted by the Education Department of Ontario.

" 4. A certificate of having passed the senior Arts matriculation conducted by any chartered university of Canada.

" 5. A certificate of having passed the joint university examination for junior matriculation in Arts, as conducted by the Education Department of Ontario, with an advanced percentage, as follows: 40 per cent. minimum on each subject, and 50 per cent. on the aggregate.

" 6. A certificate of having passed the joint university examination for junior matriculation in Arts, as conducted by the Education Department of Ontario, with honors in any two departments.

" The matriculation fee will be $20."

The case of Thos. J. Gray, of Kingston, who personated James McDowall, also of Kingston, at the recent examinations, was dealt with. Gray was suspended for two years, and McDowall for three years. This means that these gentlemen will be prevented from writing on any examination under the Council's jurisdiction for the term of their respective suspensions. It is not likely that any criminal prosecution will take place. Evidence was given that Gray had personated McDowall in the primary, intermediate and final written examinations this year, and in the oral examinations for primary and intermediate. In the latter he was caught, and confessed.

The Executive Committee reported the case of Owen B. Van Epp, a qualified practitioner of Ohio, who resides on Pelee Island, in the County of Essex, and who had a bill passed by the Legislature admitting him to practise medicine in that township only, on petition of seven hundred of the residents thereof. He is the only practitioner on the island. He passed the final examination of the Medical Council. Chairman Hon. Dr. Sullivan remarked: " I never heard of a doctor being chained upon an island before."

The matter of a complaint received of fifth-year students practising the art of healing, was brought up in the report of the Prosecution Committee, but no action was taken. Two cases of unprofessional conduct were referred to the Discipline Committee for consideration.

The report, after referring to these and several minor cases, went on to say:

" Besides the above cases, I have had a large number of complaints against osteopaths, Christian Science healers, magnetic healers, and others of that kind, but owing to the fact that they prescribe no medicines, I have been unable to do anything further than giving their cases as much publicity as possible, and, until the Legislature in their wisdom see fit to amend the Ontario Medical Act so as to cover this class of ' healers,' I am unable to protect the public against them."

The Property Committee reported that, as directed, they had made enquiries of real estate experts as to the value of the College of Physicians' building at the corner of Bay and Richmond Streets. Pearson Bros. had reported to them that the land, eighty-seven feet, five inches on Bay Street, by ninety-five feet on Richmond Street, was worth $500 a foot, equal to a valuation of $47,708; the building was worth $58,000; total, $101,708. In case the Council wanted to sell, therefore, they ought to be able to count on $100,000. The report was adopted, but no decision was reached as to whether the Council would sell or not.

The Examination Committee reported that at the spring examination in the final year, 142 candidates had presented themselves, 93 of whom passed, and 49 failed.

Notice of motion was given that the subjects of medical jurisprudence and sanitary science should, for examination purposes, be made separate, and that separate examiners be appointed for each subject. Also that certain members of the Council be appointed to attend every examination and act as censors or assessors.

At the morning session a committee was appointed to consider the composition of various patent medicines and report at the present session with the view of laying before the Legislature the necessity, in the interests of the public, of having the formula of all remedies printed on each package.

Dr. Bray said that there was a general agitation for temperance, which was right. But if people were not to be allowed to drink lager beer, which contained only about 2½ per cent. of alcohol, it was a great wrong to permit the sale of medicines containing alcohol running from 15 to 40 per cent. Lydia Pinkham's Compound is said to contain 20 per cent. of alcohol; Ayer's Sarsaparilla, 26 per cent.; Paine's Celery Compound, 21 per cent.; Peruna, 27.5 per cent.; Parker's Tonic, 41.6 per cent.; Hostetter's Bitters, 44.3 per cent., and Warner's Safe Tonic Bitters, 45.7 per cent. Worse than alcohol were the opium and morphine found in some patent medicines, which were the cause of forming the opium habit in the cases of many women in Outario. If the formula were printed on every package, the public would know what they were buying.

The manner in which some medical men in various parts of the province are said to issue orders (and which we do not credit) to liquor dealers, authorizing them to sell liquor to persons who would otherwise not be able to obtain it, has caused the Provincial License Department some concern. Of late the evil, they think, has become aggravated, and, with a view to preventing, or at least minimizing it, Mr. Eudo Saunders, chief officer of the Department, sent the following letter to Dr. R. A. Pyne, M.P.P., Registrar of the Ontario Medical Council, during its session on June 29th:

" The Provincial License Department has recently received a number of complaints from various parts of the province that medical practitioners in the districts in question are in the habit of giving prescriptions, or orders, to hotel-keepers or shop licensees to supply liquor to the holders of the orders, sometimes for indefinite periods, and often in absurdly large quantities, and it was thought probable that the Medical Council might see fit, if attention were called to the matter, to make an effort to minimize this evil.

" The Department would prefer not to give any names for publication, lest it should be prejudicial to the practitioners without being correspondingly beneficial to the public. I may, however, say that within the last few days three complaints have been received of this character. In one instance thirty orders had been given within ten days in a small place, mostly to persons whose maladies appear to have reached an acute stage on two successive Sundays. In another locality seventeen orders were given for alcohol, chiefly by the quart, and, what is worse, many of these orders were to bearer. In Woodstock, recently, a curious order was presented to a hotel-keeper, signed by a medical practitioner, authorizing him to supply the bearer, whose name was mentioned, with three or four glasses a day, in order that he might ' wean off.' The weaning-off process, as I understand it, is not generally accomplished in this way. This particular order was not subject to any limitation in point of time, and the hotel-keeper appears to have thought that it would hold good for several months. It should be stated, in this connection, that a notice had previously been served upon the hotel-keeper under section 125 of the Liquor License Act, forbidding him to supply the person in question with any liquor whatever.

" If you think it would be of any benefit to bring this matter before the Council, will you kindly do so?"

Third Day's Session.

The members of the Medical Council spent the major portion of their third day's session in considering the question of disposing of the College's building at the corner of Bay and Richmond Streets. The members were practically unanimous as to the wisdom of selling the property, but there was a diversity of opinion as to the value of the property, the estimates placed on it running as high as $150,000. The land and building cost originally about $88,000, but owing to the increased value of the land and the rise in cost of building operations, there has been a decided advance in the value of the building.

The matter was brought before the Council by a resolution moved by Dr. Henry, and seconded by Dr. Griffin, that the Property Committee sell the property at as early a date as possible, the resolution fixing a minimum price.

This motion was vigorously discussed. Dr. A. A. Macdonald, the Vice-President, objected to the fixing of a minimum price on the building. He thought the property was worth fully $150,000. In this he was supported by Dr. E. E. King, who pointed out, however, that at present the income from the building was only $4,743 per annum, while the maintenance charges, taxes, and interest amounted to $7,733. He favored selling the property, and erecting a suitable building which would be devoted solely to the purposes of the College and the profession. He then moved, in amendment, that tenders for the purchase of the property be invited by advertisement. After further discussion, the motion was withdrawn, and the amendment was carried unanimously.

Dr. C. T. Campbell's motion that certain members of the Council be appointed to attend every examination to act as censors or assessors, was referred to the Education Committee.

Dr. Campbell also moved that the Finance Committee consider the fixing of salaries and allowances for the members and officers of the Council. This was carried.

The Registration Committee brought in a number of recommendations regarding unqualified candidates, which were adopted.

Dr. A. J. Johnson, chairman of the special committee appointed last year to consider a general tariff for professional services, brought in a report setting forth minimum and maximum fees. As the Council has no legal right to fix a tariff, it simply approved of the report, which contained also a recommendation that the practitioners of each division form separate associations, and adopt a general tariff.

The morning session was largely taken up with the consideration of the report of the Matriculation Committee, which was presented to the Council on Wednesday afternoon. Among the criticisms levelled at the report were that it did not go far enough; that experimental science was not made compulsory; that senior matriculation should have been recommended.

The report was adopted on a division of 20 to 4.

Mr. Eudo Saunders' letter complaining that medical practitioners issued orders for liquors in large quantities for patients, was laid on the table, after being characterized by Senator Sullivan as an impertinence.

At 1 o'clock the members of the Council sat down as guests to luncheon, tendered them at the new Medical Building by Dean Reeve and the faculty of the school. The dean, in proposing the health of President Sullivan and the Council, expressed his conviction that that body would deal fairly by both the public and the medical institutions in the matter of medical education. The faculty of the school had been increased, but this was made necessary by the larger number of students in attendance since' the amalgamation.

Senator Sullivan, in replying, referred to the advance of the profession, which was largely due to the improved facilities for acquiring knowledge. He proposed the health of Dr. J. H. Richardson, emeritus Professor of Anatomy, and the veteran teacher was honored with an outburst of hearty cheers when he rose to make a brief but sincere reply. He said he had always tried to retain the friendship of his students and fellow-professors, by treating them like gentlemen, and if he had succeeded in doing so, he felt amply repaid.

Fourth Day's Session.

The Ontario Medical Council celebrated Dominion Day by remaining in session all day, and evolving ideas for the welfare of the public health and the medical profession.

The use, or rather the abuse, of patent medicines, was one of the chief matters considered. The report of the special committee appointed to consider the best methods of dealing with injuries resulting from the public's excessive use of proprietary medicines, declared that, in view of the large and rapidly increasing sale of patent medicines, including snuffs and cosmetics, and the unwarranted statements contained in advertisements of the same, steps should be taken to memorialize the Dominion Government, asking that a law be passed making it compulsory to have displayed on each and every bottle a complete and correct formula of ingredients. It should also be made a misdemeanor to state in any advertisement that an article was a cure for any specific ailment, which statement the formula did not warrant.

The report further went on to state that the excessive amount of alcohol contained in the greater proportion of proprietary medicines made them injurious to the health of the public, and conducive to the alcoholic habit. Of some ninety-one separate tonics and bitters recently analyzed by the Massachusetts State Board of Health, seven contained below 10 per cent. of alcohol, fifty-four contained an average of 22.5 per cent. of alcohol, and twenty-seven contained over 30 per cent. of alcohol.

The Council unanimously endorsed this report.

The report of the Finance Committee showed a cash balance of $5,120 on deposit in the bank. During the year, $7,500 was paid off the mortgage on the Council's building. The estimated receipts for 1904-5 were placed at $29,627, with an estimated expenditure of $22,009. The total assets amounted to $137,427, including $125,000 for building and site. On the latter there is at present a mortgage of $47,500. The Registrar's salary was placed at $2,500, and the Treasurer's at $600.

The Committee on Complaints reported that of forty-nine students unsuccessful at the recent examinations, twenty-four had appealed. Only one appeal was allowed, that of F. A. Aylesworth.

The date of the annual spring examinations at Toronto and Kingston was made the third Tuesday in May, instead of the second Tuesday, as heretofore. The subjects of medical jurisprudence and sanitary science were divided, for examination purposes, into two separate subjects.

The Committee on Discipline reported that Dr. H. B. Lemon's application for reinstatement had been granted, while that of Dr. H. E. Shepard had been refused. The charges of unprofessional conduct against Dr. H. E. Hett, of Berlin, and Dr. A. Crighton, of Castleton, were referred to the committee to investigate.

·The special committee appointed to consider the communication from the Provincial Secretary respecting reciprocity in registration with Great Britain and France, reported that they had not sufficient information on the subject at present to bring in an intelligent report.

An address of appreciation was passed to Dr. Thorburn, who is retiring from the Council after many years of service.

FIFTH DAY'S SESSION.

The Ontario Medical Council concluded their sessions at 12.45 p.m., July 2nd.

The meeting was chiefly given up to the reception of reports.

An Executive Committee of the Council was appointed, consisting of Drs. Sullivan, Macdonald, and Henderson.

A motion was made by Dr. Klotz, seconded by Dr. Mearns, that the attention of the Dominion Medical Association and the various councils be called to the action of the Ontario Medical 'Council in relation to the desired restrictions on the sale of patent medicines. The motion was carried.

The report of the Education Committee was received. A change was made in the regulations by which fifth-year students will be allowed to practise under physicians for information and clinical experience.

An amendment was moved to allow fifth-year students to receive a certificate for having been one year in a hospital of over fifty beds, or for one year assistant to a doctor, instead of taking the fifth-year lectures. After some warm discussion, this was carried by a vote of 18 to 9.

Dr. Johnson's motion to provide separate instruction for medical jurisprudence and sanitary science was rejected.

Four months of clinical work was added to the four months' course in gynecology.

The Board of Examiners appointed for the coming year was as follows: Descriptive Anatomy, Dr. McKay, Oshawa; Theory and Practice of Medicine, Dr. Ryan, Kingston; Midwifery, etc., Dr. McCabe, Strathroy; Physiology and Histology, Dr. A. Primrose, Toronto; Surgery and Operative, Dr. W. T. Parkes; Medical, etc., Dr. Middleborough; Chemistry, etc., Dr. R. A. Pyne; Materia Medica, Dr. J. A. Sprague; Medical Jurisprudence, Dr. A. J. Sinclair; Assistant Examiner, Surgery and Diseases of Women, Dr. R. Ferguson, London; Assistant Examiner, Clinical Surgery, Dr. O'Reilly, Toronto; 1st Assistant, Medicine, Diseases of Children, Dr. A. Haig, Kingston; 2nd Assistant Examiner in Medicine, Dr. G. H. Field, Cobourg; Homeopathic Examiner, Dr. W. McFall, Peterboro'.

The Council then adjourned.

❧ *School Hygiene.* ❧

CONTAGIOUS AND SCHOOL WORK IN NEW YORK.

A VERY important branch of nursing is that of the " contagious nurses " in New York, and one that should be highly commended.

The staff is small, only four at present being in the field, but a great amount of work is accomplished. One nurse takes the diphtheria cases, and while it may seem almost impossible for one to look after all the needy patients suffering from this disease, still, if we consider that with the use of antitoxin very much less nursing is required, she can manage very well.

Two nurses devote their time to scarlet fever and are kept busy. Many complications are found, and the disease is long-drawn-out on account of the desquamation. A short time ago a girl, nine years of age, was found working on fancy braid that was being prepared for sale, and after being warned not to do so still persisted. The child was removed to the hospital at once until the " peeling " had stopped, and the house fumigated. This shows how watchful the nurses must be and how numbers of people, maybe many miles distant, are protected from contagion by their efforts.

The fourth nurse looks after those suffering with measles, and all precautions are taken, but the patients are never so ill as with scarlet fever.

The Department of Health provides this essential service for the sick poor of the city, and will increase it as the needs arise. This branch of service comes under the same supervision as the school work.

The school nursing continues to increase both in staff and area. A nurse has been placed permanently on Staten Island; one has been assigned to the Bronx and one in Long Island City, Borough of Queens. It was thought by some that the new administration would not be as much in favor of the work as was previously shown, but Dr. Darlington, our new Commissioner, is much interested, and has shown his efforts to continue its success by adding six more nurses.

The appropriation this year is $47,000, an increase of $17,000 over last year.

The number of schools now covered is 150. Some among these are parochial and industrial schools.

Communications are constantly being received from the principals, and from the local School Boards asking to have nurses sent to their schools. One quite recently came from the secretary of the Board of Education.—*The American Journal of Nursing.*

H. McM.

The Canadian
Journal of Medicine and Surgery

J. J. CASSIDY, M.D.,

EDITOR,

43 BLOOR STREET EAST, TORONTO.

W. A. YOUNG, M.D., L.R.C.P.Lond.,

MANAGING EDITOR,

145 COLLEGE STREET, TORONTO.

Surgery—BRUCE L. RIORDAN, M D.,C M , McGill University; M D University of Toronto; Surgeon Toronto General Hospital; Surgeon Grand Trunk R R.; Consulting Surgeon Toronto Home for Incurables; Pension Examiner United States Government: and F. N. G. STARR, M B., Toronto, Associate Professor of Clinical Surgery, Toronto University; Surgeon to the Out-Door Department Toronto General Hospital and Hospital for Sick Children.

Clinical Surgery—ALEX. PRIMROSE, M B., C.M Edinburgh University; Professor of Anatomy and Director of the Anatomical Department, Toronto University Associate Professor of Clinical Surgery, Toronto University; Secretary Medical Faculty, Toronto University.

Orthopedic Surgery—B. E McKENZIE, B A., M.D., Toronto, Surgeon to the Toronto Orthopedic Hospital; Surgeon to the Out-Patient Department, Toronto General Hospital; Assistant Professor of Clinical Surgery, Ontario Medical College for Women; Member of the American Orthopedic Association; and H. P. H. GALLOWAY, M.D, Toronto, Surgeon to the Toronto Orthopedic Hospital; Orthopedic Surgeon, Toronto Western Hospital; Member of the American Orthopedic Association.

Oral Surgery—E H. ADAMS, M.D., D.D.S , Toronto.

Surgical Pathology—T. H. MANLEY, M D., New York, Visiting Surgeon to Harlem Hospital, Professor of Surgery, New York School of Clinical Medicine, New York, etc , etc

Gynecology and Obstetrics—GEO. T. McKEOUGH, M D, M.R C.S. Eng , Chatham, Ont.; and J. H LOWE, M.D., Newmarket, Ont.

Medical Jurisprudence and Toxicology—ARTHUR JUKES JOHNSON, M.B., M.R C.S. Eng : Coroner for the City of Toronto; Surgeon Toronto Railway Co., Toronto; W. A. YOUNG, M D., L.R.C.P. Lond.; Associate Coroner, City of Toronto.

Pharmacology and Therapeutics—A. J. HARRINGTON M D., M R C S Eng., Toronto.

Medicine—J J. CASSIDY, M D., Toronto, Member Ontario Provincial Board of Health; Consulting Surgeon, Toronto General Hospital; and W. J. WILSON, M.D. Toronto, Physician Toronto Western Hospital.

Clinical Medicine—ALEXANDER McPHEDRAN, M D., Professor of Medicine and Clinical Medicine Toronto University; Physician Toronto General Hospital, St Michael's Hospital, and Victoria Hospital for Sick Children.

Mental and Nervous Diseases—N. H. BEEMER, M D., Mimico Insane Asylum; CAMPBELL MEYERS, M.D. M.R C S., L R C P. (London, Eng.), Private Hospital, Deer Park, Toronto; and EZRA H. STAFFORD, M.D.

Public Health and Hygiene—J. J CASSIDY, M D , Toronto, Member Ontario Provincial Board of Health; Consulting Surgeon Toronto General Hospital; and E. H. ADAMS, M D., Toronto.

Physiology—A. B. EADIE, M.D., Toronto, Professor of Physiology Woman s Medical College, Toronto.

Pediatrics—AUGUSTA STOWE GULLEN, M D., Toronto, Professor of Diseases of Children Woman's Medical College, Toronto; A. R GORDON, M D., Toronto.

Pathology—W. H. PEPLER, M.D., C.M., Trinity University; Pathologist Hospital for Sick Children, Toronto; Associate Demonstrator of Pathology Toronto University; Physician-to Outdoor Department Toronto General Hospital; Surgeon Canadian Pacific R.R., Toronto; and J. J. MACKENZIE, B.A., M B., Professor of Pathology and Bacteriology, Toronto University Medical Faculty.

Ophthalmology and Otology—J. M. MACCALLUM, M D., Toronto, Professor of Materia Medica Toronto University; Assistant Physician Toronto General Hospital; Oculist and Aurist Victoria Hospital for Sick Children, Toronto

Laryngology and Rhinology—J, D. THORBURN, M D., Toronto, Laryngologist and Rhinologist, Toronto General Hospital.

Address all Communications, Correspondence, Books, Matter Regarding Advertising, and make all Cheques, Drafts and Post-office Orders payable to "The Canadian Journal of Medicine and Surgery," 145 College St., Toronto, Canada.

Doctors will confer a favor by sending news, reports and papers of interest from any section of the country. Individual experience and theories are also solicited Contributors must kindly remember that all papers, reports, correspondence, etc., *must be* in our hands by the fifteenth of the month previous to publication.

Advertisements, to insure insertion in the issue of any month. should be sent not later than the tenth of the preceding month. London, Eng. Representative, W. Hamilton Miln, 8 Bouverie Street, E. C. Agents for Germany Saarbach's News Exchange, Mainz, Germany.

VOL. XVI.   **TORONTO, AUGUST, 1904.**   **NO. 2.**

Editorials.

STRANGULATION OR INHIBITION.

" IT is scarcely necessary to state, that all marks of violence on the body of a supposed strangled person should be accurately noted, as the questions respecting them, however slight the marks may be, are material. A witness will be expected to state whether they were inflicted before or after death; if before, whether they were sufficient to account for death, or whether they were such as to be explicable on the supposition of an accidental, suicidal, or homicidal origin." (Taylor's "Medical Jurisprudence.")

The above remarks apply very well to the circumstances of the case we are about to relate. At the Assize Court, held at Sarthe, France, March 17th, 1904, a one-handed shoemaker, named Dézélée, was tried for murdering, by strangulation, a girl, eighteen years of age, named Emilienne Meunier. The result of the trial turned on a radical difference of opinion between experts as to the interpretation which might be put on the marks of violence found at the necropsy.

Dr. Blaise, a medical•expert, had been instructed by the legal authorities to make the necropsy, and the external and internal marks found on the cadaver had enabled him to reach the conclusion that death had been caused by strangulation. According to this witness, the accused must have squeezed the neck of the deceased girl four or five minutes. Her tongue was swollen, and protruded beyond the teeth. Cyanosis of the lips, white foam flowing from the mouth, and congestion of the lungs were, in Dr. Blaise's opinion, so many proofs of death from asphyxia.

A second physician, Dr. Persy, who had assisted at the necropsy, was of the same opinion, except with regard to the length of time the murderer's fingers had compressed the windpipe of his victim. Dr. Persy fixed this period of time at from thirty to forty seconds.

Professor Brouardel, who also gave expert evidence at the trial, had not seen the cadaver; but, after a study of Dr. Blaise's report, he reached the conclusion that in this case death had not resulted from strangulation, but that it was a sudden death from inhibition. According to him, the deceased girl's death had resulted from a violent compression of the neck, which had produced a sudden stoppage of the heart's action. Evidently, if Dézélée had not throttled Emilienne Meunier, she would not have died when the assault was made, but her death was not caused by strangulation. According to Professor Brouardel, congestion of the lungs, white foam flowing from the mouth, cyanosis of the lips, a swollen tongue protruding beyond the teeth are not proofs of death from strangulation.

Dr. Persy closed the discussion between the medical experts by the following remark: " After what Professor Brouardel has said, all we need do is to make a bonfire of the medical books placed at our disposal, because they contain scarcely anything but errors."

The court and the jury, however, adopted Professor Brouardel's opinion. The charge of murder was withdrawn, and, after an affirmative verdict on the subsidiary question that blows and wounds, inflicted by the accused, had caused the death of the deceased girl, without any intention on the part of the accused, Dézélée was sentenced to three years in prison.

The defence appears to have rested on solid ground. The deceased girl was probably of a delicate frame, or of a timid disposition, so that, according to Professor Brouardel, her heart's action was inhibited shortly after Dézélée's fingers clutched her throat. A sudden death then intervened, and prevented the full development of the classical marks of a death from strangulation.

According to Tardieu ("Ann. d'Hygiene," 1859, Vol. 1, p. 132), in a case where death resulted from strangulation, the lining membrane of the larynx and windpipe was more or less reddened from congestion. Sometimes it was livid, or of a dark red color. There was bloody froth extending into the air-tubes. The state of the lungs was variable. Contrary to what is generally alleged to be characteristic of death by asphyxia, Tardieu found these organs to contain but little blood. Sometimes they were congested; at other times normal. There were ruptures of the superficial air-cells, producing patches of emphysema, which were seen singly or in groups. This condition, which was rarely absent, gave to the surface of the lungs the appearance of being covered with white layers of thin, false membrane. When these patches were punctured, air escaped. There was an absence of that condition of the lungs which he observed in death from simple suffocation, namely, dotted ecchymosis on the surface immediately below the investing membrane (the pleura). Throughout the substance of the lungs, effusions of blood, varying in size, were, however, generally found, provided an early inspection of the body was made. When some days had elapsed, the lungs were found pale or congested, without any ecchymosed or mottled appearance. The ruptured air-cells, with air beneath them, were still visible on the surface. The heart presents no uniform condition; it is sometimes quite empty, and at others it contains dark fluid blood. The brain is occasionally congested, but more commonly in its natural state. In one instance blood was found diffused in the brain, but this is an unusual appearance. It has also been stated that a congested state of the sexual organs, both in males and females, was one of the appearances connected with strangulation, but this has not been confirmed by careful observers. M. Tardieu met with nothing to call for notice in this respect in the numerous cases which he examined. The involuntary discharge of feces, urine, and seminal fluid, described as one of the characteristics of death by hanging, may equally occur in death by strangulation. No importance can be attached to this as a sign of death from asphyxia in any form. It frequently occurs in sudden and violent death from any cause, and there are many instances of death from asphyxia in which it is not observed.

In the act of strangulation a much greater degree of violence is commonly employed than is necessary to cause death, and hence the marks on the skin of the neck will be, generally speaking, more evident than in hanging, where the mere weight of the body is the medium by which the windpipe is compressed. If much force has been used in producing the constriction, the wind-pipe, with the muscles and vessels in the fore part of the neck, may be found cut or lacerated, and the vertebræ of the neck may be fractured. The face is commonly livid and swollen, the eyes wide open, prominent, and congested, and the pupils are dilated. The tongue is swollen, dark-colored, and protruded; it is sometimes bitten by the teeth, and a bloody froth escapes from the mouth and nostrils. The principal external signs of strangulation are seen in the marks on the neck, produced either by a cord or manual pressure. Tardieu also describes numerous small spots of ecchymosis upon the skin of the face, neck and chest, as well as on the conjunctivæ of the eyes. These parts present a dotted redness, which has, however, been met with in other cases besides death from strangulation. ("Annal. d'Hyg.," 1859, Vol. 1, p. 125.)

Several instances of laceration and rupture of the windpipe in death from strangulation are quoted by Dr. Chevers. (Taylor's "Medical Jurisprudence.")

A summary of the signs of death by homicidal strangulation,

according to Tardieu, would be: Reddening from congestion of
the larynx and windpipe; bloody foam, extending into the air-
tubes; patches of emphysema on the pulmonary surfaces; effusion of blood in the substance of the lung; marks on the skin of
the fore part of the neck, and severe injury to the larynx, with
sometimes fracture of the vertebræ of the neck; face livid and
swollen; eyes. wide open, prominent and congested, with dilated
pupils; tongue swollen, dark-colored and protruded.

Some of these marks were discovered at the necropsy of
Emilienne Meunier, but not all, and the more important ones
were not mentioned by the witnesses for the prosecution. That
a certain amount of choking had been done to the deceased girl
was admitted; that death had resulted from strangulation was
denied; and the verdict of the jury was based on the latter
opinion.   J. J. C.

RAISING THE MATRICULATION STANDARD OF THE COLLEGE OF PHYSICIANS AND SURGEONS OF ONTARIO.

Up to the present time the junior matriculation in Arts of the
University of Toronto has been accepted as the standard for
matriculation in the Ontario College of Physicians and Surgeons,
the minimum in each subject, for a pass, being $33\frac{1}{3}$ per cent. At
the meeting of the College in June of last year, the matriculation
standard in medicine was very fully discussed, and so dissatisfied
was the College with it, that a resolution was adopted, by a large
majority, declaring that senior matriculation in Arts should be
made the standard in future instead of the junior one. The
resolution meant, in effect, that a medical matriculant in Ontario
would require to receive a training in non-professional subjects
equal to that possessed by a student who has passed the first year's
examination in the department of Arts.

Consternation immediately began to prevail among Ontario
High School masters and their pupils who were preparing for
the matriculation examination in medicine. After much discussion between medical men and educational authorities, the Executive of the College of Physicians and Surgeons decided that the
obnoxious resolution should not be enforced at the examinations

8

of 1904. The Educational Committee of the College, who had been responsible for the resolution, were also instructed to reconsider the question and to report again in 1904. This committee consists of Drs. Britton, Spankie and Macdonald, and their report was presented June 29th, 1904. It provides for a 40 per cent. minimum in each subject, and 50 per cent. in the aggregate. A regulation was also added that honors would have to be obtained in two subjects of the examination. The fee for the examination is $20. The report was adopted by the College by a vote of 20 yeas to 4 nays.

As this matter now stands, therefore, the would-be medical matriculant will have to obtain a minimum of 40 per cent. in each subject, instead of $33\frac{1}{3}$ per cent., and an aggregate of 50 per cent. Honors are required in two subjects, and as third-class honors range from 50 to 66 per cent., the matriculant must also obtain at least 50 per cent. in two subjects. The outcome of this regulation will probably be that with the advent of stiff papers a few more rails will be added to the neat fence which guards the approach to the temple of Esculapius in Ontario. Probably the fence will be made as high as it ought to be in reason. No one will question the wisdom of making the Ontario medical students a scholarly class of men. Even the least cultured people expect that a medical student should be well educated, in the common, everyday acceptance of that term; and if he has learned something about the language and literature of Rome and of Greece, if he has sound knowledge of his native language, as well as fair acquirements in history, geography, arithmetic, algebra, geometry, physics and chemistry, so much the better.

By carrying out the new standard mentioned above, the Ontario College will secure a fair measure of non-professional education in their matriculants; and it seems to us, that further than that they have no right to go. If a medical student wishes to obtain a complete Arts course and the B.A. degree, the road is open; but even though he should be quite successful in his educational venture in Arts—a prize winner, even—his subsequent success in medicine may prove to be mediocre. " Poeta nascitur non fit," and the Latin proverb is just as applicable to the doctor as to the bard. The present-day leaders of the medical and surgical professions in Toronto, the men who earn the large fees, are not remarkable for knowledge of ancient or modern languages. Not one of them has ever attained fame for any achievement in literature, art, or mechanics outside of what falls within the category of a medical career. They have achieved success, by earning it, in their chosen vocations, and it is very doubtful, that more Greek and Latin, greater fluency in French and German, a more accurate knowledge of mathematics, would advance their prospects among their patients in the slightest degree, or place them in a more advantageous light in relation to their professional brethren.

To put spokes in the wheels of incompetent medical students is one thing; to design a scheme of study which may help to evolve a Pepper or an Osler, is beyond the might of the best committee of the Ontario College. J. J. C.

EDITORIAL NOTES.

A Strange Form of Parasitism Carried by the Larvæ of Insects.—It is well known that the eggs of insects are deposited in flowers and vegetables. Thus the female of a little fly of the group Anthomyzinæ and the species Anthomya canicularis, deposits its eggs on certain vegetables or on the earth. This insect also frequents all kinds of flowers, but has a predilection for the synantheræ and the umbelliferæ. These vegetable families include a certain number of plants—artichoke, lettuce, parsley, dandelion, chervil, carrot, etc.—which are often eaten in the raw condition. One can thus understand how the larvæ of the fly, which may have been laid on the vegetable, may be swallowed with it when the raw vegetable is eaten. Last summer Dr. Lorber, a French physician, practising at Fesches-le-Chatel, treated a young lady for a strange form of parasitism caused by the larvæ of the insects mentioned above. For a considerable time the patient complained of pain of an obscure character in the region of her stomach. These pains began when she rose in the morning, sometimes lasting for a few minutes, and sometimes for several hours. During the attacks she became pale, nerveless, and had a strong inclination to vomit, and looked as though she were going to faint. She complained, besides, of a continual itching of the skin, a slight cough, and an excessive secretion of saliva. These symptoms lasted up to September 15th, 1903, when, after repeated attacks of vomiting, the patient brought up a considerable quantity of living insect larvæ. These larvæ, preserved in spirit, were subsequently examined by M. Florentin, Professor of Zoology in the University of Nancy, who identified them. The eggs of Anthomya, which are deposited in vegetables used as food, not being noticed owing to their small size, are swallowed with the leaves or roots in the uncooked condition. These eggs, swallowed in great number and at a time when they were near the hatching period, produced the larvæ, which, being provided on the surface of their bodies with a multitude of small sharp thorns, attached themselves to the walls of the mucous surface of the stomach, or of the esophagus, and were thus enabled to maintain their position without being carried away by the passing food. Their prolonged sojourn in the digestive tube of the patient was said to be due to the fact that the larvæ possess considerable reserves of fat, which enable them to subsist without seeking for food, and also because of their tracheal system of respiration which enables them to resist asphyxia. Dr. Lorber ascertained that, some time before his patient began to complain of the first symptoms of her trouble, she had eaten a considerable quantity of salad made from dandelions, which she had gathered in the fields.

Typhoid Fever Mortality in Toronto and Filtration of the Water Supply.—The mortality from typhoid fever in Toronto is remarkably low. The population of Toronto is 225,000 souls, and the mortality from typhoid fever during the first six months of the current year was as follows: January, 1; February, 3; March, 1; April, 3; May, 2; June, 3; total for the half year, 13. Just as in other cities situated on the shores of a lake or river, from which the water supply is taken, Toronto citizens run the risk of drinking contaminated water. More particularly is this true in times of flood, when excremental filth is washed along the natural declivities and the streets, and carried far out by rain or melting snow to the source of the civic water supply. The simplest way to rectify the difficulty would be to purify the water taken from Lake Ontario by sand filtration. At the present time there seems to be an arbitrary standard in the methods of water purification. That is to say, methods are extensively used which make the cost of purifying a million gallons of water, including interest and sinking fund charges, somewhere in the neighborhood of $10, and which are sufficient to remove 99 or 99½ per cent. of the bacteria of the applied water. This may fairly be called the best practice to-day. A purification like this serves to furnish a water from the Merrimac or from the Hudson in every respect as good, and perhaps better, than is obtained from the best upland sources. The daily cost of filtering 30,000,000 gallons of water for Toronto would, therefore, amount to $300; the annual cost of the same would be $109,500. Quite an expense, indeed! Admitted; but consider the result. The triumphs in the past have been great. The typhoid fever death rates in a number of American cities have been reduced by the installation of filters by 70 or 80 per cent., or more. The general death rates have also been reduced by amounts which correspond to much more than the reduction in the typhoid fever rates. It is true that the Toronto water supply of to-day is not a bad one; but it will not improve, if left severely to the alchemy of nature, particularly in flood time. With the growth of a desire for cleaner and purer water, the consideration of the filtration of the water supply of Toronto will come to the front, and the practical application of water filtration will be accompanied with the greatest benefit to this city.　　　　　　　　　　　　　　　　　J. J. C.

The Prevention of Consumption.—The fifth general meeting of the members of the National Association for the Prevention of Consumption and other Forms of Tuberculosis was held on March 10th, afternoon, at 30 Hanover Square, London, Eng. Sir William Church, in seconding the adoption of the annual report, said that the whole medical profession was watching with extreme interest the results of compulsory notification at Sheffield, as they were watching with great interest what might come out of the voluntary notification which was going on in many other parts of the country. Many persons who had an unreasonable dread of the infectiousness of tubercle, kept themselves at a distance from the tubercle bacillus, imagining that that was all they need do, and neglected the proper hygienic measures, which placed them in a condition to resist the attacks of the enemy. The Association had placed these two lines of defence side by side and hand in hand, as they should. General hygienic measures had always been recommended, but, at the same time, they had indicated the means by which they might specially protect themselves and the public from the dangers of infection. He had been pleased to see how very strongly the Association had expressed the view that sanatoria should be inexpensive buildings; and he thought a useful purpose might be served if the Council could become a sort of advisory body for county councils, boards of guardians, and other public bodies, upon the construction, site, and situation of sanatoria. It was regrettable that large sums should be spent on bricks and mortar, when inexpensive buildings would not only fulfil the same object but, in his opinion, fulfil it very much better.

The Inefficiency of Filters.—The Chicago *Bulletin of Health,* May 26th, 1904, says: " The common tap filters are not only worthless, but are actually harmful, because they do not stop any of the bacteria—only the organic matter, such as vegetable and animal detritus. Now, when the water is shut off, a few bacteria remaining upon this animal matter find it to be a suitable food, and, as a result, they increase enormously in numbers, so that the next water drawn through the tap filter washes them out, and the longer such a filter is used the more bacteria are found in the water which it filters. Stone or porcelain filters are of value, but only if properly cleaned. During the first few hours such a filter is used, the bacteria, being so small, pass through the pores of the filter. These pores finally become clogged with bacteria. Then, after a number of hours, depending upon the pressure, the water will be free from bacteria, but after a day or so the bacteria grow through the filter, and the water is again contaminated. Therefore, the first water coming from such a filter should be rejected, and the filter itself should be boiled and thoroughly cleaned every two or three days." From these remarks it can readily be seen that even the best filters are worthless, unless properly cared for. The trite old instruction given by sanitarians in times of typhoid epidemic, " to boil the water," is productive of most satisfactory results in the matter of rendering water safe to drink. At the second quarterly meeting of the Provincial Board of Health for this year,

Dr. Amyot, bacteriologist of the Board, gave the results of the analysis of water that had been passed through an ordinary hot-water boiler, attached to a range. The bacterial counts were, he said, decidedly altered for the better, the water being nearly always practically sterile, although it may not have boiled.

Relations between the Ear and the So-called Naso-Genital Zone in Women.—A. Heiman (*Gaz. lek.*, 1903, No. 38) has treated several unmarried young women, of ages ranging from eighteen to twenty-seven, and whose complaint consisted of obstinate ear-ache of unknown origin, which could not be relieved by any of the numerous means employed for the purpose. One of the patients having drawn his attention to a coincidence in her case between the pain in the ear and the occurrence of the menstrual period, Dr. Heiman examined her nose, and, finding that the mucous membrane of the part was swollen, he swabbed it with a 20 per cent. solution of cocaine. Immediately the pain in the patient's ears diminished, and after a few more treatments completely disappeared. Cauterization of the inferior turbinated bones by means of the galvano-cautery not only cured the ear-ache, but also the abdominal pains which accompanied the menses. Similar results were obtained in two other cases. On the contrary, in cases in which neuralgia was not of menstrual origin, swabbing the nasal mucosa with cocaine produced no effect. Dr. Heiman concluded that if ear neuralgias are cured by the use of cocaine, the trouble is seated in the naso-genital zone. When this treatment fails, the cause must be looked for in another direction.

Is it Dangerous to Get Out of Bed in a Hurry?—Lauder Brunton mentions, in *The Action of Medicines,* that he was consulted once by a physician about what he thought was an epileptic fit. "One morning he had jumped up suddenly out of bed to pass water, and the first thing that he knew afterwards was that he was lying on the floor of his bed-room, with the chamber pot broken in pieces. He thought this was an epileptic fit, and he was in a state of great anxiety about it. It was not an epileptic fit, but it was simply a condition of syncope brought about by suddenly jumping up from the horizontal to the upright position; the effect of this being still further increased by the diminution in the blood pressure in his abdomen through his emptying his bladder." We notice in an editorial in *The Indian Lancet,* April 18th, 1904, that a middle-aged man who had sprung out of bed very quickly, almost immediately staggered and fell to the ground. He died from heart disease, and a physician stated that if the man had got out of bed quietly, instead of with a rush, he would be alive still.

PERSONALS.

DR. BURNHAM, 134 Bloor Street East left the city on July 6th, and will return to resume his practice on September 2nd.

CONGRATULATIONS are in order to our esteemed confrere and collaborator, Dr. J. M. MacCallum, on the birth of an heiress on July 3rd.

CANADIAN MEDICAL ASSOCIATION.

THE thirty-seventh annual meeting of the Canadian Medical Association is to be held this year in Vancouver, on the 23rd, 24th, 25th and 26th inst. Victoria joins hands with her sister city in extending the hospitality of the Pacific Province to all the members of our great national medical organization. In the thirty-seven years of its history, this is the first time a meeting of the Canadian Medical Association has been held in British Columbia; and the opportunity to visit Victoria, an Outpost of Empire, and Vancouver, the Pride and Glory of the West, should not be lightly passed by. Indeed, the entire West is a " panorama of beauty " and a " scene of bustle."

There will be no special train. No arrangements are in force to return *via* California, Salt Lake City and Colorado, as none could be secured, so far as the Canadian Medical Association is concerned, but below will be found information which will cover that route in returning, same being an open rate not requiring special certificate for purchasing transportation. Under the arrangements made, tickets will be good going *via* Canadian Pacific Railway direct, *via* Port Arthur, *via* Sault Ste. Marie, St. Paul, thence Soo-Pacific Route, Great Northern or Northern Pacific, or Grand Trunk *via* Detroit or Port Huron to Chicago, St. Paul, thence Soo-Pacific Route, Great Northern or Northern Pacific, returning same route or any other of the above routes. Lake route, Owen Sound to Port Arthur, may be taken one or both ways on payment of $4.25 additional each way. Boats leave Owen Sound, Tuesdays, Thursdays and Saturdays.

It is also proposed to allow variation to St. Louis *via* St. Paul and Chicago on return trip, when tickets are routed on return trip *via* those points, on payment of $10 additional. Secure return tickets if return is to be made other than Canadian Pacific Railway *via* the Northern Pacific Railway to St. Paul; Chicago and Northwestern, from St. Paul to Chicago; Wabash, Chicago to St. Louis or Chicago to Detroit, either Wabash or Grand Trunk; Illinois Central, Chicago to St. Louis and return. Through sleeping car accommodations from St. Louis *via* Chicago to all points in Canada on Grand Trunk Railway; or from St. Louis *via* Wabash to Detroit direct, or to Chicago and thence to Detroit.

The Intercolonial Railway joins in the arrangements in force for the Maritime Provinces and also in Quebec.

Transportation arrangements are as follows: To Vancouver and Victoria, from Port Arthur, Fort William, Rat Portage, $50.00; from Winnipeg, Emerson, Gretna, Portage la Prairie, Brandon, Indian Head, Winnipeg to Boissevain, Winnipeg to Carrol, Brandon to Hartney, and Weyburn to North Portal, $45.00; Rapid City Junction, $45.85; Gladstone, $46.05; Neepawa and Minnedosa, ·$46.85.

The above blankets pretty nearly all of the important points in Manitoba, but to make rates from points not shown above the one way first-class rate to the nearest point shown is to be added, but not to exceed the rate from a point more distant on the direct line. From points in the North-West Territories and British Columbia, Qu'Appelle and west, round trip tickets to Vancouver and Victoria will be issued at single fare. Passengers ticketed at stations Medicine Hat and east have the option of going *via* the main line, and returning Crow's Nest, or *vice versa,* as they may decide when purchasing their tickets. Tickets will be issued to either Vancouver or Victoria, where the same rate applies to either place; but if, as is the case from some far western points, the rates are higher to Victoria than to Vancouver, then tickets to Victoria will be issued only at the Victoria rate.

From all points in Ontario and Quebec, tickets will be on sale from the 15th to the 21st of August, inclusive, and from points east of Vanceboro', Me., August 14th to the 20th. The final return limit is October the 23rd, which means that all must be home on that date.

Stop-overs will be granted west of Port Arthur on going and returning journey, and west of St. Paul when tickets are routed on return journey by that point.

The Calgary Medical Association is desirous of extending an entertainment during the course of one day on the way out to Vancouver. This entertainment will be a typical Western one, and will take the form of an Indian gathering in costume, Indian races and games, roping and cowboy feats. Those who would like to stop over at Calgary for this entertainment so kindly offered through the Calgary Medical Association, should notify the General Secretary without any delay, so that if there would be sufficient number, same could be forwarded in time for proper preparation of the entertainment.

In Vancouver arrangements have been made for various excursions, yachting trips; steamer, rail and tram to surrounding points of interest; receptions, private and public; a dinner or a ball. On one of the days of the meeting the delegates will be taken by tram to New Westminster, visit the asylum there and other points of interest, then take the boat down the mighty Fraser to Steveston, visit some of the canneries, so that visitors will have the opportunity of verifying the stories of the salmon industry; then take the train back to Vancouver—a trip of great interest from start to finish.

In Victoria a committee is arranging a series of entertainments there, viz., reception at Government House, conversazione at the Parliament Buildings, a visit to Esquimalt and William Head Quarantine Station, beside other excursions to points of interest in and about Victoria.

For those who would like to extend their visit, special rates are arranged for to Nanaimo, where they will have an opportunity of seeing the vast coal fields of British Columbia. Arrangements can be made for stop-overs at Kaslo and Golden, the Board of Trade of the latter having issued a special invitation to the members of the Association to visit that thriving city. Other side trips have been arranged for to Skagway, Atlin, *via* Yukon and White Pass Railway to Dawson City.

For those who would like hunting excursions, full information can be secured from the local secretary at Vancouver as regards game laws, and excellent sport is promised. Hunting parties can be made up at Vancouver, and reliable guides furnished.

Guides can also be supplied for those who want to do mountain climbing.

The following are the rates for hotel accommodation: Vancouver Hotel, $3.00 to $5.00 per day; Badminton Hotel, $2.00 to $3.00 per day; Leland Hotel, $2.00 to $3.00 per day; Commercial Hotel, $2.00 to $3.00 per day; Metropole Hotel, $2.00 to $4.00 per day; Dominion Hotel, $1.00 to $2.00 per day.

Board and rooms can also be arranged for at private houses, a complete list of which can be obtained from the local secretary.

The Pullman rate from Toronto to Vancouver is $17.00 each way; from Montreal, $18.00 each way. Meals for five days about $12.50.

Yellowstone National Park is situated mostly in the State of Wyoming, in its north-western corner. Those contemplating visiting this "Wonderland" after the meeting in Vancouver, should see that their tickets are routed on return journey *via* the Northern Pacific Railway. From Vancouver the return trip is made over the Canadian Pacific Railway to the boundary where

the Northern Pacific is taken at Sumas. Thence through
Auburn and Spokane to Livingston, where change is made for
Gardiner, at the entrance to the Park. A six-days' trip by stage-
coach through the Park, including meals and lodging at the
hotels, which are all first-class, will cost $49.50. The Park is
sixty-two miles from north to south, and fifty-four miles wide.
The General Secretary will be glad to hear from all those intending to take in this trip on return journey, having been assured
that a party of from twenty-five to fifty will receive better attention than smaller ones.

As announced above, the Canadian Medical Association has
no arrangements in force for return *via* California. For the
benefit of those, however, who wish to return that way to St.
Louis, the information may be tendered that there will be in force
at the same time as our own convention an open rate of $70.25
from Toronto to San Francisco, good going *via* Canadian Pacific
Railway to Vancouver, allowing liberal stop-overs in each direction; final return limit, 23rd of October. No certificates are required for this trip, as it is an open rate to all. In taking this
trip, members of the Canadian Medical Association going to
Vancouver should be routed on return *via* Southern Pacific, Portland to San Francisco or Los Angeles; Southern Pacific, San
Francisco or Los Angeles to Ogden; Union Pacific to Kansas
City and St. Louis. Mr. H. F. Carter, T.P.A., Union Pacific
Railway, 14 Janes Building, Toronto, will supply any further
information regarding this route.

The fee for membership is $2.00, and may be paid to the
Treasurer, Dr. H. Beaumont Small, Ottawa, when registering
at the meeting. For the information of those who have not been
elected to membership, the same rates apply to them as well, and
they are instructed to ask for application forms when registering.

All delegates must have for themselves, their wives and
daughters, if going, a special certificate from the General Secretary, in order to secure reduced transportation rates.

Should any one require any further information as to accommodation at Vancouver or Victoria, side trips, hunting, etc., they
will kindly address the Local Secretary, Dr. W. D. Bryden Jack,
Vancouver, B.C. For certificates and general information,
address the General Secretary.

The following are some of the papers to be read:

President's address—Simon J. Tunstall, Vancouver.

Address in Surgery—Mr. Mayo Robson, England.

Address in Medicine—Dr. —— ——.

Address in Gynecology—Dr. E. C. Dudley, Chicago.

Paper, title to be announced—Dr. A. McPhedran, Toronto.

Paper, title to be announced—Dr. J. H. Elliott, Gravenhurst, Ont.

Surgical Treatment of Trachoma—Dr. G. Sterling Ryerson, Toronto.

Paper, title to be announced—Dr. A. Armstrong, Arnprior, Ont.

Paper, title to be announced—Dr. A. E. Garrow, Montreal.

The Operative Treatment of Spina Bifida—Dr. E. R. Secord, Brantford, Ont.

The Business Aspect of the Medical Profession—Dr. James E. Hanna, Ottawa, Ont.

Paper, title to be announced—Dr. D. J. Gibb Wishart, Toronto.

Paper, title to be announced—Dr. J. W. Stirling, Montreal.

Paper, title to be announced—Dr. B. E. McKenzie, Toronto.

Hernia of Bladder Complicating Inguinal Hernia—Dr. Francis J. Shepherd, Montreal.

Gastric Ulcer and its Treatment—Dr. J. B. McConnell, Montreal.

La Syphilis Canadienne et Différents Facteurs et Gravite— Dr. D. E. LeCavelier, Montreal.

Case Reports—Dr. Robert H. Craig, Montreal.

Paper, title to be announced—Dr. James S. Edwards, Grand Rapids, Mich.

Paper, title to be announced—Dr. Henry Howitt, Guelph, Ont.

Chronic Cystitis—Dr. J. O. Camirand, Sherbrooke, Que.

Iniencephaly, with a Report of Three Cases—Dr. Maud E. Abbott, and Dr. F. A. L. Lockhart, Montreal.

Actinomycosis—Dr. James Bell, Montreal.

Paper, title to be announced—Dr. Ingersoll Olmstead, Hamilton, Ont.

Prostatectomy Under Local Anesthesia—Dr. H. H. Sinclair, Walkerton, Ont.

High Frequency Currents in Functional Disease, more particularly Functional Neuroses—Dr. S. F. Wilson, Montreal.

Therapeutic Hints from Bacteriology—Dr. G. R. Cruickshank, Windsor, Ont.

Paper, title to be announced—Dr. C. H. Mayo, Rochester, Minn.

In addition there will be a number of papers from Western men, whose names have not yet been received.

Any further particulars required will be gladly furnished by the General Secretary, Dr. George Elliott, 129 John Street, Toronto.

ITEMS OF INTEREST.

Honors for Canadians.—On the occasion of the visit of the British Medical Association to Oxford, on July 27th, the honorary degree of D.S.C. will be conferred, among others, on Dr. Roddick, of Montreal, and Dr. Wm. Osler, of Baltimore.

A Splendid Booklet.—The firm of C. J. Hewlett & Son, 35 to 42 Charlotte Street, London, E.C., England, have recently published a splendid surgical instruments and druggists' sundries list, and are prepared to send a copy of it, free, to any Canadian physician on application.

Resident Physicians.—The following have been appointed resident physicians at the Hospital for Sick Children for the year commencing 1st July, 1904: Dr. Bruce Courtney Whyte, of Millbrook; Dr. Melville H. Embree, of Parkdale; Dr. K. D. Panton, of Milton, and Dr. Walter W. Wright, of Toronto.

Milk in Typhoid Fever.—A booklet bearing this title has recently been issued by the firm of Smith, Kline & French, Philadelphia, Pa., and is intended for free distribution among the medical profession. It will be sent by the publishers on application, and is worth while having, as it is most interesting, and written in a thoroughly scientific manner, showing that the constituent properties of milk are such that it is even a more valuable form of food in many diseases than some practitioners think. We would recommend our readers to secure a copy and peruse it.

The Mississippi Valley Medical Association.—The Thirtieth Annual Session of the Mississippi Valley Medical Association will be held at Cincinnati, Ohio, October 11th, 12th and 13th, 1904, under the presidency of Dr. Hugh T. Patrick, of Chicago. The headquarters and meeting places will be at the Grand Hotel. The annual orations will be delivered by Dr. Wm. J. Mayo, of Rochester, Minn., in Surgery, and Dr. C. Travis Drennen, of Hot Springs, Ark., in Medicine. Request for places upon the programme, or information in regard to the meeting, can be had by addressing the Secretary, Dr. Henry Enos Tuley, Louisville, Ky., or the Assistant Secretary, Dr. S. C. Stanton, Masonic Temple, Chicago, Ill. The usual railroad rates will be in effect.

The Physician's Library.

BOOK REVIEWS.

Progressive Medicine. A Quarterly Digest of Advances, Discoveries and Improvements in the Medical and Surgical Sciences. Edited by HOBART AMORY HARE, M.D., Professor of Therapeutics and Materia Medica in the Jefferson Medical College, Philadelphia. Assisted by H. R. M. LANDIS, M.D. Philadelphia and New York: Lea Brothers & Co. $6.00 per annum.

Volume I., 1904, issued March 1st, 1904, includes articles on Surgery of the Head, Neck and Thorax; Infectious Diseases, including Acute Rheumatism, Croupous Pneumonia and Influenza; the Diseases of Children; Laryngology and Rhinology; and Otology.

Volume II., 1904, issued June 1st, 1904, contains articles on Surgery of the Abdomen, including Hernia; Gynecology; Diseases of the Blood; Diathetic and Metabolic Diseases; Diseases of the Spleen, Thyroid Gland and Lymphatic System; and Ophthalmology.

It is impossible in a short review to refer to the many excellent points contained in the several chapters of each volume. It may be sufficient to state that, on the whole, the articles are short and practical, and that they contain the latest information available, presented in a most readable and satisfactory manner.

A. E.

Special Diagnosis of Internal Medicine. A Handbook for Physicians and Students. By DR. WILHELM V. LEUBE, Professor of Medicine and Physician-in-Chief to the Julius Hospital at Würsburg. Authorized translation from the sixth German edition. Edited, with annotations, by Julius L. Salinger, M.D., late Assistant Professor of Clinical Medicine in the Jefferson Medical College, and Physician to the Philadelphia Hospital. With five colored plates and seventy-four illustrations in the text. New York and London: D. Appleton & Co. 1904. Canadian agents: Geo. Morang & Co., Limited, Toronto.

Dr. v. Leube's work, dealing as it does with special medical diagnosis, is very useful to the true lover of medical science, for diagnosis being truly made, treatment suggests itself.

We have referred to it in a case of traumatic neurosis, hemiplegia, and have been gratified with the manner in which that difficult subject is presented, the clearness with which the diagnostic points are brought out. The work is clearly not a rival to well-known works on the practice of medicine, but it may be fitly regarded as complementary to the best of them—an authority on internal medicine, which a practitioner will consult with eagerness and will resort to as a friend in times of difficulty. The translation has been so well done that one would think the original work had been written in the English language. Dr. Leube should be pleased at the considerable number of friends and patrons in the English-speaking world who will be enabled, through Dr. Salinger's work, to avail themselves of the storehouse of knowledge which he has created.

The publishers' work has been very satisfactorily done.

J. J. C.

The Doctor's Recreation Series. By CHAS. WELLS MOULTON, General Editor. Arranged by Porter Davies, M.D. 1904. Akron, O., Chicago and New York : The Saalfield Publishing Co. Vol. I., " The Doctor's Leisure Hour," facts and fancies of interest to the doctor and his patient.

As announced in our columns a few months ago, Vol. I. of this exceedingly interesting series has just come out and each will follow the other at intervals of one month. Though only in our hands ten days, and we have not had time to read more than halfway through the first volume, we bespeak for the series a very hearty reception. It is just what the profession wants, especially during the holiday weather, there being too great a tendency to stick to heavy medical literature. To read " The Doctor's Leisure Hour " is a great rest to one who leads a busy life, many parts of the book refering to the relations of the doctor and patient being very amusing indeed and highly entertaining. The series consists of twelve volumes in all, and is sold by subscription only. It can be secured in two bindings, cloth and half morocco, at $2.50 and $4.00 respectively. Doctor, if you are going away for a vacation add to its enjoyment by taking " The Doctor's Leisure hour " in your grip.

W. A. Y.

Golden Rules of Anesthesia. By R. J. PROBYN-WILLIAMS, M.D., Anesthetist to London Hospital, etc. " Golden Rules " Series, No. XIV. Bristol: Jno. Wright & Co. London: Simpkin, Marshall, Hamilton, Kent & Co., Limited.

A very handy vest-pocket volume, a *vade-mecum,* in fact, full of " pointers " as to anesthetics and their administration.

W. A. Y.

The Canadian
Journal of Medicine and Surgery

A JOURNAL PUBLISHED MONTHLY IN THE INTEREST OF
MEDICINE AND SURGERY

| VOL. XVI. | TORONTO, SEPTEMBER, 1904. | NO. 3. |

Original Contributions.

REPORT OF A CASE OF BILATERAL, CONGENITAL DIS-LOCATION OF THE HIP TREATED BY THE LORENZ BLOODLESS METHOD—A BRIEF REVIEW OF THE PRESENT STATUS OF THE LORENZ METHOD.*

BY H. P. H. GALLOWAY, M.D.,

Surgeon to Toronto Orthopedic Hospital: Orthopedic Surgeon to Grace Hospital and the Western Hospital ; Member of the American Orthopedic Association.

E. L., aged two years and four months. I first examined this patient on February 26th, 1903. The parents sought advice because the child's gait had been peculiar from the time she began to walk, and was not improving. The waddling gait and the characteristic deformity of a patient with bilateral, congenital dislocation of the hip were very apparent, and the diagnosis could be easily and positively made by examination. Fig. 1 is reproduced from an X-ray picture taken a couple of days before treatment was commenced. While this is an exceptionally clear skiagraph, it is unfortunate that it was taken with the limbs rotated outward, so that the head, neck and trochanter are viewed in antero-posterior perspective, which makes it difficult to appreciate the proper shape and true relations of these parts of the femur. The fact that the head of the bone is not in the acetabulum, however, can be seen with perfect distinctness.

Fig. 2 shows the position of right-angled abduction in which the limbs were placed and retained by the plaster-of-Paris dressing. This first dressing was not disturbed for six months,

* Read before the Ontario Medical Association, June, 1904.

4

when it was cut off and immediately replaced with the limbs in the position shown in Fig. 3. Eight weeks later the third and last dressing was put on with the limbs brought still nearer the natural position, as shown in Fig. 4. This final dressing remained on about seven weeks.

While the dressings were on the child was encouraged to stand upon the feet. While wearing the last two dressings she learned to walk after a fashion with a fair degree of freedom. She has now been going about without any dressing on the limbs

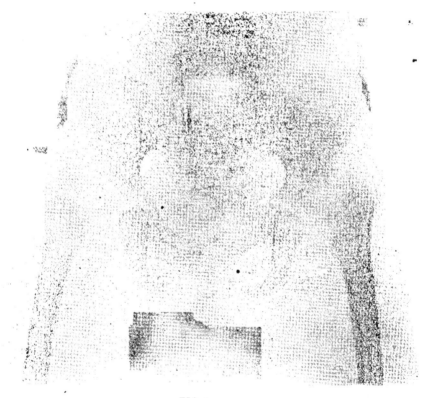

FIG. 1.

for nearly six months, and the X-ray picture shown in Fig. 5, which was taken two days ago, shows perfect anatomical replacement. The gait is improving all the time and will soon, I believe, be absolutely natural.

There is so much confusion and misunderstanding in the profession as well as among the laity regarding what has come to be known as " The Lorenz Bloodless Method " of treating congenital dislocation of the hip, that a brief review of the present status of professional opinion in relation to this subject may not be untimely.

Like most surgical procedures this operation must pass through a period of trial, and the experience of various operators in different parts of the world must be carefully reported, and the evidence derived therefrom judicially weighed before anything approaching final judgment can be arrived at.   Inasmuch as this operation aims at the relief of a disability until recently regarded as practically beyond help, not to say cure, the importance of the matter is everywhere conceded; but unfortunately, it is likely to take an unusually long time before professional opinion can finally crystallize, owing chiefly to the relative rarity of congenital dislocation of the hip, which must make it ever impossible

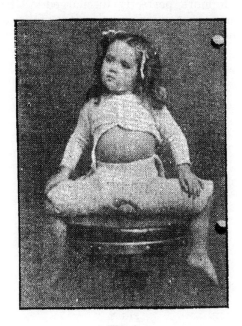

FIG. 2.

for more than a comparatively small number of surgeons to gain any large amount of experience with it.   It is only fair to state that Dr. Lorenz should not be held accountable for the exaggerated and extravagant claims regarding his methods of treatment, which for several months were so much in evidence in the lay press.   It is the business of newspaper representatives to be perpetually hungry for news, and the altogether extraordinary circumstances under which Dr. Lorenz visited this continent, gave the press an exceptional opportunity, with the result that the reporters fully sustained their reputation for enterprise and inventive power.   I personally saw and heard Dr. Lorenz refuse information to a representative of one of the Boston newspapers, who asked for a copy of his address at one of his clinical demonstrations in that city in December, 1902.

At one of his clinics in New York City, Dr. Lorenz was asked specifically regarding the results claimed by him. In effect, he replied, that he expected twenty-five per cent. of cures in bilateral dislocation, and fifty per cent. in unilateral cases. By " cure " was meant practically perfect anatomical and physiological restoration of the joint. Of those that could not be " cured " in that sense, he claimed that the vast majority were greatly improved, the location of the head of the femur being so changed by the manipulations used in the operation that the functions of the joint were much more perfectly discharged. Using this statement of Dr. Lorenz as a starting point it remains to be seen how far the experience of other operators will justify the claims made.

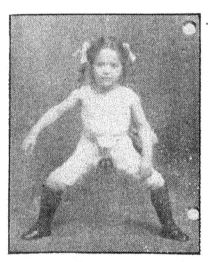

FIG. 3.

Recently Ridlon, of Chicago, in a paper read before the New York Academy of Medicine, presented an extended review of this subject based upon an exhaustive study of results in ninety-four cases operated upon; these cases included a number of those operated on by Lorenz during his stay in Chicago. His conclusion is that of the cases operated upon by this method there will be about ten per cent. of perfectly stable and anatomically perfect replacements; about fifty to sixty per cent. of " good results," and twenty to thirty per cent. of failures. Under " good results " are grouped the cases in which an anatomical replacement has not been secured, but the location of the head of the femur has been so changed that improvement in function has resulted, the shortening being diminished, the limp lessened, and the characteristic deformity largely obliterated. This changed location of the head of the femur usually means that anterior transposition has been brought about.

In the discussion which followed Dr. Ridlon's paper, Royal Whitman expressed the opinion that forty per cent. of the cases operated upon by the Lorenz method should be perfectly cured. Somewhat varying opinions have been expressed by other operators. Against Whitman's somewhat optimistic view it is interesting to balance the following statement by Walsham, of St. Bartholomew's Hospital, a surgeon of wide experience in general and in orthopedic surgery: " No one has yet demonstrated a definite and permanent improvement by this method, but it may

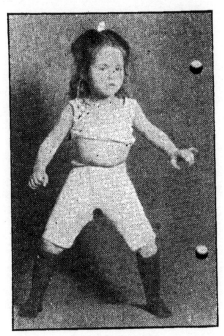

FIG. 4.

be held that the arrest of the increasing adduction is valuable." This quotation can be found on page 1150 of the last edition of Walsham's " Theory and Practice of Surgery," published last fall. It is well known that Lorenz was not enthusiastically received in England, but it is difficult to understand how such a pessimistic opinion could be arrived at by so able an observer as Walsham.

In a paper read before the American Orthopedic Association in Atlantic City last June, Prof. Albert Hoffa, of Berlin, Germany, claimed 30 per cent. of anatomical cures in unilateral cases, and 7.7 per cent. in bilateral, when operated upon by his bloodless method of reduction, which differs somewhat from the az method. At the same meeting various members of the iation reported results of treatment in a considerable number ses treated by Lorenz during his American tour, and the general feeling was one of disappointment at the results secured. n at Philadelphia last June the writer saw a number of cases had been operated upon by Lorenz and other surgeons, who

FIG. 5.

had followed his methods, and the average result was certainly disappointing.

Dr. Harry Sherman, of San Francisco, read a paper at the meeting above referred to, in which he very ably advocated operation by open incision, in preference to uncertain bloodless methods. He argued that we are not justified in submitting our patients to the primary dangers, and the subsequent prolonged after-treatmen of the Lorenz method when we know that not more than one in ten of those treated will realize a perfect anatomical cure. He was satisfied from his study of the anatomical conditions present in nearly thirty cases, upon which he had operated by open incision, that an anatomical cure was mechanically impossible by any purely manipulative method, except in a very small proportion of cases; and strongly urged that it was much better practice for the surgeon to open the joint, remove the mechanical obstructions to reduction, and thus work with certainty and precision.

Few operators on this continent have yet had sufficiently extended experience to reach final, independent conclusions. Without extending the scope of this paper so as to review the available evidence in detail I shall simply formulate a number of conclusions which I believe correctly represent the general trend of the most reliable professional opinion in regard to this important subject:

1. A certain proportion of cases of congenital dislocation of the hip are intrinsically incurable, owing to anatomical obstacles which are hopelessly beyond the surgeon's control. The acetabulum may be too shallow to retain the head in position; the head and neck of the femur may be so imperfect or deformed as to be quite unsuited for articulation; or there may be such contraction of the soft tissues as to form an insurmountable obstacle to reduction. The X-ray is of great value in many cases in determining the actual anatomical conditions.

2. Subcutaneous or open division of tendinous, muscular and ligamentous tissues which obstinately oppose reduction may be resorted to with benefit in certain cases when reduction by manipulation alone is impracticable.

3. In about ten per cent. of the cases treated by the Lorenz bloodless method, a perfect anatomical and physiological cure will be obtained.

4. In some of the cases of apparently perfect cure, redislocation may occur, even several months later. A repetition of the operation will be followed by ultimate success in some of these relapsed cases.

5. In probably sixty per cent. of the cases treated by the Lorenz method a true anatomical replacement is not secured, but an anterior transposition of the head of the femur is brought about. In a considerable proportion of these cases the condition of the patient is greatly improved, the shortening being diminished, the limp lessened, and the characteristic deformity largely or completely obliterated. In a word, there is a large and distinct functional gain.

6. The ideal age for operation is from three to five years. Under three years of age replacement is easy but the difficulty of

keeping the plaster dressings from becoming very foul is almost insuperable. After five years reduction is often very difficult, but success may sometimes be attained up to the age of thirteen years, and even beyond. Within reasonable limits the age of the patient *per se* has less to do with success or failure than the anatomical conditions in and about the joint in the individual case. One may fail in a patient of seven years and succeed in another of ten or twelve.

7. The operation usually is perfectly safe. Accidents have occurred, however, both in the hands of Lorenz and other surgeons. The possible accidents are thus summed up by Ridlon: Paralysis from over-stretching; fracture of the neck of the femur; fracture of the shaft of the femur; fracture of the ramus of the pubes; fracture of the ischium; tearing of the perineum; rupture of the femoral artery; gangrene from cutting off the circulation through stretching the femoral vessels. He somewhat facetiously adds: " There may be others, but these are sufficient for the surgeon who has experienced one or more of them."

8. The results in the cases operated upon by Lorenz himself and by his followers on this continent have on the whole proved disappointing.

9. Open methods of operation, which permit some of the obstacles to reduction to be discovered and removed; and which afford the surgeon the opportunity to satisfy himself that his manipulations have really placed the head of the femur in the acetabulum, are likely to be largely adopted in the future, the bloodless method being reserved for very young patients, and cases where objections to the use of the knife cannot be overcome.

12 East Bloor Street, Toronto.

THE DIAGNOSIS OF MODIFIED SMALLPOX (SO-CALLED).*

BY CHARLES A. HODGETTS, M.D., L.R.C.P. (LOND.),

Secretary of the Provincial Board of Health of Ontario ; member of the Sanitary Institute of Great Britain.

THE term "modified smallpox" given in the title is somewhat misleading, for heretofore the word "modified" has been reserved for cases of smallpox occurring in vaccinated persons only; it has, in short, been considered a synonym of varioloid. The continuance of variola in a mild form for the past five years has led to the application of the term "modified" to all cases where the course has been considered in any way atypical. By the setting up as a clinical standard a certain chain of symptoms, which has for many decades been considered diagnostic of variola, there has become engrained into medical practitioners the idea that these are the only symptoms which could be found in a case warranting the diagnosis "smallpox."

The infallibility of this doctrine has, like many other of the "sure things" of this world, been proved to be fallacious. Like others of the group exanthemata, we know, as indeed have all writers of authority upon the subject, that smallpox is capable of every degree of modification, from the initial stage through each successive stage, until that of complete recovery is reached.

That this long continuance of smallpox in so mild a form is perhaps unprecedented, is true, certainly, as far as modern medical history is concerned; but a careful study of the writings of those who have discussed the subject at any length, cannot fail to convince one that in outbreaks where the mortality was high, atypical (mild cases) were always to be seen. Most cases were severe, and so the description recorded corresponded with the type. In like manner one writing now would describe in detail the progress and symptoms of the type of case as observed, incidentally referring to the severe or very mild ones as atypical of this epidemic.

Again the modified cases have for the past one hundred years been considered as those upon which vaccination has had a controlling influence, and at this date to apply the term "modified" to a large series of cases upon which the beneficial effects of vaccination cannot claim to have exercised any modifying influence, is most misleading.

It is, therefore, preferable to consider all cases which occur in the unvaccinated as smallpox, no matter of what type, reserving the terms "varioloid" and "modified smallpox" for

---
* Read before the Ontario Medical Association (by request), June 15th, 1904.

those cases happening in persons who have derived any immunity from a successful vaccination or re-vaccination, or previous attack of smallpox. The possibility of an inherited immunity derived from vaccination in a line of ancestors as being a factor in the cause of the mild type characterizing the recent epidemic, is not substantiated by observations extending over the whole period of its presence.

For the past five years perhaps no subject has called forth more discussion than that of smallpox, chiefly from the fact that the mild type, which characterized the first cases of the disease, has been almost constant throughout that period. True it is that individual instances have not been wanting where all the virulent symptoms have been present, but these typical cases have been like oases in the desert, and their appearance has cheered the heart of many an anxious medical health officer, whose diagnosis had at last been confirmed, his hope being often realized that virulence would be followed by public alarm, which would result in precautionary measures being taken with more alacrity.

Before considering the differential diagnosis, the presentation of a brief review of the symptoms which have characterized the disease as it has occurred in Ontario, is desirable.

History.—Some five years ago the first cases appeared in Essex County, and in the following year the disease became widely scattered in the lumber camps of Northern Ontario before its presence was known. In both instances it came from the State of Michigan. At first considerable difference existed as to the diagnosis. By some it was considered to be chickenpox; while others were as confirmed in their opinion that it was impetigo contagiosa; and a number expressed the opinion that it was some new cutaneous disease without a name; and for a time, at least, the opinion was expressed that it was of a syphilitic character.

This latter opinion was, no doubt, due to the fact that male adults seemed to be the chief persons attacked, but soon it became apparent that it was not limited either by age, race or sex; and, although it spread somewhat insidiously, yet those unvaccinated became its victims when brought into contact with it. Usually it required more than a passing exposure, but frequently cases occurred where the contact was but slight. When it occurred in schools, unchecked, it was particularly interesting to observe that a period of several weeks would elapse between the appearance of the first case and the general outbreak, the first cases being those occupying seats contiguous to the initial one, it being clearly evident that the infection was of a mild character. A very noticeable feature, and one that was emphasized as the cases became more numerous, was the immunity of those who had been vaccinated, the disease pursuing an almost unaltered course through thousands of unvaccinated persons, at times presenting slight exacerbations in those who, from personal susceptibility, developed the old-fashioned type of smallpox.

Climate and season.—The disease has continued from year to year, with a maximum number of cases in January, and a minimum in the summer months. The type presented no variation in the cold of winter as compared to those happening in the heat of summer.

Contagiousness.—It would appear that the virulence of the contagion is in direct relationship to the severity of the attack. During the early stages preceding pustulation, the infection is not as great as subsequently, and the mere entering a room or house wherein is a mild case during the pustular stage, is not always followed by an attack. Often persons live for weeks in the same house with a mild case before they develop it. I have not known of a case due to convection; indeed, on this point I am somewhat sceptical.

Incubation.—The usual period of twelve full days from the date of one receiving the specific infection of smallpox is, as a rule, the correct one; but the exceptions have been so numerous during the past five years, where fifteen, sixteen and eighteen days have elapsed, that for mild cases the period may safely be extended to fifteen days. For the reason of prolonged incubation, the period of quarantine has been extended to eighteen days, and in some of the neighboring districts three weeks is the statutory period.

Initial symptoms.—While in many cases the onset, although slight in character, is often sudden, yet many patients have suffered so little discomfort, that it has been hard for them to fix any time for the onset. Mild and insidious, indeed, have been his prodromata, from a passing malaise to headache and backache, accompanied by nausea and vomiting; children and adults alike have had the same experience, and the latter have often followed their usual occupation throughout the whole progress of the disease. Many have described this group of symptoms as simulating la grippe more than anything else. The temperature has averaged from 100 F. to 102 F., while the instances have been as many below the minimum as above the maximum quoted.

The fever continues, as a rule, for twenty-four hours to seventy-two hours, although it frequently passes unnoticed by the patient; the temperature drops to normal or subnormal with the appearance of the eruption, and thus ends for many their sickness, and the usual occupation is resumed. Because the onset is severe it does not follow that the attack will be severe, nor does it hold true that the mild onset will be followed by a slight attack.

The Eruption.—This appears from a few hours to seventy-two hours after the onset, and consists, in the first instance, of minute red macules that disappear on pressure. They are not hard to the touch nor perceptibly raised above the surface. The distribution conforms very much to that of the more severe type of the disease, being more marked upon the face and extremities than on the trunk. Often within a few hours the maculæ become papules, when the shotty feel is first noticeable. This is frequently the first stage noticeable in mild cases, and this time some of them may show distinct signs of beginning vesiculation. Thus it is stated by the patient that they began as vesicles, whereas the correct way to state it would be, the eruption was first noticed when vesiculation began. This is a fruitful source of error in diagnosis, and leads the practitioner to call the attack one of chicken-pox.

The rash may appear in one crop, but more frequently, even in very mild cases, from one to three days may elapse before it has fully come out.

During vesiculation, which continues for about three days, rarely five, as seen in previous outbreaks, the rash increases in size until many of them become as large as a pea, pearly in appearance, and either filled or partially filled with serum. The more typical will be found to be multilocular and different to the others; will not collapse on being transfixed by a needle. Some, but not all, of the vesicles will present umbilication.

The change to a pustule may begin as early as the fourth day, and usually, in most cases, is markedly noticeable on the fifth day. The rash on the face, usually shrinking and drying up into thin crusts, is shed from the face and neck often as early as the tenth day. Not so, however, is the course of the lesions on the other portions of the body and the extremities. The course here is prolonged, and the pustules present a more typical appearance, and on the sixth to the eighth day of the eruption there will be found a circular pustule presenting a dome-shaped appearance, and surrounded by a marked areola. These pustules shrivel, and subsequently rupture or are broken, and the contents form a dry crust, or they become inspissated, presenting a brownish appearance. Particularly is this the case in the feet and hands, where the epidermis is thickened. The stage of incrustation continues for a longer period in the latter case than where simply thin crusts form. In the majority of cases there is no dermatitis, and if present, is but slight. Intumescence, if present, is not only slight in degree but is evanescent in character, and lasts for two or three days.

The average duration of this atypical form of smallpox is slightly under twenty-one days. The chief difficulties met with have been as follows: 1. The frequently mild form of the onset. 2. The abortive character of the eruption, as observed chiefly on the exposed parts. 3. The entire absence of constitutional depression after the appearance of the rash, thus permitting of many persons resuming their usual calling. 4. The absence of secondary fever, even in more markedly typical cases. 5. The extreme mildness of the infection, as shown in many instances. 6. The brevity of the period of isolation as compared with former outbreaks. These, and possibly a few others of a minor character, have thrown many a physician off his guard, and led in the past to rather widespread outbreaks in some portions of the Province.

Of the foregoing, the abortive character of the eruption is the greatest source of diagnostic mistakes, for it is found that the eruption, when once out, does not pass through the successive stages even in an imperfect manner, but it pursues an abortive course; given a case with a definite number of maculæ, there will be found to be an aborting of numbers of these, the remainder developing into papules, of which in turn, a number will also abort before becoming even slightly pustular. It will be further found that the papules have developed into solid conical elevations, crowned by small vesicles containing sero-purulent or sero-sanguino-purulent fluid, which vesicles desiccate early, leaving the solid portion which remains for some time as a warty-like excrescence of the skin. This is most frequently noticed on the face, but disappears without leaving any permanent disfiguration.

The size of the pustules or the aborted vesicles will be briefly referred to before leaving this portion of the subject. Usually circular in size and of the size of a split pea, yet in many instances it is found that the greater number are smaller in size, some not larger than a good-sized pin-head. The apex of many will present a dark appearance similar to an acne, though without any marked dermatitis or intumescence. In such cases some few typical pustules will be found, possibly, on the abdomen or extremities or along the hair line. Again, early rupture of the vesicles or pustules produces, where such has occurred, an irregular outline, somewhat simulating chicken-pox.

The affections with which smallpox of the present type has been, and unfortunately still is, most frequently confounded, are chicken-pox, impetigo contagiosa, pustular syphiloderm, urticaria papulosa and acne. Of these chicken-pox is the most common, chiefly owing to the fact that the premonitory symptoms have been so mild that the patient has misrepresented them to the physician; and coupled with these mis-statements there is found on looking at the exposed parts only a few, often only one or two, abortive vesicles or pustules. The examination is not pushed any further. Both parties concerned are satisfied; the patient particularly so from the knowledge of the fact that isolation will not be necessary, although he may be well aware that had the physician stripped him, an altogether different condition of affairs would have been found on the "hidden parts." The blame is in most instances to be laid at the door of the patient rather than at that of the medical attendant for the mistake, for had the one been honest, the other would have been more painstaking in his examination. In smallpox, believe nothing you hear, doubt much you see on first appearances, but carefully note all that the surface of the body has to reveal to both touch and sight.

The chief characteristics which distinguish chicken-pox from the present mild form of smallpox are: 1. It is a disease chiefly confined to childhood, being only occasionally seen in adults. 2. It rapidly runs its course in a week, passing through the stages of pimple, vesicle and scab often within a few hours; certainly within twenty-four hours after the first appearance of the papular rose spot the vesicle develops. 3. The premonitory symptoms are but slightly marked; indeed, are frequently wanting altogether. 4. The temperature accompanies or follows the appearance of the rash. 5. The vesicles of chicken-pox are ovoid or irregular in appearance, and attain their maximum development much quicker than do those of smallpox. 6. The eruption, as a rule, appears first on the portions of the body covered by clothing. 7. After the crusts fall off they leave a red instead of a pigmented spot.

With these marked differential symptoms, it must be stated that many cases of smallpox of the present type occur, making it extremely difficult to correctly place them.* "It may, however, be stated in a general way, that a mildly febrile eruption, appearing without prodromal symptoms, being distinctly vesicular from the beginning, and commencing to desiccate on the second or third day, should be regarded as chicken-pox; and on the other hand, an acute exanthem, preceded by an initial stage of forty-eight hours, in which the temperature was distinctly elevated, beginning as papules and ending in vesicles and vesico-pustules, even though the period of evolution be short, should be regarded as smallpox."

Impetigo Contagiosa.—The chief points in the differential diagnosis of this disease are: 1. It is a skin affection, rarely accompanied at any stage of its progress by an elevation of temperature. 2. There is no initial stage. 3. It does not begin as a papule, but as a vesicle, or vesico-pustule, or growth of the

---

* Wm. W. Welch, M.D., *Philadelphia Medical Journal*, Nov. 18th, 1889.

same upon an apparently normal skin. 4. It appears chiefly on the face, head and hands—the exposed parts. 5. It is usually unsymmetrical and superficial, and spreads from the periphery, often attaining the size of a ten-cent piece. 6. The crusts are of differing degrees of thickness, are varied in color from straw to a brownish hue. They are friable, crumbling very easily. On removal, the base is covered with pus, which on healing leaves no scar. 7. Fresh inoculation may occur in the same individual, the infecting material being generally carried by the finger nails to any part of the skin.

Pustular Syphiloderm.—Although few mistakes have arisen from the diagnosis of cases of smallpox for pustular syphiloderm, yet there is a greater resemblance between these two diseases than is generally supposed. This stage of syphilis is ushered in by fever and accompanying pains and aches, very similar to smallpox. There then follows the papular eruption, which subsequently ends in the pustule. The chief distinguishing points are: 1. The absence of the shotty feel of papules. 2. The formation of small vesicles at summit of the papules. 3. The large indurated base of the vesicles. 4. The appearance of the rash in successive crops. 5. Umbilication is absent. 6. The tendency of some of the lesions to ulcerate. 7. Examination reveals other symptoms of syphilis. 8. A history of the initial syphilitic lesion is confirmatory.

Urticaria Papulosa.—In this disease the papules are small, the size generally of a split pea; in color a dull white. They attain their full size in one to two hours. The initial symptoms are absent.

Acne.—This skin affection occurs chiefly at puberty, and the chief points in the diagnosis are: 1. The absence of initial symptoms. 2. The pustules are acuminated with a black central dot or comedo. Base is indurated. 3. The face, shoulders and back are chiefly affected. 4. The rash will be found in all stages in the different portions of the body. 5. The chief diagnostic difficulty is found in the rash as it affects the face, as in these mild cases it often simulates acne. An examination of the whole body will assist in clearing up the diagnosis. There is no necessity to refer to the rashes which happen in the initial stage, for in this type of smallpox they do not occur.

A CASE OF GASTROSCHISIS OR FISSURA ABDOMINALIS.*

BY JOSEPH H. PETERS, M.D., HAMILTON, ONT.

THE specimen presents the condition known as gastroschisis, or fissura abdominalis. The abdominal organs have no covering, except the peritoneum and the chorion and amnion continued from the placenta. There is a hernia of the liver and intestines, if not more of the abdominal organs, into the sac so formed. The pubic bones do not unite in the middle line. There is complete absence of the anterior wall of the bladder, and one can see its posterior wall continuous with the skin. Just posterior to the bladder will be noticed a projection of mucous membrane, which is found to be the rectum slightly prolapsed. The genital organs are completely absent with the exception of a rudimentary scrotum, which is cleft, each lateral half being attached to the corresponding nates. It will be noticed that the right leg is rotated inwards through an angle of 180 degrees, so that the foot looks directly backward. There is a spina bifida in the lower dorsal region.

It will be remembered that in the process of development, the visceral arches (splanchno-pleures) grow forward, and for the most part coalesce in the middle line. The neural arches unite behind in a similar fashion. Non-union sometimes occurs and gives rise to various forms of clefts, such as those illustrated by this case.

The incomplete closure is said to be caused by the abnormal protrusion of the viscera, preventing closure in front. " The cause of such protrusions may be dropsical accumulations, more especially in case of the thorax and abdomen, but it may be due to interference, by adhesions, or otherwise, of the amnion or allantois."—*Coates.* The child was alive at birth.

---

*Read at the Ontario Medical Association, Toronto, June, 1904.

PROGRESS IN THE TREATMENT OF ECZEMA.

BY PROF. KROMAYER, BERLIN.

THE province of eczema treatment shares with the remaining provinces in therapeutics, the questionable lot, that at brief intervals new remedies or novel compositions are ever being advanced and recommended as particularly effective in their action. In spite of these recommendations, however, but few remedies have been proved to represent real progress. The majority have met with a well-merited fate: in a short time they have become forgotten and been replaced by new ones.

As against all these passing appearances, which prove the need of a new system of treatment, there stands fast, like a *rocher de bronce,* the old method of the Hebra school: Hebra ointment, tar, sulphur and soft soap (sapo viridis). Not that I mean to say, there has not been considerable progress made in the treatment of eczema since Hebra's time, quite the contrary; but despite such progress, the Hebra treatment in all essentials has maintained its position; it constitutes, as it were, the foundation upon which later improvements have been built up, without, however, rendering the foundation either unnecessary or superfluous.

If, therefore, the progress which has been made in eczema treatment is to be rightly judged, we must go back to this foundation and get a clear idea of the principles upon which the Hebra treatment is based; and it is, of course, a matter of indifference, whether Hebra himself worked according to these principles, or whether he, our most genial clinical dermatologist, created the treatment, as a poet his song, without any theoretical speculations.

At all events, I am unable to discover in Hebra's works any theoretical expositions on the point. Nevertheless, such are not to be dispensed with, if we wish to arrive at a proper understanding of the treatment of eczema.

There are three principles underlying the treatment of eczema:

1. *Removal of the irritation of the skin.*—All inflammatory

5

processes which have not yet brought about any considerable alteration in the histological structure of the skin, are again reduced to the normal (acute eczema).

2. *Removal of the chronic inflammatory processes* (which have led to deep-seated alterations in the histological structure) by means of a reducing agent (chronic eczema).

3. *Destruction of the tissue-changes* which do not return to the normal, either through removal of the irritation of the skin, or by means of a reducing agent (chronic eczema, obstinately complicated with acute, inflammatory outbursts).

If we consider these three indications which come in question in the treatment of eczema, and the progress which has so far been made, we shall not only obtain a clear opinion of them, but also be able to judge their value in the treatment of eczema itself.

1. *Indication of the removal of the irritation of the skin.*— For this indication we find Hebra employed: water dressings, dressings treated with ointment, and dusting with powder. An essential improvement has been the introduction of ointments, which, as is well known, were first recommended by Lassar; whilst the mulls treated with ointment, as proposed by Unna, have not been able to maintain a permanent position, and painting with gelatine, as recommended by Pick in the treatment of eczema, has been given up after a very short time.

Ointment, as prototype of which I may cite Lassar's (zinc oxide 10, amyl 10, vasel. 20), protects the skin better, not only from external injuries, by reason of its very suitable consistency, but it is also far better adapted to absorb the secretions, so that the ointment treatment must be regarded as a great advance. Furthermore, the ointment is perfectly adapted for absorbing the medicaments in solid, soft or liquid form, so that it likewise forms an extremely convenient method of application for all medicaments.

2. *The second indication*, removal of chronic inflammatory alterations (inflammatory infiltrations), is effected, according to Hebra, essentially by means of tar, soft soap and also red or white precipitate-ointment. Strange to say, Hebra thinks little of sulphur in the treatment of eczema. To understand this, it is necessary to make a further division of " chronic eczema," under which we generally understand two altogether different conditions:

1. Acute eczema, which has persisted for a considerable time, and by frequent recurrences has caused chronic inflammatory infiltration of the skin, whereby the latter has become thick, red and swollen.

2. True chronic eczema, which from the commencement appears as red, scaly papulæ, and which is variously designated sehorrheic, psoriatic, or parasitic eczema.

Whereas the first group of eczemas is, it is true, but little, if at all, accessible to treatment with sulphur, the latter is one of the chief medicaments for the group of so-called "seborrheic" eczemas. Tar, on the contrary, has its domain in the first group of chronic eczemas. This is a distinguishing feature in the application of tar and sulphur, which should be clearly understood, since other medicaments in their action are grouped around these two remedies, and it is in this direction that much progress has been made in therapeutics.

As tar, owing to both color and smell, is disagreeable to the patient, many attempts have been made to find a substitute, but without complete success. The derivatives of tar: phenol, naphthol, salicylic acid, greatly allay irritation, and in this respect render admirable service also in eczema, especially in a cooling ointment of the following composition:

R Naphthol,
Acid. Carbol.,
Acid. salicyl ....aa. 0.5—1.0
Lanolin,
Vaselin. alb. amor.,
Aqua dest................................aa.   30.0

Nevertheless, there is not the reducing action on the inflammatory infiltrated connective tissue. The same must be said of tumenol, which is likewise only a good palliative for the itching irritation. The experiments hitherto made with a view to improving the tar itself have also been but partially successful.

The preparations from pit-coal tar, by their number alone, show that they have not fully met the reasonable demands made of them: liquor carbonis detergens, liquor anthracis simplex, tinctura lithantracis (Leistikow), solutio lithantracis (Sack), liantral (Troplowitz).

Recently, a really great advance in the purification of tar, and thus in the tar treatment, appears to have been made, Veith having succeeded in distilling both from pit-coal and wood tar, a colorless product, *anthrasol* (Knoll),[*] which, according to my observations (extending over a period of nine months), proves admirable in its purely tar effect. The absence of color is not only agreeable to the patient, but also no small advantage to the physician, since he can observe the action of the tar with much more exactitude, and can far more readily remark any irritation on the just commencing redness, not hidden by any brown color.

[*]A. Sack, M.D., Ph.D., and H. Veith, Ph.D., *Munchener Med. Wochenschrift,* 1903, No. 18
Dr. Sack, *Alleg. Medic. Centralzeitung,* 1903, No. 44.
Report of the Eighth Congress of the German Dermatological Society, Sarajevo. *Monatshefte fur prakt. Dermatologie,* Vol. 37, No. 9, p. 390.
Dr. Veith, *Therapie der Gegenwort,* 1903, No. 2.
Karl Hercheimer, M.D. (Senior Physician, Station for Skin Diseases, Municipal Hospital (Frankfort-on-Main). *Deutsch. Medic. Wochenschrift,* 1904, No. 5.

With the second group of chronic eczemas (seborrheic and psoriatic), the therapeutic progress which has been made since Hebra, has been much more considerable; here pyrogallic acid and chrysarobin have made a triumphal entry.   With them or their derivatives, especially eugallol, with its pronounced action, cures in these forms of eczema can be effected so quickly, that sulphur would appear to be altogether left in the shade.   And yet sulphur cannot be altogether dispensed with: it works much slower and more quietly, but, on the other hand, it has not the disagreeable properties of the two new medicaments, viz., their poisonous character and tendency to slightly irritate.

A special province remains for it, viz., that of seborrhea, pityriasis, acne.   The following preparations exhibit essentially the action of sulphur: ichthyol, thiol, thiocol, but without having any essential advantages over sulphur itself, and thus not constituting any appreciable progress in the treatment.

3. The most difficult is the third indication, in which case Hebra has recommended liquor potassæ and soft soap.   It is here generally a case of extremely irritating eczema, which has persisted for a long time, failing to give way under the ordinary treatment adopted for the removal of the inflammation, since the tissue-changes have already progressed too far.   Even the reducing treatment with tar and its substitutes cannot here be usefully employed, as they are liable to cause further irritation. For this obstinate eczema, which is exceedingly difficult to treat, and in which the red, infiltrated, edematous skin usually exhibits numerous superficial or deep-rooted vesicles, running places and scurf, Hebra reserved as *ultimum refugium* liquor potassæ, with which in 30 per cent. solution he cauterized the whole of the eczematous surface, and thus simply destroy the, for the most part, altered and inflamed tissue.   Such cauterization must be undertaken several times, at intervals of one week, before it is of any definite effect, as, even after the cauterization, new inflammatory outbreaks take place.   One of the chief advantages to be noticed immediately after the cauterization is the disappearance of the tormenting itch, since the liquor potassæ destroys the covering of the vesicles, so that the inflammatory secretion can escape and run over the surface of the skin.

Since this cauterization, however, is attended with no inconsiderable pain, Hebra, before having recourse to this extreme measure, first employed soapy ablutions, by means of which he likewise disturbed the covering of the vesicles, naturally without producing so intense a cauterizing action.

So excellent the prescriptions of Hebra are in themselves, they have one drawback, which was acknowledged by him himself, viz., that the application is by no means easy, and that a certain degree of experience is necessary to apply the cauterization and the soapy ablutions at the right moment and in the proper strength. Otherwise, these measures may bring about irritations and change for the worse.

These are the reasons why Hebra's method has not found its way into ordinary practice, at all events, not amongst general practitioners, and, so far as I am aware, not even among all specialists. There is thus a real want in the therapeutics of eczema, and it is owing to this void that all other, however well-chosen, measures in the treatment so frequently fail.

This want has been met in recent years by lenigallol.* This is a chemical compound of acetic acid and pyrogallic acid. It is a white powder, insoluble in water, which, in contact with the diseased skin, gradually splits up into its compounds, acetic acid and pyrogallic acid, by reason of the former exercising a slightly macerating effect, and owing to the pyrogallic acid having a mild, cauterizing action. This latter action, however, is so slow and moderate that no pain or irritation is caused. Lenigallol is usually applied in 10 per cent. zinc ointment:

> R Lenigallol (Knoll)........................10.0
> Past. zinci......................... ad 100.0

and is used in the same manner as the latter. As lenigallol is not decomposed on the healthy skin, it exercises no irritant action on such. Hence it is that, in spite of its cauterizing action, it belongs to the almost non-irritant remedies, and can thus be employed in all cases where there is danger of irritation being caused by other cauterizing agents.

Owing to these properties, it is a remedy *par excellence* for eczema, where all irritation must be carefully avoided. All eczemas, with the exception of acute, irritant eczema, can be treated with lenigallol.

Its most brilliant action is seen naturally in those cases where, on chronically altered and inflamed skin, acute inflammatory outbursts are ever making their appearance anew; that is to say, where, in addition to the thickened skin, there are running places, vesicles and scurf, where an excruciating itching always tempts the patient to scratch, thus calling forth a new outburst of inflammation. In such cases lenigallol acts like magic. Whereas the patient, in consequence of the persistent itching, for weeks and months can get no sleep at night, rest is obtained after the first application of a dressing with lenigallol zinc ointment. When the dressing is removed after twelve hours, innumerable brown and black places, spots and points on the skin

---

*Prepared by Dr. Veith, chemist to Messrs. Knoll & Co., Ludwigshafen-on-Rhine, and introduced into dermatological practice.

will be observed, where the lenigallol has been decomposed and has exerted a mild cauterizing action. On the eczematous province the irritation is allayed; whereas, otherwise, one is shocked at the effects caused through the patient scratching himself, and through the signs of a new outburst of inflammation the acute inflammatory swelling will now be seen to be diminished, the province of the eczema is more sharply defined, the scurf readily loosens, the wet places become dry. After the lenigallol treatment has been continued for some days, for the purpose of increasing the cauterizing action and rendering it more permanent, the lenigallol will have done its work. It is not advisable to continue the lenigallol treatment for any great length of time, as finally, in consequence of the liberation of pyrogallic acid, irritation may be caused, and for the treatment of this eczema there are other steps to be taken before cure is effected.

I have already stated several times, that the first group of chronic eczema comprises acute and chronic processes of inflammation. When the acute have been overcome by means of superficial cauterization with lenigallol, it remains to remove the chronic processes with the aid of tar.

This can be done by employing, instead of lenigallol zinc ointment, a tar zinc ointment:

> Anthrasol (Knoll)..........................10.0
> Past. zinci. ....ad 100.0

or by continuing the lenigallol treatment, but at the same time applying tar, by means of the following ointment:

> R   Lenigallol (Knoll)......................... 10.0
> Anthrasol................................. 10.0
> Past. zinci..................... ....ad 100.0

D.S. Lenigallol anthrasol ointment, only concluding the cure with the tar treatment, gradually increasing in strength.

This therapeutic scheme suits nearly all ordinary eczemas, as the majority consist of chronic and acute inflammatory changes, with the sole difference, that in the one the chronic and in the other the acute symptoms predominate; and that in the one considerable, and in the other slight, irritation is present, which, of course, must be carefully observed in treating.

If, during the tar treatment, new outbursts occur, the tar must be desisted from, and the lenigallol treatment again commenced, the tar only being returned to cautiously later on.

In this manner, the treatment being adapted to the various individual requirements, even the most obstinate eczemas can be cured, such as hitherto could not be done without the aid of liquor potassæ.

Naturally lenigallol is no panacea. As it practically acts only on the surface, deep-rooted alterations are not reached by it. Vesicles and pustules which have formed beneath a thick corneous layer, remain uninfluenced, as the horny layer is not penetrated by the remedy. If cauterization is here to be undertaken, resource must be had, after all, to liquor potassæ.

But even in these cases a preliminary treatment with lenigallol is of the greatest value, as all superficial inflammatory processes are in this manner cured, and the field thus prepared for the more convenient and certain application of liquor potassæ. For the latter now no longer has to attack the superficial seat of inflammation and eat deep holes, but penetrates gradually into the deeply located seat of inflammation and destroys the parts there, where the fresh outbursts and recurrences most frequently commence. The action of the liquor potassæ is rendered much more intense and thorough, but at the same time less extended and painful, and thus more certain in its effect.

Every physician who has had experience in the treatment of eczema, knows that there is no other cutaneous disease in which it is so important to have the parts under strict observation, and to control the course of treatment; knows that definite prescriptions for the treatment even in any particular case, can only be given for a short time. Here it is necessary, as in no other skin disease, in each case to observe continually how the skin reacts to the therapeutic measures adopted. That physician will be best able to cure eczema who is best in the position to observe and judge the effect of the treatment.

If, therefore, in the above I have endeavored to set forth a scheme of treatment in eczema, it is only intended for quite general application, since it must be modified to suit each particular case.

I am, therefore, of opinion that it may be profitable to describe a concrete case, which was a difficult one to treat and frequently led to total changes in the treatment, but which, for this very reason, is instructive and to a certain degree typical.

F. K., railway official, 50 years of age, suffering from eczema for over six months. Status: both hands and forearms, both thighs and legs, attacked *in toto,* and in patches, the back and head (well haired). Taken into my private clinic. Character of the affection: arms and legs much swollen and edematous, intensely red and bluish red (legs), surface covered, for the most part, with dirty, crusty scurf, partly running, partly drier, scaly, places covered with the effects of recent scratching.

Treatment.—I should have preferred to have put the man into a bath at once, in order thus to soften the scurf, scales and dirt in the mildest manner; since, however, the affected parts were very extended, and would be converted from dry, and at all events crusted over places, into running patches, whereby general irritation might easily be caused—and I was, as yet, wholly ignorant of the condition of the patient's skin—I decided to proceed with caution, and commenced the treatment on the same evening by application of a dressing with lenigallol zinc ointment. Next morning, the whole of the parts effected were cleansed with liquid paraffin; the crust, as far as soft, removed; dressing renewed. This treatment continued for four days in succession, morning and evening. The result was brilliant; the itching almost entirely ceased; the edema disappeared with the exception of mere traces; the skin dry all over, and now that the edema is gone, it can be seen how intensely infiltrated and thick it is. On closer observation numerous groups of vesicles can be seen, especially on the backs of the hands.

On the fifth day of treatment: Bath and ablution with soap, for the purpose of disturbing the covering of the vesicles, thereupon anthrasol in lenigallol zinc paste. Evening, dressing renewed, result good, no irritation.

Sixth day of treatment: The same; result good, no irritation.

Seventh day: Same treatment. Evening, irritation. The patient had, during the day, for the first time left the clinic, and, in view of the fine weather, had made a walk, had perspired, and scratched himself. Evening, dressing renewed, only with zinc ointment.

Eighth day: Irritation persisting; cooling zinc ointment of the following composition: lanolin, vaselin, paste zinci, each 30.0; aceti, aqua, each 15.0.

Ninth day: Irritation less, but still considerable itching. Patient longs for bath, which is allowed. After the bath, immediately rubbed over with cooling zinc ointment. Notwithstanding this, increased irritation, which only disappears after two days under treatment with cooling zinc ointment and wet dressings with acetic acid clay (1:200).

Eleventh day: Previous experience thus shows that the skin of the patient is extremely sensitive, and inclined to prolonged irritation, so that great caution is requisite in the treatment. Very characteristic, also, is the fact that once the irritation has arisen, the skin has now become altogether more irritable, and not even a simple bath, which was at first taken without complaint, can be well borne, despite the mildest subsequent treatment with cooling zinc ointment.

Twelfth day: Lenigallol zinc ointment again; result good, no bath.

Thirteenth and fourteenth days: Anthrasol zinc ointment; result good, no bath.

Fifteenth day: Both hands and forearms cauterized with officinal 15 per cent. liquor potassæ. This proved necessary, firstly, on account of the numerous groups of vesicles on the backs of the hands, and, secondly, because of the several seriously infiltrated knots on the forearms, which are ever itching anew. Result good, itching disappeared.

Fifteenth to eighteenth days: Dressing with anthrasol zinc ointment, below which, on the formerly uniformly deep red patches, lighter places and stripes now form, a sure sign of commencement of healing.

Sixteenth to twentieth days: Anthrasol zinc paste, further healing; every other day a soap bath, no irritation.

Twenty-first day: Hands cauterized again with potassium.

Twenty-second to twenty-fourth days: Healing progressing under the anthrasol treatment and baths.

Without the preliminary treatment with lenigallol it would have been absolutely impossible in this case to have obtained such rapid results.

It was only through the softening of the crusts, and simultaneous drying of the wet skin below, in consequence of the mild cauterizing action of the lenigallol, that the possibility was presented of the tar treatment being successfully employed, and for the application of the baths and liquor potassæ.

I have for now some six years, in over one thousand cases of eczema, tried lenigallol, and should be sorry to miss it from amongst my medicines.

If, now, in concluding, I sum up the chief progress which has been made in eczema treatment since Hebra's classical treatment, for acute eczemas and as a form of application of medicaments, the first advance to be mentioned is the ointment treatment. For chronic psoriatic forms of eczema, chrysarobin and pyrogallic acid represent an essential improvement in therapeutics; the tar treatment has been greatly enriched through the preparation of anthrasol, and finally in lenigallol* a remedy has been discovered which must be classed as almost ideal for all forms of eczema which are to be attacked by the mildest superficial cauterization in the rapidest manner possible.

---

*F. Kromayer. M D.. and H. Veith. Ph.D.. *Monatshefte fur prakt. Dermatol.,* Jol. 27, 1898.
H. Bottstein. M.D. (Dr A. Blaschke's Clinic, Berlin). *Therapeut. Monatshefte.* Jan., 1899.
Paul Grueneberg. M.D.. *Dermatol. Zeitschrift,* 1899, Vol 6.
E. Kromayer, M.D , and P. Grueneberg, M.D.. *Munch. Medic. Wochenschrift,* 1901, No. 6.
Franz von Poor. M D , *Orvosi Hetilop,* 1901, No. 43.
Friedr. Lnithlen, M.D., *Therapie der Hautkrankheiten,* pp. 40 and 99. (Vienna: Alfred Holder, 1902)
S. Jessner. M.D. *Dermatol. Voitroge fur Praktiker,* No. 8, pp. 55. (Stuber, 1902).
Walther Nic. Clemm M.D. *Therapeut Monatshefte.* 1902, No. 9.
Ernst Heuss, M.D, Zurich, *Paracelsus Fahresbericht,* 1899, pp. 78 *et seq.*

AN ORATION DELIVERED BY DR. W. P. C. BARTON IN 1821.
WITH EXPLANATORY NOTE.

BY WILLIAM PEPPER, M.D.,

Instructor in Medicine in the University of Pennsylvania.

(Continued from the July Issue.)

"Can it be possible," thought I, "that this man, whose physiognomy bespeaks rather extreme benevolence, intermingled with correct judgment, than keen intellect—can it be possible that he, too, is a professor in the same school?" I awaited an answer to these mental queries, in further opportunity of observation. During this period I found the professor—for such his preparations for an anatomical lecture discovered him really to be—characterized by a kind, very urbane, and conciliatory attention, a considerate, patient and willing instruction, to the pupils who were dissecting, and a remarkable degree of modesty and suavity of demeanor toward all around him. At his invitation I took a seat near the table containing the subjects for his lecture, which was at the bottom of an immense circular room, with benches rising gradually above each other to a great height, and crowded with students, the same I had seen in the field, the laboratory, the surgery and the hospital.

A profound silence reigned on the appearance of their beloved preceptor; and the pleasant countenance beaming with kind greeting, which each student presented to my view, gave goodly assurance that they were accustomed to hear from his lips strains of useful instruction. He began with great modesty after a courteous salutation; and when he became animated with his subject, a greater degree of eloquence did I never hear! Fluent, clear, concise, impressive, full of fire and enthusiasm, he taught me the useful lesson that physiognomy is not always to be trusted. Never shall I forget the effect which his demonstrations had upon me and his class! All were silent as the tomb, riveted with attention, and all evidently disappointed when a long lecture was terminated. Such a man, thought I, must make the study of anatomy a pleasure, and the hour of his prelection a mental repast.

I crossed the table, accosted my sage guide, and entreated him to give me a view of the exterior of the building, within the walls of which these eloquent and instructive lessons in the various departments of medicine were delivered. He obligingly did so.

I found it a massy structure of plain doric architecture, elevated considerably in the air, and even towering, and supported by five huge moonstone columns or pillars, deeply embedded in a solid mass of enormous stones, resembling small rocks. He informed me that they had been brought there by great labor performed by the five professors, aided by one who was dead,* and by the pupils, who occasionally lent a helping hand. That perseverance, probity, a conscientious discharge of their duties, as lecturers and preceptors, added to their learning and talents, endeared them to their pupils, and thus rendered the latter willing to impose this subsidiary help on themselves. That under the whole mass two worthies had been interred,† and, being converted into granite, were the foundation stones, giving a steadfastness and strength to the superstructure which the professors themselves had laid. He modestly said that four of the moonstone pillars were, in fact, professors; that he told me this because he would not deceive me for the world, never having, in a long life, willingly done that to any man. He directed my attention to a closer examination of the materials of these columns; and they suddenly presented to my view, strong though coarse resemblances of the professor I had seen in the fields, he in the cavern or laboratory, the one in the hospital, and that one who dissected in the anatomical theatre; and when I turned around to inquire why the fifth pillar appeared solid rock without resemblance to human kind, a mist had enveloped him, he faintly pronounced " Farewell;' and, on imploringly asking him in the grief of separation if I should never again see him, his finger alone was visible, pointing to the fifth pillar of moonstone; then, with a faint ejaculation of the word " There," the finger disappeared, and all vanished from my view. Chagrined and distressed, I voluntarily looked toward the column to which my lost guide's finger pointed, and, to my astonishment, found it a strong, unspeaking resemblance of himself! I became spellbound and bewildered, with mingled emotions and conflicting thoughts; then faint with sickheartedness, and on turning around to look for a seat, from which

---

* James Hutchinson, born in 1752, had been Professor of Materia Medica from 1789 to 1791, and Profesor of Chemistry from 1792 to 1794. He was in medical service in the patriot cause in America. He was a trustee of the University, 1779 to 1789. He also was one of the incorporators of the College of Physicians of Philadelphia. He died in 1793, aged forty-two years.

† John Morgan and William Shippen, who may well be called the foundation stones of the first medical school in America. Morgan died October 15, 1789, aged fifty-three years. Shippen died July 11, 1808, nearly seventy-two years old. Morgan was the first Professor in the Medical School, being elected to the Chair of Theory and Practice of Physic, May 3, 1765. Shippen, the second to be elected, only a few months later, September 23, 1765. So much has been written of these two young men, who on beginning their professional duties were but thirty and twenty-nine years old, respectively, that I shall add nothing further.

:ny eye could dwell on the petrified countenance of my benefactor
and guide, the scene suddenly changed.

The great massy structure had vanished from my view, while
a prospect of totally different description was presented before me.
An unbounded expanse of open sea here broke upon the sight, the
horizon only terminating the view in front. I thought myself at
the White seat of Mount Edgecumbe, in England; and from the
commanding spot where I stood the whole circumjacent country
was expanded at my feet. I could completely and distinctly over-
look Hamvaze, and the whole course of the river Tamar, as high
as the town of Sattark; the ship in the harbor, dock-yard, and
town of Dock, the fortifications and Government house; the church
and village of Stoke; the Military Hospital; the Stonehouse, with
the Naval Hospital and Marine Barracks; the citadel and
churches of Plymouth; Saltrem; Catwater, with its shipping,
enclosed by Mount Baten; St. Nicholas Island; the Sound and
Stratton Heights beyond it, the whole view bounded by a range
of lofty hills, among which the round top of Kingston Down, the
peaked head of Brent-Tor, and the irregular summits of Dart-
moor, all in rapid succession, presented themselves to my glance.*
At this moment I was hailed from the beach below by a midship-
man of a boat, who told me he had come to carry me on board the
frigate to which I belonged, and which I now found had not been
shipwrecked!

After six years' foreign service I sailed for my native country,
and thought myself, when in sight of it, again shipwrecked on the
same shores where many years before I had fallen and been
wounded, and met with relief from my chirurgical guide.†

The entrance from the landing-place, where I was thrown
into the traversable grounds, was at the end of a double avenue
of finely spreading elms. The arcade of foliage thus formed
gradually widened, and on reaching the foot of the hills it dilated
into a spacious lawn, irregularly bordered by poplar and dogwood trees, the gay Judas tree, and the flowering Aronias. Groves
of stately chestnut and other trees were scattered along its margins, and formed a natural enclosure laid out in irregular beds
of shrubs and flowers. Between this a deep valley presented
itself. Its sides above the road were planted by nature's hand,
with various fragrant shrubs, the lower part thickly overspread
with wild plants, and down the centre was a grassy walk. At
the upper end I descried a picturesque building, dedicated to
Flora, composed of moonstone arches, niches and pinnacles, and

---

* This may refer to some visit Dr. Barton made to England. .

† I take it that Dr. Barton is now describing the affairs in connection with the Medical
School a the time the wrote this oration, namely, in 1821.

overgrown with ivy. Its portal was illuminated by rays of fas-
cination, and its entrance strewed with flowers. The most perfect order, subordination and arrangement characterized each
department of this temple. The coppices which surrounded it, the
lawns which were spread before it, and even the waters which
irrigated the meadows of its neighborhood, were decked with
Flora's charms, checkering their surface with the various hues of
fragrant shrubs and trees. From a seat in the portal I could look
down on the irregularly formed vale in front, beyond the opening of which no object whatever appeared, but a wide expanse of
sea.* I soon discovered a young man at a distance digging roots
and culling flowers, shrubs and twigs of trees.† He seemed
deeply engrossed with the objects of his search, and a few seconds
after I overheard him instructing, with much ardor, a few youths
who had been concealed from my view by a thicket. He dilated
on the properties and characters of the plants before him, with an
enthusiasm which showed that he had a real love for the subject.
I approached him, and, apologizing for my intrusion, stated that
a few years before I had observed an older man deeply engaged
in the same pursuit, but with a larger train of pupils, and begged
to be informed if he were still living.‡ He replied, with an air
of sadness, that he presumed I alluded to one of the five moonstone pillars of their academy, which had fallen by the hand of
time. That three others had been prostrated by the same cause
almost simultaneously,** and the superstructure had well-nigh
tumbled to the earth. That though these pillars had been renewed,†† they were not of moonstone, but of softer material, and
the cement by which they were fixed to the base and capital of
the old columns had never thoroughly dried, owing, he presumed,
to the heterogeneous nature of the new and old materials. That
a pernicious moisture was exhaled from the still soft mortar,
which blighted all the plants in the neighborhood, and so subtle,
chilling and damp was its vapor that it insinuated itself into
the lecture-room appropriated for teaching botany, there killed

---

* Is he, perhaps, describing Bartram's Garden?

† This is Dr. W. P. C. Barton himself at this time, 1821, Professor of Botany in the
University of Pennsylvania.

‡ Dr. Benjamin Smith Barton, who died in 1813.

** Woodhouse, who died in 1809, Rush in 1813, and Wistar in 1818.

†† Dr. Woodhouse had been succeeded in 1809 by Dr. John Redman Coxe, who held the
Chair of Chemistry until 1818, and was then succeeded by Robert Hare. Dr. Coxe is
evidently the man of softer make. Dr. Rush had been succeeded in 1813 by Dr. Benjamin
Smith Barton, who held the Chair of Theory and Practice until his death in 1815, when Dr.
Nathaniel Chapman was elected. Chapman is one of those he refers to as the softer
material. Dr. B. S. Barton had been succeeded in the Chair of Materia Medica by Dr J. S.
Dorsey, who held it only two years, and was followed in 1818 by Dr. J. R. Coxe, mentioned
above. Dr. Wistar's successor will be explained later.

the plants, chilled the professor's zeal, and drove his pupils out. That, resolved never to be overcome in his pursuit, he was obliged to seek this sequestered spot (I now found it was to the professor I was speaking) with a few pupils, who avoided standing under or leaning against the new and chilling pillars, and consequently escaped the effects of the vapor-damp which emanated from them.

He further informed me that a sixth pillar had been added to the building which supported the apartment above it, destined to the cultivation of obstetrical knowledge;[*] that it was very solid and well shaped, stood somewhat apart from the new ones, and did not send forth the noxious effluvium which blighted plants near the others, because its cement had acquired solidity; but that being alone it could afford very little protection, yet what support it could yield, by occasionally suffering a twining plant to cling to it, was given; and it was evident, from the kindness with which it lent its single aid, that with a plurality of pillars of the same material, and equally innocent with itself toward the plants, much good to botany could yet be done. This young man further said that *one* moonstone pillar of the original five still remained, and to this one all the others, by one consent, and all the pupils and friends of the building, looked as its only remaining prop.[†]

"But join in my train," said he, "and I will cheerfully conduct you to a further acquaintance with this interesting subject." Eager to learn whether this remaining pillar of moonstone bore any resemblance to my former guide who dressed my wounds, I gladly accompanied him. In our walk he spoke of the surrounding scenic beauties, and called my attention to the richness and variety of the herbage and shrubbery. He told me that beside the purposes of decoration, and the joy they imparted to the beholder, the surrounding plants, shrubs and trees were not only useful, but many of them indispensable in satisfying the multifarious necessities of man; that they supplied his numerous daily wants, and in the aching hour of sickness and sorrow yielded those medicines which ministered to his comfort and relief. "Yet the study of all this," said he, "is decried as useless, and I daresay I shall have occasion to show you some of those most active in disseminating this idea, industriously at their work."

---

* Dr. Thomas Chalkley James, elected Professor of Midwifery in 1810, the first man of this country to occupy a Chair devoted solely to the teaching of Obstetrics. He was born in 1766, and graduated in 1787 from the Medical School. He was a Fellow of the College in Physicians, a member of the Philosophical Society, and one of the Medical Staff of the Pennsylvania Hospital. He died in 1835, having held his position in the University for fourteen years.

† Dr. Philip Syng Physick, who lived until 1837, being at the time of death sixty-seven years old.

We had not gone far before he descried someone in the perspective, and pointed out to me, on a nearer approach, a very elderly, gray-headed, and grave-looking man,[*] deeply engaged in girdling dogwood and tulip trees, and throwing into a burning pile large quantities of roots of Indian physic and wild ipecacuan. "Who is that, and what is the meaning of his occupation?" asked I. "Is he substituting those roots for barilla and kelp to make soda, that he should thus burn them? · And why does he kill the dogwood and tulip trees?" "Alas!" said this second botanist, "there is no rational way of accounting for his conduct, which justly excites your astonishment as it often has mine. He will not leave my medicinal ·trees and flowers to myself;· but, though he will not himself use nor recommend them, and though these grounds are none of his, nor does he know the riches they contain, he unkindly intrudes on my premises, lays waste my domains, burns my roots, and girdles my trees to kill them, saying they are useless; that we have enough medicines from foreign countries. He supplies the place of one of the fallen moonstone pillars of our school, and has ample opportunity to instigate his pupils to enter my field and tear down my flowers, as you now see him doing himself.

"The pupils, however, of that institution are characterized by their manly and correct behavior, and I really do not think I have seen a single instance of one of them injuring these products of nature, by a rude footstep or a wanton blow. They, on the contrary, walk through these vales and lawns in the heyday of spring, admire and gaze with evident pleasure on their charms, and would woo them were they not taught to believe it is against their interest. This cannot be doubted, for the natural ebullition of youthful feeling is in strict harmony with a cultivation of every department of natural history, but particularly botany."

I contrasted this information with the interesting story told me by my sage guide of the first botanist he had introduced me to, and I asked why the successor of that teacher ·in one of his branches had so much power over the interests of another chair, which he had also held. To my sorrow and chagrin I learned that a little corner only in the great building was appropriated to botany.[†] And as neither immunities, privileges, encourage-

---

[*] Dr. John Redman Coxe, born in 1773. He was a graduate of the Medical Department of the University, and also a Trustee before being elected Professor of Chemistry in 1809. In 1818 he resigned from that Chair to take that of Materia Medica. He served in this capacity, until in 1835 the Medical School went through that riotous time, so aptly termed by some wit its "attack of Coxalgia," which resulted in the forced retirement of Professor Coxe. He lived to be ninety-one years of age, dying in 1864.

[†] Dr. Barton again refers here to his chief cause of complaint, the fact that his own chair had been separated from the Medical Faculty.

ment nor reward attended the discharge of its duties, and as the room suffered greatly from the damp exhalation before spoken of, and the incumbent took cold whenever he went into it, it was not surprising that labor was vainly applied to contend against the bulls of excommunication which medical popery was perpetually throwing out from those walls. He concluded this account by telling me that the delightful spot on which we were enjoying the beauties of nature belonged to the institution, and had been purchased for a botanical garden.* But, though nature had done everything for it, the governors of the medical castle (though willing) could not appropriate funds to improve it, being sedulously taught that such an establishment would be unpopular amongst students—thus incorrectly attributing their apathy to a natural dislike of the subject, while in fact it arose, in every instance where shown, from too near an approach to the subtle and freezing vapor-damp arising from the new pillars.

"Yet," he added, "I will not deceive you. That teacher whom you have seen girdling trees has his virtues.† He conscientiously does his best. He labors and toils with increasing assiduity, and is willing to give more than his pupils bargain for. So that I am surprised he withholds his influence in favor of botany. He is reputed to be, and I believe he is, a man of great, nay, exemplary probity; yet, strange to tell, he defrauds me of my just rights, and enters my grounds with no other view than wantonly to devastate the seedling products of my soil. He is a master director of those young gentlemen whom you see hard by pounding drugs and compounding medicines. And, after a certain probation in his terms, they are taught the means of emptying the bottles and drawers of that long range of shops of nearly all their contents. The useful simplicity of this novel mode of instruction is particularly conspicuous in this country, he contends, because, in his opinion, extensive as is its territory, and rich as you have seen it is in vegetable productions, it cannot possibly be supposed capable of yielding any active medicines or drugs! The few which he has been told are so he directs them to burn and girdle, as he himself is now doing. Yet this gentleman finds too ready assistance in his views from a coadjutor of very different and very remarkable character.‡ See yonder, he is near the

---

* In 1817 the Trustees of the University did purchase a botanical garden, and the Medical Faculty subscribed $600. The ground was sold, however, shortly afterward.

† Dr. J. R. Coxe.

‡ The Faculty in 1821 was composed of:
  Dr. Coxe, Professor of Materia Medica.
  Dr. James, Professor of Midwifery.
  Dr. Chapman, Professor of Theory and Practice.

foundation of that huge mill digging a grave, and throwing medical books, essays and opinions into it, thus burying them from sight, as well as the reputation of their authors.

"Possessing a mind of keen and native power, and educated in adversity, he knows men's hearts and frailties well. He is, perhaps, the most pleasant man alive. No sternness can withstand the point of his satire, his mirth, his pleasantry and his facetiousness. Care, pain, anger, resentment, distress and mortification all fly before the shafts of his adroit colloquial talents. Need I say that to these he owes his influence? He is, too, in the main, magnanimous and forgiving, or seems so, and really possesses, or seems to possess, an uncommon share of the charities and benevolence of this life. He is not without brilliant and very subtle talents. His mind is quick in its conception, though for this reason often faulty in its views, vehement in its decisions, and consequently often indiscreet in judgment, and, finally, it acts with the celerity inseparable from dangerous errors. His mansion you perceive faces the north, and its portal opens on the path straight in that direction, which it is expected he will pursue. A few crooked and diverging lanes, all leading from the object of his life, strike out of the path directly south of his home. And, though it is quite as easy to travel to the north as to the south, the man will turn his steps that way; this strange gentleman flirts occasionally through the crooked south ways. In one of these he has imbibed notions prejudicial to the science of plants, and consequently inimical to the interests of liberal medicine. He has, fatally for that science, so far as connected with the institution over which he holds a mystic kind of influence, as well as for the real interests of enlightened medical education, not hesitated to use his utmost efforts, and successfully, to crush it. Yet he has at times planted flowers in his own garden, and reared medicinal plants there.* And, though conscious that he has gained credit for so doing, and embellished his little favorite spot, he still

---

Dr. Hare, Professor of Chemistry.

Dr. Physick, Professor of Anatomy.

Dr. Gibson, Professor of Surgery.

As Dr. Barton has spoken of Coxe, James, and Physick, the other three names are left to choose from, and, as Chapman had been connected with the school since 1810, and because Dr. Barton's description fits him better than Gibson or Hare, I believe without any doubt that he is here meant.

Dr. Nathaniel Chapman, born in 1780, of an old Virginian family descended from a Captain of Cavalry in the British army, who was a cousin of Sir Walter Raleigh, graduated in 1801 from the Medical Department of the University of Pennsylvaina. He published a book on Therapeutics and Materia Medica, and was Professor of the Theory and Practice of Medicine from 1816 to 1850. In 1848 he was by acclamation elected the first President of the American Medical Association; he was also one of the Philosophical Society. He died in 1853.

*Referring to the time (1813-16) that Dr. Chapman had been Professor of Materia Medica.

6

strangely turns in moments of slumbering perception as to what
is really useful, rudely treads down the poor innocent herbs,
plucks up the flowers by the roots, and throws the physic to the
dogs.

" The pillar, therefore, which supports his department is one
of those which sweats the same kind of subtle, insinuating, pernicious moisture which has been mentioned. It even seems,
though not so visible, to penetrate farther than the exhalation
from the others. This strange man, with all his genius, is a
schemer. He has expended much of his time in erecting and
superintending a huge Mill."[+] Here I interrupted the young
man by an ejaculation of surprise, to know what a Mill could
have to do with a medical school. The only answer I could obtain from him was the remark, attended with a significant shrug
of the shoulders and very meaning look, " that on that subject he
would not presume to speak. But he supposed, of course, it was
to grind something. And as it was near the great building, he
also thought it likely the grist came thence. The common people
supposed it was to grind physic out of dead men's bones," he
said ; " while shrewder people, namely, doctors, had openly declared it was to grind doctors themselves. All that I know
on the subject," continued he, " is that the Mill stands
where the hospital used to be ; and you must examine for
yourself, and judge accordingly. More than one miller attends
the grinding, whether this grinding be of physic or doctors. Certain is one thing, that lots of dissension have been laid out in the
neighborhood of the Mill. Discord, medical anarchy, jealousy,
suspicion and distrust have all sprung up wild weeds in the exposed parts of those lots. As, however, in the whole course of a
long study of botany I have not met with a single plant referable
to any one of the genera distinguished by these names, I am
wholly ignorant of them or their uses, nor do I wish to be further
informed on the subject." Here our conversation was interrupted
by a sudden arrival at the building itself, and the young botanist
vanished with his class, fearing, I suppose, the deadly effect of
the vapor-damps from the new pillars. I saw him no more.

I was affected with a mixture of pleasure and pain on behold-
ing once more this structure—pleasure at recognizing in the upright fifth moonstone pillar my old friend, the sage guide who
dressed my wound ; pain at discerning the evident shock and
cracks the building itself had received. The principal alterations

---

* I do not understand this allegory of the huge mill. Does it refer to the Philadelphia
Medical Institute which Dr. Chapman founded in 1817, and in which he delivered his
famous summer lectures?

I could discover were marks of removal in the fifth stone pillar
a little to the left of where it formerly stood.* And as I used to
think its old place was exactly right, I was lost in amazement to
understand why this change had been made. Indeed, I could not
help exclaiming to myself, " I would have thought no power on
earth could have achieved so miraculous a change of position."
" True," replied a voice from a crack in the wall, near the most
showy of the new pillars,† " it was a Herculean labor. But we
have a talismanic power attached to this structure, which alters
its arrangements at a moment's warning. Yet you must not suppose this pillar has been changed to another part of the building
without reason, or, at least, a semblance of it. It was not at first
contemplated to remove it. On the loss of the moonstone pillar
which last fell,‡ it was determined to supply its place by a material
of the strength and excellence of which exalted expectations were
justly formed.§ But no sooner was this done than an unexpected
blow levelled it with the earth, and again it was to be removed.
At one time a rock of schistus beset with rubies, emeralds and
topazes from a mineralogist's collection was contemplated.** At
another it was supposed a sparkling gem from the practical de-
'partment would be placed there, under the impression that the
glory-rays surrounding it would dazzle and allure, though they
could not afford a tangible support.††

" It was at length determined to supply its place by a Scotch
pebble, and a huge one was imported for the purpose. But it
was declared to have a flaw, and consequently disused.‡‡ Indeed,
after much faultfinding with the materials, some being too little,
and some too great, some from their solid nature not likely to

---

* Dr. Physick had in 1819 resigned the Chair of Surgery that he had so gloriously filled
for fourteen years, and had accepted the Chair of Anatomy; this fact had naturally
excited comment.

† Dr. William Gibson.

‡ Dr. Caspar Wistar, who died in 1818.

§ Dr. John Syng Dorsey, born in Philadelphia in 1783. He graduated from the Medical
Department of the University of Pennsylvania at the age of eighteen years, by special per-
mission from the Trustees. In 1807 he was elected Adjunct Professor of Surgery; in 1815
Professor of Materia Medica, and in 1818, on the death of Dr. Wistar, he was elected
Professor. He delivered but his introductory lecture, and was then the same evening
taken violently ill and died the same week, at the early age of thirty-five.

**In the minutes of the Board of Trustees the names given as applicants for the vacant
Chair of Anatomy are Dr. T. T. Hewson, Dr. W. E. Horner, Dr. G. S. Patterson, and Dr.
George Watson.

††Which of these Dr. Barton refers to in these two allusions I am not able to say.

‡‡Is this Dr. Granville Sharpe Patterson? In the minutes of the Board of Trustees of date
April 6, 1819, there is mention of their having received a letter dated Glasgow from him.

unite with the peculiar cement employed in keeping the building together, the present plan was adopted.†

"All the contemplated materials were easily got rid of except this huge Scotch pebble, owing to the trouble at finding a place for it in the purlieus of the building; until at length a coach, drawn by four professors, arrived from a neighboring place and carried it away, and it was found to fit well in the place allotted to it. It has since, by the handsome manner in which it is displayed in the front elevation of a building, vieing with this for solidity, brilliance and duration of materials, produced some unpleasant feeling in those who decided that it would not fit here."

The distant sounds of drums, fifes and other martial instruments of music here suspended the invisible communicant's remarks. Volumes of smoke rolled through the skies in the direction whence the sounds came. These drew nearer and nearer, became harsh, discordant and grating. A large body of men, strangely accoutred, now rapidly approached, and I could discern a troop of mounted soldiers, armed with a novel kind of warlike weapons. These were huge lancets, scalpels and gorgets. Large sheets of printed paper, stamped with opprobrious epithets in five-line pica, answered the purpose of flags, and, on a nearer inspection, it seemed to be a regiment of surgeons.

The doors of the great building were now violently thrown open, and a similar procession emerged from its apartments. A hostile disposition was soon evinced, and the combatants proceeded to immediate and desperate battle. It was, however, soon over.

Desirous to render what assistance I was able to the wounded, I approached the field of battle. Many had been slain, but I found a great number only wounded. On washing away the blood I observed that each one of the killed and wounded was marked by his name on an engraved breast-plate. I particularly remarked among the names of the slain those of Professional Dignity and Harmony. The first appeared to have been killed in the onset, and the other had evidently fought desperately before he yielded, being covered with wounds. Among the names of the wounded I read those of Propriety, Integrity, Truth, Decorum and Justice. But so desperate were the wounds that I hastily left the field to seek some other and more experienced aid. Breathless I retraced my steps to the building, hoping to find a physician or surgeon whose humanity would induce him to lend assistance; but what was my astonishment to find stains on it, from the gush of blood issuing from this fatal contest. The first assault had been made with great guns, and a few shots had penetrated two of the

---

† Namely, that of transferring Dr. Physick to the Chair of Anatomy.

pillars of the building. A dense mist from the reeking battle-ground obscured the whole structure. I found myself alone, and called loudly but vainly through the empty halls on Humanity and Decorum for aid; when, at length,. observing a crowd of physicians and surgeons standing at a distance, I beckoned their approach. They, however, obstinately resisted all solicitations to enter the field. Believing it possible that they had not understood my signals, I approached and inquired querulously who and what they were that so sullenly looked on this devastating carnage, and why they did not afford succor. They were, they said, the physicians and surgeons of the city in which these feuds originated; but to my second interrogatory coolly replied that they were mere lookers-on, and would not enter into disputes, which their hearts and heads taught them were unnecessary and ruinous,. and of which they most cordially disapproved. And as each one had a larger or smaller volume in his hand, bound in black, and containing, I found on inquiry, more or less personal complaint, which he was receiving to lay at the door of the great medical edifice, I could not blame them for their determination.[*]

I returned to the building and invoked its inhabitants, who had now entered it, by all the names of its founders to send for some healing balm for these deadly wounds. But, instead of succor craved, I had proscription thrown on my head from one window,. hatred from another, cold water from a third, and from the angry group which looked out of all I was received with frigid suspicion and distrust. " Begone ! intruder," cried they, with one voice; " we desire no balm for these feuds. It is only on terms of utter extermination of our enemies we are willing 'to make peace."

Indignant as I may naturally be supposed to have felt at this unjust and impolitic denunciation, and conscious that good motives alone actuated my conduct, I was on the point of recriminating, when I thought my path was crossed by the shadow of the venerable man I had once seen in the hospital giving clinical lectures, and imploring *" still one minute more for instruction."*

He was habited, not as he then was, but in the costume of a

---

[*] This all refers to the truly troublesome condition of Medical Education in the early twenties. Almost every practitioner of any prominence unconnected with the University of Pennsylvania had his private school for medical students, and many were the squabbles and fights. Dr. W. P. C. Barton, while Professor of Botany in the University, applied to the Legislature during the session of 1818-19 for a charter, intending to start up a rival medical school; this attempt was very nearly successful. Such affairs must have caused very strained relations between a great many of the physicians in Philadelphia. In the Philadelphia Medical Society the discussions were very warm and lengthy, and the daily press was also used by the contestants to air their views. From all this fomenting sprang (in 1825) the Jefferson Medical College, to which Dr. Barton changed his allegiance, which, for the University, had become very slight by this time.

prophet, and it was only by his peculiar physiognomy that I recognized him. A large black cowl was drawn carelessly over his head and shoulders, while his silvered locks strayed from under it, and by separating on the forehead discovered a wreath of green and imperishable holly twined round his wrinkled brow. A sackcloth robe drawn tight to his waist by cincture of scintillating gems invested his aged frame and tottering limbs. His sorrowful eyes were fixed on the building, while the furrows of his keen visage were filled with floods of galling tears. Overcome withal by his mysterious appearance, I did not venture to address him, not knowing, indeed, whether he was a sprite of the glens, a being of this, or a spirit of the other world. A deep, sepulchral voice soon convinced me that he was the latter. He waved a wand of mistletoe which he carried in his left hand, while with his right he grasped mine and drew me rapidly away.

"Come, young man, from the vicinity of that tottering pile," said he; "see ye not that it is falling?" And here sobs of grief choked his utterance. When a little recovered, he addressed me in these prophetic words: "Some of the inhabitants of that structure are academicians of Laputa and Balnibari. They are projectors of so wild a cast that they seem to verify the old observation 'that there is nothing so extravagant and irrational which some philosophers have not maintained for Truth.' They possess the power or claim the prerogative of extensive monopoly, and edicting bulls of excommunication and ruin. They act, in some of their freaks of self-aggrandizement and fame, like harlequins of a fair, before a mixed and tumultuous concourse of people, who, according as they are directed by minions in the crowd, evince a pandemic impulse in their favor and applaud them for their charlatanical tricks. They domineer with ill-judged intolerance over all without their walls, and then wonder that they are jealously watched. They set themselves up, though but two or three of a whole body, as umpires of merit and awarders of just praise, taking care to foster or protect none but those willing to be trammelled by subserviency to their will. Yet scrutinize this self-appointed caucus—this fag-end of a distinguished public assembly. It has not even the aspect of a deliberative association nor the physiognomy of an impartial tribunal of professional merit, equity, or justice—*nec color imperii, nec frons erat ulla senatus.* They have power, but, like the evil genius, they blindly use it to destroy themselves. Tyranny produces, in a country and a profession like theirs, the most ruinous effects. Dissolute monopoly and extravagant thirst for unearned fame will abuse a cause which, judiciously conducted, would produce an influx of solid reputation. The spring of that spirit which should move such a body is relaxed by intolerance or snapped by arbitrariness. They, by intemperate exercise of their ill-used talents, sophistically confound their power with a sense of justice and prudence. And they will perceive too late that it is only when power and justice are the same that they can exert the former to the stretch they have extended it, consistently with wisdom or even self-interest itself. They will find that vain and idle speculation and purloined effulgence will never penetrate beyond the mist which envelops the community.

" Be assured, then, that such measures are as certainly ruinous as they are manifestly impolitic and unjust. Where there is such repeated confiscation of character to satisfy self-interested views the treasury may grow rich, but it will groan ere long, with its ill-acquired wealth burst its enclosures, and waste its coin on the greedy onlookers who cry ' *scrambles,*' and each catches what he can get!

" Already rival institutions are performing this part, and it will be surprising if the natural and just causes of blame at home, united with the force of novelty and exaggerated odium abroad, do not eventually seduce away the youthful concourse which in my day filled that mansion.

" Where there is no dignity there can be no philosophy, and where sophistry reigns truth cannot stay. Wonder not, then, if ere a few short years rapacity after fame, inveterate deafness to the merits of others, and a sordid desire to accumulate wealth at the expense of duty shall raze with the earth this once gorgeous structure in which you have taken so much interest. And that such will be the result *I prophesy!*

" Once earnestly engaged·in decorating it by my toil, I have not ceased to haunt its walls with parental solicitude. I have heard the discourses delivered in it, and insinuated myself into its secret council chambers. Though I confess I have found several occupying the places of dignity, truth and science, and honestly and perseveringly pursuing their ways, some who occupy the *highest* seats in the synagogue remind me of Burke's pathetic reflection on the state of philosophy and learning in France during the period of its cabalistic anarchy. ' Alas! the age of chivalry is done, that of sophisters and self-aggrandizing calculators has succeeded, and the glory of Europe is extinguished forever!' " And having said this he struck me with his wand, the darkness was dispelled, the building became visible, he mysteriously pointed to the fifth moonstone pillar, saying, " Observe, think and judge for yourself," and vanished into air!

A tumult arose from the lobbies of the building, which I found occasioned by the pupils running hastily, some to the north and others to the south to finish their studies. The sudden noise of their footsteps and vociferations awakened me, I presume, for I found myself in the act of taking leave of them as I now, gentlemen, do of you.

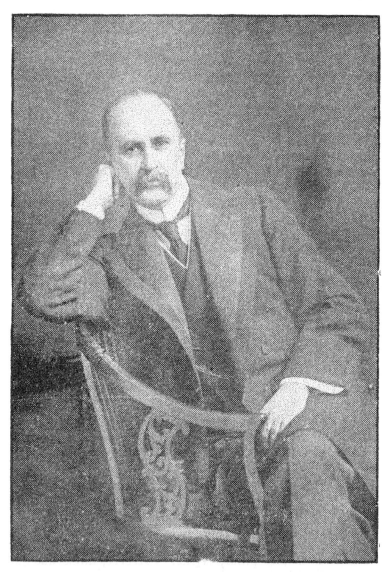

DR. WILLIAM OSLER, RECENTLY APPOINTED BY KING EDWARD VII.
REGIUS PROFESSOR OF MEDICINE, OXFORD UNIVERSITY.
(*Vide* page 205.)

The Canadian
Journal of Medicine and Surgery

J. J. CASSIDY, M.D.,
EDITOR,
43 BLOOR STREET EAST, TORONTO.

W. A. YOUNG, M.D., L.R.C.P.Lond.,
MANAGING EDITOR,
145 COLLEGE STREET, TORONTO.

Surgery—BRUCE L. RIORDAN, M D.,C M., McGill University; M D University of Toronto; Surgeon Toronto General Hospital; Surgeon Grand Trunk R R.; Consulting Surgeon Toronto Home for Incurables; Pension Examiner United States Government: and F. N. G. STARR, M B., Toronto, Associate Professor of Clinical Surgery, Toronto University; Surgeon to the Out-Door Department Toronto General Hospital and Hospital for Sick Children

Clinical Surgery—ALEX PRIMROSE, M B., C.M. Edinburgh University; Professor of Anatomy and Director of the Anatomical Department, Toronto University Associate Professor of Clinical Surgery, Toronto University; Secretary Medical Faculty, Toronto University

Orthopedic Surgery—B. E MCKENZIE, B A., M.D., Toronto, Surgeon to the Toronto Orthopedic Hospital; Surgeon to the Out-Patient Department, Toronto General Hospital; Assistant Professor of Clinical Surgery, Ontario Medical College for Women; Member of the American Orthopedic Association; and H. P. H. GALLOWAY, M D., Toronto, Surgeon to the Toronto Orthopedic Hospital; Orthopedic Surgeon, Toronto Western Hospital; Member of the American Orthopedic Association.

Oral Surgery—E H. ADAMS, M.D., D.D S, Toronto.

Surgical Pathology—T H MANLEY, M D., New York, Visiting Surgeon to Harlem Hospital, Professor of Surgery, New York School of Clinical Medicine, New York, etc, etc.

Gynecology and Obstetrics—GEO. T. MCKEOUGH, M.D., M.R.C.S Eng, Chatham, Ont.; and J. H LOWE, M.D., Newmarket, Ont

Medical Jurisprudence and Toxicology—ARTHUR JUKES JOHNSON, M.B, M R.C S Eng; Coroner for the City of Toronto; Surgeon Toronto Railway Co., Toronto; W. A YOUNG, M D, L R C.P. Lond.; Associate Coroner, City of Toronto.

Pharmacology and Therapeutics—A. J. HARRINGTON M D., M R C S.Eng, Toronto

Medicine—J J. CASSIDY, M D, Toronto, Member Ontario Provincial Board of Health; Consulting Surgeon, Toronto General Hospital; and W. J. WILSON, M D. Toronto, Physician Toronto Western Hospital.

Clinical Medicine—ALEXANDER MCPHEDRAN, M D., Professor of Medicine and Clinical Medicine Toronto University; Physician Toronto General Hospital, St Michael's Hospital, and Victoria Hospital for Sick Children.

Mental and Nervous Diseases—N. H BEEMER, M. D. Mimico Insane Asylum, CAMPBELL MEYERS, M.D M.R C S L R.C P (London, Eng), Private Hospital Deer Park, Toronto; and EZRA H STAFFORD, M.D.

Public Health and Hygiene—J J CASSIDY, M D, Toronto, Member Ontario Provincial Board of Health; Consulting Surgeon Toronto General Hospital; and E. H. ADAMS, M D., Toronto

Physiology—A B EADIE, M D., Toronto, Professor of Physiology Woman s Medical College, Toronto

Pediatrics—AUGUSTA STOWE GULLEN, M D., Toronto, Professor of Diseases of Children Woman s Medical College, Toronto, A. R GORDON, M D., Toronto.

Pathology—W. H PEPLER, M D., C.M, Trinity University; Pathologist Hospital for Sick Children, Toronto; Associate Demonstrator of Pathology Toronto University: Physician to Outdoor Department Toronto General Hospital; Surgeon Canadian Pacific R R., Toronto; and J J MACKENZIE, B.A., M B, Professor of Pathology and Bacteriology Toronto University Medical Faculty.

Ophthalmology and Otology—J M. MACCALLUM, M D., Toronto, Professor of Materia Medica Toronto University; Assistant Physician Toronto General Hospital; Oculist and Aurist Victoria Hospital for Sick Children, Toronto

Laryngology and Rhinology—J D. THORBURN, M D., Toronto, Laryngologist and Rhinologist, Toronto General Hospital.

Address all Communications, Correspondence, Books, Matter Regarding Advertising, and make all Cheques, Drafts and Post-office Orders payable to "The Canadian Journal of Medicine and Surgery," 145 College St., Toronto, Canada.

Doctors will confer a favor by sending news, reports and papers of interest from any section of the country. Individual experience and theories are also solicited Contributors must kindly remember that all papers, reports, correspondence, etc, *must be* in our hands by the fifteenth of the month previous to publication.

Advertisements, to insure insertion in the issue of any month should be sent not later than the tenth of the preceding month. London, Eng Representative, W. Hamilton Miln, 8 Bouverie Street, E. C. Agents for Germany Saarbach's News Exchange, Mainz, Germany.

VOL. XVI.   TORONTO, SEPTEMBER, 1904.   NO. 3.

Editorials.

QUACK ADVERTISEMENTS.

On August 2nd, one of the closing days of the last session of the Federal Parliament of Canada, Sir William Mulock introduced an amendment to the Post Office Act in order to restrict quack advertisements. The amendment reads as follows: " It shall not be lawful to transmit by mail any books, magazines, periodicals, circulars, newspapers, or other publications, which contain advertisements representing marvellous, extravagant or grossly improbable cures, or curative or healing powers, by means of medicines, appliances or devices referred to in such advertisements."

In speaking to the amendment, Sir William said that it was necessary to put a stop to the methods of scoundrels who advertise marvellous cures and make fortunes out of the unfortunate sufferers. Only the other day one advertisement claiming supernatural powers and shocking in its nature was published. This method of making fortunes was one of the greatest frauds allowed by the law of the land.

The amendment was adopted and the bill reported. On the following day, August 3rd, however, at the request of the leader of the Opposition, Mr. R. L. Borden, the bill to further amend the Post Office Act was referred back to the Committee of the Whole for the purpose of striking out the clause inserted at the suggestion of Sir William Mulock, prohibiting the passage through the mails of newspapers, magazines and periodicals containing advertisements of marvellous, curative medicines, etc. Mr. Borden said that very little consideration had been given to the clause, which was far-reaching in its effects. He had received many representations in reference to the matter, and thought it might well be left over till next year without any great evil being done. Sir William Mulock accepted the suggestion of Mr. Borden and the bill was amended accordingly. Mr. Borden's first statement, that very little consideration had been given to the clause, which was far-reaching in its effects, coupled with the second statement, that he had received many representations in reference to the matter, and thought it might well be left over till next year without any great evil being done, meant a good deal which does not appear on the surface. In the first place it meant: That the patent medicine advertisers of Canadian newspapers did a good deal of consideration after Sir William Mulock's amendment had been adopted by the Committee of the Whole in the Canadian Parliament on August 2nd; in the second place it meant that they sent many representatives to the leader of the Opposition in reference to the amendment; so many, indeed, that as the Government had announced a wish to prorogue on Saturday, August 6th, Mr. Borden had only to indicate his determination to fight Sir William Mulock's amendment to a finish in order to show that the retention of the dangerous amendment in the Civil Service Amendment bill would mean a considerable prolongation of the session.

As Sir William did not wish to injure his bantling's health, he picked it out of the ring and retired it for the present. Thanks, Sir William Mulock. We shall keep an eye on the Civil Service Act and expect to see your amendment in the forefront of the fight next session.

We cordially approve of the amendment outlined above, and hope that it will become law in Canada. Our readers will recall that in several issues of this journal we have drawn attention to the shameless quack advertisements which deface our leading newspapers, and we feel gratified that our strictures have evoked a very telling protest. The editors of our newspapers, the leaders and formers of public opinion, forsooth, know full well that these quack advertisements are all a pack of lies; but they print them all the same, because it pays them to do so. One of these papers had the effrontery to turn on this journal and endeavor to prove a *tu quoque,* stating that the real reason why we object to the lucrative traffic between the owners of proprietary medicines and newspapers is because we want to do it all ourselves.

Let us say, once for all, that this argument is baseless. The newspaper reading public contains in its ranks a great many credulous, unskilled, uneducated persons, quite unable to form a valid opinion as to the diseases or ailments from which they suffer, and incapable of differentiating between good, bad or indifferent remedies for the same. Proprietary medicines which are advertised to the medical profession in reputable medical journals are offered to keen critics, who believe in facts and know exactly what they seek; *i.e.,* understand the diseased condition they are treating and know what they may expect from a remedy. The owner of a proprietary medicine who sets out to please the medical profession must be perfectly sure of his ground, be accurate in his statements, and must, if he wishes to receive the financial backing of his patrons, supply a first-class article.

Is there any comparison between advertising of this kind and the shameless, blatant advertising of the general press? None whatever. We repeat that we are delighted with the stand taken by the Canadian Postmaster-General for repressing quack advertisements, and think we voice the opinion of Canadian physicians when we say that Sir William Mulock deserves the highest praise at our hands for the contemplated amendment to the Post Office Act.

NEW RESEARCHES IN DIPHTHERITIC PARALYSIS.

Dr. Leo Babonneix has just published at Paris a thesis, in which he details some new researches made by him to elucidate the origin of diphtheritic paralysis. An abstract of this thesis appears in *La Presse Médicale* (June 4th, 1904). In the first pages reference is made to the notions prevalent to-day about the nature of diphtheritic paralysis, which may be summarized as follows: Anatomico-pathological examinations reveal cellular lesions in the spinal marrow, especially in the anterior horns and neuritis, ordinarily of the Wallerian type, and sometimes of the peri-axial type. Experimentally he succeeded in reproducing these legions, but whether the question related to human paralyses or experimental paralysis, the lesions of neuritis may exist alone, or be accompanied by central lesions. From these anatomico-pathological facts it results that some authors explain diphtheritic paralysis as a pure neuritis, while others believe in the coexistence of medullary and peripheral lesions. This coexistence leaves involved the question whether the lesions have developed in a concomitant fashion or if some have appeared as a consequence of others; peripheral lesions secondary to central ones, or *vice versa;* the partisans of the theory of ascending neuritis are much less numerous than the partisans of the other theory. Respecting the *modus faciendi* of the lesions, two theories offer interpretations: that of Roux and Yersin, who attribute their production to the toxin brought by means of the blood, and the theory of Beaulieu, who places these lesions under the dependence of a direct action of the bacilli carried to the nerve tissue. In presence of these pathogenic uncertainties the author remarks that one cannot dream of establishing a one-way pathogenesis, because it is not a case of *one,* but of *several* diphtheritic paralyses, and because in what concerns more particularly experimental paralyses, those which he has reproduced up to the present time differ profoundly from human paralyses. Experimentation ought, therefore, to aim at realizing paralyses approaching as closely as possible to the paralyses observed in man.

The most important clinical character of human paralyses consists in the remarkable relation which, in the majority of cases, exists between the seat of the primitive diphtheritic inoculation and that of the consecutive paralysis; pharyngeal diphtheria, for instance, followed by paralysis of the velum palati. In certain cases even a unilateral paralysis succeeds a unilateral angina. This is the leading idea which the author has followed in his experiments when diphtheritic toxin has been introduced into the dog and the rabbit. By intra-venous injection of strong doses of toxin he has succeeded in reproducing, as Roux and Yersin and many others have done, subacute intoxication without paralysis; by subcutaneous injection of strong doses of toxin acute ascending paralysis has resulted, followed by death in a few days. These results bear no evolutionary or symptomatic analogy to what is observed in man. To reproduce paralyses exactly similar to human ones, it is necessary to operate with very small doses of an attenuated toxin, and then one gets a monoplegia strictly localized in the paw of the animal, where the injection was made. By augmenting the dose a little, one gets paralysis, beginning in the inoculated region like the generalized form observed in man and which increases slowly in the sequel. In spite of everything one obtains in these experiments only an analogy, and the experimental reproduction of generalized human paralyses remains yet to be realized.

Localization of paralytic phenomena in the injected member makes one ask if the toxin follows the blood route, or the nerve route, in causing these lesions. The experiment made to settle this question, and which consists in injecting toxin into the sciatic nerve, brings about a paralysis of the corresponding paw, but the paralysis does not always remain localized in the same paw and may extend to the opposite one.

Experimentally, therefore, one may realize all the intermediate conditions between subacute intoxication without paralysis and strictly localized paralysis; the relation between primitive diphtheritic localization and consecutive paralysis appears to be explained by the ascending propagation of the toxin along the peripheral nerves. This is a new idea, which permits us to place diphtheria alongside of certain infectious diseases, such as rabies and tetanus.

From the experimental point of view the researches of Dr. Babonneix make him conclude that, like Landry's paralysis, experimental paralyses are due to central lesions; localized paralyses appear equally to spring from central lesions, although they are less marked. Finally certain distant paralyses obtained by injection of toxin into the sciatic nerve appear to be connected with an ascending neuritis.   . J. J. C.

OUR REPORT OF THE VANCOUVER MEETING.

As the current issue of THE JOURNAL goes to press before the Canadian Medical Association adjourns at Vancouver, B.C., it is impossible for us to publish our special report till next month.

From appearances at time of writing, the 1904 session of our National Association is going to be a huge success from every standpoint, and, notwithstanding the fact that to attend the Convention means a trip across the Continent, we understand that, in point of numbers, it will almost beat the record.

We hope to give our subscribers the benefit of a splendid report in detail in next issue, thinking it wiser to do so than to disappoint them by not coming out, as is our wont, sharp on the first of the month.   W. A. Y.

TORONTO'S NEW MEDICAL LIBRARY.

A MEDICAL library in a University City the size of Toronto is a necessity. For years we have had one, good enough in its way, but hardly adequate to the demands of the present. The value of the library as a factor in medical education cannot be over-estimated. We feel we cannot do the subject more graceful justice than by reprinting a paragraph from the interesting paper of Albert T. Huntington, of Brooklyn, N.Y., published in the *Medical Library and Historical Journal,* of April, 1904. He writes: " As Dr. Spivak has pointed out, the medical school course is merely preparatory for what is to follow. Real knowledge of the science and art of medicine is post-graduate. . . . Private practice is the first institution, a teacher grim and morose, but of the highest order, if one only knows how to take advantage of its chastising lesson. Hospital practice is an institution wherein instruction is more systematized, the observations more certain, and the results better noted. Unfortunately there are but few in a city and less in the country. . . . who can utilize it. Medical societies are valuable means of education, fostering and encouraging thought. But they have their drawbacks—the stated meetings that one is unable to attend; the subject that one is obliged to listen to in which he is not interested; the idle and empty discussions from which there is no escape even in the best societies, etc. There is but one grand institution that stands above all, that has

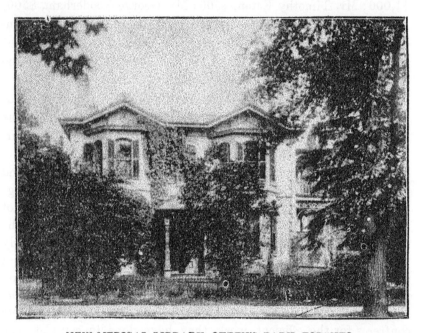

NEW MEDICAL LIBRARY, QUEEN'S PARK, TORONTO.

all the virtues and none of the defects of those enumerated, and that is the *library*. . . . On this shelf is my physiological laboratory, on the other my biological institute; here is my anatomical theatre, there my lying-in hospital."

A library near the circle of student life, and yet not too far from the centre of the city, where the members of the profession could peruse some " latest edition," or meet and chat over things medical amid comfortable and pleasant surroundings has been a longed-for oasis in the Sahara of the Toronto doctor's daily round. But, alas, the project was only a longing, until three men, good and true, saw this new harvest moon over their left shoulder, and

wished, and (with apologies) a goose laid a golden egg, and then
other geese who wanted to peck at the oats in the new barnyard followed the example of the leader, and, presto! birds of a feather,
" the house is yours." The site is a beautiful one, consisting of
No. 9 Queen's Park, worth about $12,000.

The acquisition of the Thorne residence was rendered practicable by the generosity of the Massey estate, which subscribed
$5,000 towards that purpose. Other generous friends then came
forward, including Dr. Wm. Osler, of Philadelphia, who subscribed
$1,000; Mr. Timothy Eaton, $500; Mr. George Gooderham, $500,
and Mr. E. B. Osler, $500, and others, the medical profession con-
tributing the balance. The property has been put in the hands of
the following trustees: Dr. J. F. W. Ross, President of the
Association; Dr. R. A. Reeve and Dr. N. A. Powell.

The library housed at present in the Medical Council Building, on Bay Street, consists of about 8,000 volumes. But the
Association intend, upon removing to their new building, to encourage the use of it as a meeting place for the profession.

The Toronto Medical Society, the Toronto Clinical Society and
the Toronto Pathological Society will hold their regular meetings
there as soon as the necessary alterations are made. Sufficient of
the funds now in hand will be invested in order to yield the
small charge per annum for the leasehold, which still has nearly
twenty years to run and is renewable. It is proposed to put a
competent librarian in charge, who will catalogue the books and
make the library of the greatest possible use to the profession.
Dr. J. F. W. Ross and his Associates deserve the thanks of their
confreres for the efficient work they have done to complete the
purchase of this beautiful property, of which the profession has
every reason to feel proud.

We hope the city authorities will unhesitatingly consent to
the new medical library being exempt from taxation. As medical men, we feel we are in this not begging any favor; but that, as
the building is to be used for scientific purposes, it rightfully has
a place on the honor roll of institutions free from the payment of
taxes. The new building is to be unhampered by cliquism,
devoid of University control, and free to the profession throughout Ontario. Let the City Council do their duty in this matter
and thereby earn at least the gratitude of the medical profession
in Toronto.

In these days of rapid and cheap travel by boat and train what a boon the Toronto medical library may prove to the physiciaus living in the country, who often sigh regretfully and justly envy the privileges enjoyed, or, perchance, unappreciated, by the city doctors. We understand the door of the new building is ever to be on the latch, and the old clock on the stairs is to each hour " chime," " Welcome."   w. a. y.

HONOR CONFERRED ON DR. WILLIAM OSLER.

Just as we go to press we learn with great pleasure of the appointment of our distinguished confrère and fellow countryman, Dr. Wm. Osler, of Johns Hopkins University, Baltimore, Md., as Regius Professor of Medicine at the University of Oxford. Perhaps King Edward has, since his accession to the throne, done no more gracious act than this one, in so honoring a Canadian scientist, than whom none stand higher in the profession the wide world over.

We understand that Dr. Osler has accepted the offer made him, but does not intend to remove to England for a year or so.

Dr. Osler's appointment as Prefessor in one of the greatest Universities in the world is a severe blow to Johns Hopkins, and it will be found very difficult to fill the position he has occupied there.

We extend our heartiest congratulations to, not only the recipient of this honor, but to Oxford University who will, through the appointment, find still added strength and increased prestige in the eyes of the scientific world. We fully concur in what the *Telegram*, (Toronto) says Editorially in this connection.

" Greatness on the line of Dr. William Osler's genius is difficult of attainment and unapproached in the blessings it conveys to suffering humanity.

Such greatness is not honored with the applause that rewards other and cheaper types of human greatness.

But Medical Science has her heroes no less renowned that those of art or literature, sport or finance, and William Osler is a sovereign figure in the realm of modern medicine.

There is perhaps no greater living Canadian than Dr. William Osler, if Greatness is measured by its humane and helpful qualities. Canada is honored in the honor that comes in King Edward's appointment of Dr. Osler to the place of Regius Professor of Medicine at the University of Oxford."   w. a. y.

EDITORIAL NOTES.

Bulletin No. 96, Adulterated Jams and Jellies.—Out of a total of 74 specimens of jams and jellies, which were examined in the Inland Revenue Department, Ottawa, 55 were found adulterated, 5 doubtful, and only 14 genuine. Thos. Macfarlane, Chief Analyst, says: " They (jams and jellies) are, as Webster defines jam, the products of boiling fruits with sugar and water. The only word about which any doubt can exist is the word ' sugar.' This is defined by the same authority as a sweet crystalline substance, obtained from certain vegetable products, as the sugar cane, maple, beet, sorghum, and the like. This identifies sugar as the substance known to chemists under the names cane sugar or sucrose. Commercial glucose is not grape sugar, but a product of the action of acids on starch of very inde-finite composition, always containing, as well as reducing sugars, dextrine, starch, water, etc. Every grocer and consumer under-stands quite as well what is meant by sugar, and the substitution of commercial glucose for it in ordinary trade would not be tolerated. It is also to be remembered that reputable manufac-turers of jams and jellies use only cane sugar in preserving. Similar views to the foregoing prevail in other countries, and more especially among the Boards of Health in the United States. In general the rulings of the latter are to the effect that fruit jellies, preserves, canned fruits, etc., must consist of the fruit specified on the label of the package preserved only with cane sugar, and must not contain artificial flavors, coloring matter, or preservatives. If such articles contain any substitute for the fruit, or any material to make weight or bulk, they are considered to be adulterated." Now that the adulteration of jams and jellies with glucose is well known, would it not be well for the Depart-ment of Trade and Commerce of Canada to let the grocers know that they must not offer for sale any jams except those preserved in grape sugar ?

Organic Plumbing of the Upper Epiphysis of the Tibia after an Osteo-Myelitic Abscess.—Dr. Chaput presented to the Parisian Society of Surgery (March 1st, 1904), a woman, forty years of age, whom he had been called to treat over a year before for a large abscess of the upper epiphysis of the tibia, which appeared after several attacks of osteomyelitis. After trephining the epiphysis, and carefully curetting the abscess, which was about the size of a large walnut, with eburnated, congested and bleeding walls, Dr. Chaput introduced into the bony cavity a large lump of adipose tissue, got by making an incision in the iliac fossa of the patient. He afterwards stitched the soft parts over the cavity, allowing for a small orifice over the cavity. This result was satisfactory. The graft remained in place and survived, the wound contracted rapidly and closed entirely in five months. The patient has remained well since ·then· Dr. Chaput thought that this case was interesting enough to publish, for surgeons know how difficult it is. to obtain the healing of an epiphyseal osteo-myelitic abscess, particularly when the walls of the abscess are eburnated, congested and infected; the greater number of such abscesses persisting indefinitely in a fistulous condition. It was for this reason that Dr. Chaput selected, after much thought, a procedure which enabled him to obtain a surer and more rapid cure than the one usually obtained. The graft of cellular tissue, which he put into the bony cavity, immediately checked the free oozing of bloody fluid, rendered unnecessary the plugging of the cavity with gauze drains, which infect the wound, and drain imperfectly, and obtained the immediate reunion of the graft with the bony walls of the cavity· Dr. Chaput thinks that this method of organic plumbing is simpler, surer and less dangerous than metallic, mineral or medicinal plumbing, any one of which is liable to be followed by the elimination of the foreign body. Besides, it is always an easy matter to find in the gluteal region of even a thin patient enough cellular tissue to obliterate a bony cavity in a large epiphysis.

Overfeeding with Sugar.—Dr. Toulouse reported to the Therapeutical Society of Paris (June 22nd, 1904), some experiments which he had carried on in order to determine the dietetic value of sugar in different morbid conditions in which emaciation of the patient is to be prevented. He used sugar given in large doses, over and above the ordinary hospital diet or milk diet. The quantity of sugar varied from 50 to 300 grammes per diem, amounting in emaciated women to 8 grammes of sugar per kilo of body weight. The results obtained were remarkable. From the

time this regimen was begun, the patients fattened at the rate of
100 grammes per diem at certain periods, and in certain patients
the increase in weight amounted to 500 grammes, which was consequently over the daily amount of sugar taken. Patients thus
gained a third of their weight, rising in a few months from 35
to 48 kilos. During the overfeeding with sugar examinations of
the urine generally showed a lowering of the level of the nitrogenous wastes, without the proportions appearing sensibly changed.
With a milk diet of three litres of milk per diem, sugar exercised
the most intense action. Fermentation of the stomach and digestive
troubles were not observed. These high doses of sugar do not pass
off by the urine in healthy persons. The experiments show the
doses in which sugar can be used in therapeutical alimentation. It
is an exceedingly active agent, and is free from visible inconveni-
ences in conditions of profound malnutrition, especially in cases
in which the patients are not well nourished as the result of digestive troubles.

**Metallic Suture in Simple Fracture of the Femur—Perfect
Result.**—At a regular meeting of the Surgical Society of Paris
(June 9th, 1904), Dr. Dujarier presented a patient, a man about
thirty years old, whom he had treated for fracture of the femur
by means of a metallic hook-and-eye suture, and also two radiographs, one taken before and the other after treatment. The
fracture was at the junction of the upper with the middle third
of the bone, and the two fragments had been widely separated.
After an incision in the soft spots, and a complete reduction of
the fracture, together with the removal of a detached spiculum
of bone, Dr. Dujarier reunited the two ends of the femur with a
metal hook-and-eye. The result obtained is perfect. This also appears from the radiograph, which was taken two months after
the accident, in which the two fragments can be seen exactly
coaptated, end to end, without the slightest deviation. There is
no shortening and the patient walks without any appearance of
lameness.

**Branch Laboratory of the Provincial Board of Health of
Kingston, Ont.**—Arrangements have been made by the Ontario
Government for the establishment of a branch laboratory of the
Provincial Board of Health at Kingston. Dr. W. T. Connell

has been appointed Assistant Bacteriologist for Ontario, and he has arranged with the medical faculty of Queen's University for the use of the laboratories in making the necessary examinations. These duties Dr. Connell assumes, in addition to his duties as professor of pathology and bacteriology, professor of sanitary science, and secretary of the Kingston faculty of medicine. Dr. W. T. Connell announces that he will make free examinations for medical practitioners of swabs from cases of diphtheria (diagnosis or release), blood from suspected typhoid fever, sputum for tubercle bacilli or pneumococci, and pus, for its contained micro-organisms. Bacteriological examinations of water samples will be made when such are forwarded through officials of local boards of health. Urine, tumors and morbid tissues do not come under free regulations. The address is Dr. W. T. Connell, Pathological Laboratory, Queen's University, Kingston, Ont. We cordially extend our congratulations to Dr. Connell, and hope that the relations established between himself and the Provincial Health Department will be advantageous to the physicians living in the eastern part of the Province.

Contaminated Food Causes Summer Diarrhea. — Dr. Starkey, Professor of Hygiene, McGill University, reaches the following conclusions as to the causes of summer diarrhea in Montreal: First, attention to external ventilation, so that such things as blind alleys, closed-in courtyards, should never be constructed or allowed. In this way the air ventilating the house immediately around would certainly be pure and free from infectious disease. Second, the proper paving and drainage of these yards would prevent the soil becoming badly polluted, and eventually giving rise to infectious dust. Third, the removal of refuse is important, applying both to house refuse, which is found lying in the yards, in many instances forming foul heaps, and also to the removal of the liquid house refuse, namely, that associated with drains, privies and cesspools. Fourth, cleanliness; that is, frequent and efficient washing of these paved yards would lessen the incidence of the disease. Dr. Starkey thinks that the diarrhea results from the contamination of the food of the inhabitants, and his recommendations are based on the fact that they would tend to prevent the food becoming contaminated. He does not minimise the good results obtained from the sterilization of food, because, as he states, food might be contaminated elsewhere than in the homes of the people, and, under these circumstances, only sterilization before consumption would lessen the risk of disease.

Radiograph of an Old Fracture of the Patella.—Dr. Lucas-Championièrc, who has had an extensive experience of the ad vantages of silver wire suture in fracture of the patella, recently presented to the Surgical Society of Paris the radiograph of a patella, on which he had operated three and a half years ago for fracture. The bone having split into five pieces, the suturing of so many fragments would have been impossible, so that the operator contented himself with uniting them by drawing silver wires around them. The radiograph showed that consolidation of the pieces of bone had taken place under favorable conditions; the patella was a little spread out, but of a regular shape, and of sufficient depth. One of the silver wires had got loose, but had not caused any trouble, and (a remarkable fact) it is in the way of being absorbed. The patient walks very well.

Contagious Diseases of Animals (Canada.)—An important amendment to the Canada Animal Contagious Diseases Act of 1903 was adopted and a bill founded thereon passed through the Federal Parliament just before prorogation. The provisions of the amendment add " maladie du coit " to the list of contagious diseases, and provide that the compensation, if any, for slaughtered animals will be two-thirds of the value of the animal before it was infected. Maladie du coit is a contagious disease of the generative organs of the horse. It is comparatively rare, but, unfortunately, is considered incurable. In case a valuable stallion were to become infected, a compensation equal to two-thirds the value of the animal would be allowed by the new amendment. In· reference to the other contagious diseases of animals, the amendment is quite sound. The owners of animals afflicted with contagious disease are not likely to assist in depleting their byres, unless the Department of Agriculture is willing to assist them in making good the loss. As the Government is willing to increase the compensation to two-thirds of the value of the animal, we may expect that in future the owners of diseased stock will assist in giving notification of the contagious disease.

Street Telephones.—From *Literary Digest,* August 6th: That telephones at street corners, either on the telephone pole or on the same post with the mail-box, may be a future convenience of many cities and towns, is asserted in *Popular Mechanics* (July). Says this paper: " Already they are in use to a limited extent, keyless stations opened by merely turning the handle, and which contain the pay station and a directory, being the equipment. Hollow iron posts allow the necessary ground wires. In some places the agreement with the company insures that, for the privilege of placing the telephones, all emergency calls, such as police, fire departments and hospitals, may be free of charge. This makes the system a public benefaction, saving time in case of fire or accident, and to an extent protecting the citizen. These stations are paying investments to telephone companies, as they require little extra wiring and cost little to maintain. George A. Long, in the *American Telephone Journal,* says there is no reason why these stations should not supersede the so-called police telephone systems now in use. Police could send in their reports to headquarters over the public stations, and the blue police-box would no longer be needed; certain that such a system in residential sections would be of great public benefit. How often it would save persons going four or five blocks to the drug-store or grocery." May we add what an unspeakable boon to the tired workman, who often has to walk a long distance to ring the door-bell at his physician's house to summon him in the wee sma' hours to attend some ailing member of his household. The mouth piece of a public telephone is apt to become laden with disease germs which may be inhaled by healthy persons and cause in many cases severe illness. To obviate the possibility of this suggested danger, a Frenchman has invented a method which prevents any disease germs lodging in the receiver. He puts a pad of paper into the mouthpiece, containing a hole in the centre, and the the upper disk of the pad is torn off after every conversation.   W. A. Y.

PERSONAL.

Drs. W. A. Creswell and R. W. Irving, late senior house surgeons at Toronto General Hospital, left on August 3rd for the West, where they have received lucrative positions.

❧ *School Hygiene.* ❧

THE NUREMBERG CONGRESS.

THE great success which attended the First International Congress of School Hygiene, recently held in Nuremberg, may be judged by the fact that nine hundred members were present, while nearly as many more showed their interest by becoming members, although unable to be present.

The meetings were well organized, being held in a school building admirably adapted for the purpose, and the officials of the Congress had taken great pains to afford every information and assistance to members, who showed, in their turn, their appreciation of the importance of the Congress by their steady attendance and earnest discussion. Twenty European countries, also the United States and Japan, sent representatives, and no European country was unrepresented, except Italy and Turkey.

England was well represented, and this was due largely to Dr. James Kerr, the able and energetic medical officer of the London School Board, who aided in forming a special committee, presided over by Sir T. Lauder Brunton, and including representatives from the Royal College of Physicians of London, the Royal College of Surgeons of England, the London School Board, the Medical Officers of Schools Association, the Incorporate Society of Medical Officers of Health, the London School of Medicine for Women, the Childhood Society, the Child-Study Association, the National Union of Teachers, and the Sanitary Institute. At the general meeting the following papers were read:

1. "What Have Ophthalmic Surgeons Done for School Hygiene, and What Has Yet to be Done?"
2. "The Position of School Hygiene in Norway."
3. "The Hygiene and Personal Health of the Master in Relation to His Pupils."
4. "The Arrangement of Elementary Schools, According to the Mental Capacity of the Children."
5. "The Duties and Education of the School Doctor."
6. "The Prevention of Infectious Diseases in Schools."
7. What Is Most Required in School Ventilation?"

The sectional work of the Congress was divided into seven sections
1. School Buildings and Furnishing of the School-room.

2. The Hygiene of Residential Schools, the Methods of
Hygienic Investigation and Research in Schools, and the
Physiology and Psychology of Educational Methods and Work.

3. Instruction in Hygiene for Teachers and Scholars.

4. Physical Education and Training in Personal Hygiene.

5. Contagious Diseases, Ill-health, and Conditions Affecting
Attendance at School.

6. Special Schools, including Feeble-Minded, Blind, Deaf,
Dumb, Crippled, Invalid, and Exceptional Children.

7. Out-of-School Hygiene, Holiday Camps, the Relation of the
Home and School and the Hygiene of the Teaching Profession.

Among noteworthy things said were Professor Cohn's remark
that myopia might be regarded as a widespread disease produced by school life, and that the true cause was not known,
although close work, hereditary disposition and bad light produced it. Dr. Benda, Berlin, advised no matriculation examinations, no afternoon school hours, and as few home lessons as possible. Dr. James Kerr recommended " window-drills," direct
mechanical movement of air by means of large fans, and the
special ventilation of cloak-rooms and stairways in order to improve ventilation. The tendency of the Congress was in the direction of increased specialism, both in educational work and in
medical supervision.

The next meeting of this Congress will be held in London in
1907, and a short conference and exhibition of school hygiene
will be held in London, under the auspices of the Sanitary Institute, in January, 1905.   H. M'M.

INHERITANCE AND EDUCATION.

PROF. KARL PEARSON delivered the Huxley memorial lecture.
He took for his subject the " Inheritance in Man of Moral and
Mental Characters and Its Relation to the Inheritance of Physical Characters." He has spent much time in collecting statistics
with a view of elucidating the condition of the nature in these
respects. He dealt with his figures as a master, and some of his
audience must have followed him only by the closest attention and
determined effort. I can, therefore, only mention points in his
conclusion: General health he held to be inherited just as stature
and head measurements. The same law governed mental and
moral characters, consequently good qualities were in the breed
and not created by the environment, though they might be cultivated by it. But the parental stock was of the first importance,
education and other influences were quite secondary, or at least
what could be gained thereby depended very much on the stock.

I don't know that this conclusion differs very much from the popular notions of the value of good breeding or from the experience of schoolmasters. You cannot develop a genius out of a dull boy or girl by the most prolonged education. The children of the physically feeble are heavily handicapped in the struggle of life, and it may well be that mental and even moral qualities are apt to fade in the contest. But, even so, we cannot altogether exclude environment.

We have heard much of our national decadence in physical qualities, though the pessimists have not convinced the nation that it is only a dying one. Prof. Pearson seems to think we are declining in the other qualities, and he blames the intellectual classes, which, he says, for the last forty years, enervated by pleasure and leading a wrong life, do not furnish the right stock to carry on the work of the empire. The remedy would be restraining the breeding by bad stock and increasing the fertility of the good. This, of course, can be done in the breeding of animals, but how can a nation accomplish it? Education is the modern panacea for everything, but if we tell men they ought not to marry, how many will heed us? Even if we admit that physical and psychical qualities march in parallel lines it is hopeless to expect to persuade the feeble or degenerate that their duty is to die out and leave the world to a better breed. And as to this better breed, there are many who will deny its existence, and say such views, though interesting to speculate about, are unproved, and, even if true, outside of practical consideration.— London Letter of the *Medical Record.*

"Ringworm Schools."—At the meeting of the Metropolitan Asylums' Board of London in January, the report of the Downs Ringworm School for 1903 was adopted, showing 618 admissions, 208 discharges, and 1 death. Of those discharged only 153 had been pronounced cured (14 were transferred, and 41 were sent for by their guardians). Steps are to be taken to prevent children from being removed before they are cured.

Mentally Defective Children.—The first school for mentally defective children was opened in Germany in 1863, and was a successful institution, many of the children trained there being capable of supporting themselves. In Britain the first school of this character was opened in 1893 in Leicester and there are now schools in London, Birmingham, etc., to care for these children. In Birmingham about 17 per cent. of these children are practically self-supporting after leaving the school. Much interest attaches to the effort now being made by the Ontario Government to establish such a school at Orillia. The newly-appointed principal, Miss Nash, is to take up her duties at once.

Correspondence.   *The Editor cannot hold himself responsible for any views expressed in this Department.*

"NEURASTHENIA IN SOME OF ITS RELATIONS TO INSANITY."

To the Editor of THE CANADIAN JOURNAL OF MEDICINE AND SURGERY:

DEAR SIR,—I beg to submit a few suggestions cerebrated from reading the excellent paper of Dr. Meyers, on "Neurasthenia as an Etiological Factor of Insanity," and especially the prophylactic value of early treatment. I have no criticism of his dogma. Latterly the tendency of all writers upon psychiatry has been to assume that the general practitioner is ignorant of all things psychical, and this assumption naturally engenders platitudes. In thirty years' experience, with over 20,000 insane, and their former doctors—general practitioners—I can say that among the latter I have found many astute psychologists at whose feet many modern specialists might sit with profit to themselves. It is the rapid enlargement of neuro-psychical nomenclature that puzzles the busy doctor, and in fear of not using the latest term he refrains from giving verbal expression to experiences and observation of great value. Yet he recognizes facts and knows the meaning, and has observed the truth so well expressed by Dr. Meyers, of a neurasthenic basis for the mass of idiopathic insanities, for a long, long, time. Take the farmer's wife, for instance, a member of society furnishing more than her proportion of asylum population; ask her physician for the pathology and cause and note his reply: " She has worked like a mule sixteen hours each six days a week, and ten hours on Sunday, without companions, diversion, or brain food, until her nerve cells are starved, degenerate, exhansted, and don't work together." What reply could be better? Moreover, the country doctor in such a case recognizes the prophylaxis quite well, doctor, when he gets the chance, and uses all means in his power to put it in practice, but what can he do? He cannot give his patient change of environment (until she is legally insane), or rest, or any other effective treatment, except a short course of tonics until she gets temporary relief. He sees the inevitable end, but cannot avoid it, knowing full well it is avoidable. As for treatment suggested—travel, isolation, diversion, hydrotherapy, etc., it is not available to the great mass of neurasthenics. Drugs, although not useless, are only efficient as adjuncts to the course of treatment referred to. I want to make one exception to this dictum, although the product is not a drug, but an organic remedy, and its action is physiological. I have found wherever assimilation is much disordered, where systemic metabolism is faulty, and where these disorders are more or less basic to the symptom-complex, that dependence upon bioplasm in one of its forms is never displaced when I can reach the patient's toleration. It has become my individual dogma: for neurasthensia, bioplasm and elimination. I esteem it as the greatest boon to the nerve-exhausted—the victim of overwork, worry, and the many other causes.   Respectfully yours,

P. M. WISE, M.D.

New York, Aug. 3rd, 1904.

USE ANTITOXIN AS EARLY AS POSSIBLE.

To the Editor of THE CANADIAN JOURNAL OF MEDICINE AND SURGERY:

DEAR SIR,—Please allow me to correct an error in your otherwise very full and correct report of the late meeting of the Ontario Medical Association, on page 110, of August number. I am reported as saying that the mortality was greater with the use of antitoxin than without it. My opinion is the very opposite of this, for my experience teaches me to use antitoxin as early as possible, as the result of doing so is generally most satisfactory.

Yours, etc.,

J. HUNTER.

❧ News of the Month. ❧

AUTUMN POST-GRADUATE COURSES AT PARIS.

From Monday, 19th of September, to Saturday, 1st of October, courses and practical demonstrations, the details of which follow, will take place at the Hotel des Sociétés savantes (Science Societies House), rue Serpente (Serpente Street), and in several hospital services, at Paris :

At the Science Societies House (Hôtel des Sociétés savantes, rue Serpente) : Bacteriology, Dr. Veillon; Dermatological and Syphilographical Therapeutics, Dr. Leredde; Massage, Dr. Marchais; Diseases of Urinary Organs, Dr. Noguès; Electrotherapy, Dr. Zimmern; Midwifery, Dr. Dubrisay; Nervous Diseases, Dr. Sillier; Applied Therapeutics, Dr. Landowski; Hygiene and Therapeutics of Children, Dr. Lesné.

At the different hospitals : Gynecology, Dr. Arrou (St. Antoine Hospital) ; Practical Surgery, Dr. Souligoux (Lariboisière) : Auscultation, Dr. Caussade (Tenon) ; Stomachal Diseases, Dr. Soupault (Bichat) ; Oto-rhino-laryngology, Dr. Laurens (Bichat) ; Ophthalmology, Dr. Morax (Lariboisière).

The fee for every course (which will include about from 8 to 10 lessons), is 20 francs, to be paid when registering. Detailed programmes will be sent on request. For all information, apply to Dr. Marchais, Hôtel des Sociétés savantes, rue Serpente, Paris.

ITEMS OF INTEREST.

Must Leave Canada.—One hundred and thirty-five Syrian immigrants, who arrived on the 2nd ult., by the steamer *Halifax* of the Canadian line, from Havre, and landed at Grosse Isle quarantine station for medical inspection, were examined, and 105 of the lot were found violently affected with trachoma, and declared incurable. They were ordered to be deported by the *Halifax* on her return to Havre. This is the largest number of immigrants ever deported from any Canadian or American Atlantic port in the history of immigrant medical inspection.

The Physician's Library.

BOOK REVIEWS.

The Doctor's Recreation Series. Editor-in-chief, Charles Wells Moulton; Associate Editors: Nicholas Senn, M.D., Ph.D., LL.D., C.M.; Wm. Henry Drummond, M.D., LL.D.; John C. Hemmeter, M.D., Ph.D.; Wm. Warren Potter, M.D.; Titus Munson Coan, M.D.; Emory Lanphear, M.D.; Albert Van Der Veer, M.D., Ph.D.; Winslow Anderson, M.D.; W. J. Bell, M.D.; Henry W. Roby, M.D. 12 volumes, octavo. Cloth and half morocco. Akron, O., New York and Chicago: The Saalfield Publishing Co.

The aim of the editors has been to amass a great amount of useful, curious and entertaining literature pertaining to the medical profession, which has heretofore been either inaccessible to the general practitioner, or so widely scattered as to be practically unattainable when most needed. These volumes present as complete and varied a collection of the best purely literary medical literature as can be brought within the compass of a dozen volumes. As an actual encyclopedia of medical literature, they will take a place not hitherto occupied. Much good material, both prose and poetry, drifts hither and thither on the stream of fugitive literature, and, if not wholly lost, is likely to become forgotten. Many of the pieces here collected have been rescued from the oblivion that seemed awaiting them, while much of the set is original and presented for the first time.

In last month's issue, we had occasion to review Vol. I., " The Doctor's Leisure Hour." Vol. II. has come to hand recently. It is entitled " The Doctor's Red Lamp," a book of short stories concerning the doctor's life, selected by Charles Wells Moulton. It is a most interesting volume, containing short stories by different authors touching upon the daily life of the physician. The material has been selected from a large number of sources, the authors including such well-known litterateurs as Conan Doyle, Ian Maclaren, Ambrose Bierce, Lucy S. Furman, J. E. Montgomery, Maud Wilder Goodwin, Henry Seton Merriman, and Joseph Kirkland. We know of no better series of books for the busy physician to buy, with which to amuse himself on his vacation, or after a busy day's work.   W A. Y.

A System of Practical Surgery. By PROF. E. VON BERGMANN, M.D., of Berlin; PROF. P. VON BRUNS, M.D., of Tubingen, and PROF. J. VON MIKULICZ, M.D. , of Breslau. Volume III., Surgery of the Extremities. Translated and edited by William T. Bull, M.D., Professor of Surgery, College of Physicians and Surgeons, Columbia University, New York; and John B. Solley, M.D., New York. New York and Phila-delphia: Lea Brothers & Co. 1904.

The volumes of this excellent work continue to appear with great regularity and celerity. Volume III. is even better than its forerunners. The contributors are men of excellent reputa-tion, and are known to the profession the world over: Dr. M. Borchardt, Prof. Dr. P. L. Friedrich, Prof. Dr. A. Hoffa, Prof. Dr. F. Hofmeister, Prof. Dr. D. Nasse, Oberarzt Dr. P. Reichel, Oberarzt Dr. A. Schrieber, Privat-Docent Dr. M. Wilms. The work is largely free from the defects which so mark various "systems." It is not a compilation where the antiquary may search who is looking for discarded and effete methods; viewed even from the standpoint of the specialist it is exhaustive, yet concise, thoroughly modern, though conservative. The illustra-tions and mechanical execution of the work are of the best. The reviewer need only refer to such subjects as " Congenital Dis-location of the Hip," the treatment of which has made such rapid strides in the last decade, and to " The Treatment of Club-Foot," which has reached the very ideal of perfection, to be able to recognize that the author of these, as well as of the other subjects treated in this volume, has written what represents the best and latest knowledge upon the subject in hand. No better system of surgery has been published. B. E. M'K.

Small Hospitals: Establishment and Maintenance. By A. WORCESTER, A.M., M.D.; and Suggestions for Hospital Architecture, with Plans for a Small Hospital, by WILLIAM ATKINSON, architect. New York: John Wiley & Sons, 43 and 45 E. 19th Street.

At a time when so many new hospitals are being built, and when the public are becoming so interested in the care and man-agement of the ill and injured, a book of this kind is of great value, as it not only describes how the public may be interested, the arrangements of committees, and the organization of hos-pital boards, but it goes into the whole question of the difficulties which might be expected to exist where allopathy, homeopathy and eclecticism are all recognized as legitimate modes of practice. This little book contains many valuable hints with regard to the temporary hospitals, and the steps that may be taken to fit a dwelling-house to serve as a hospital until a better one can be built. It contains plans also for the building of hospitals, smaller and larger, and isolation wards, and the letterpress of these plans is full of suggestions that must be of value, not only to those who are building hospitals but to every practitioner, as from the knowledge of what is best, he may see a way to improve what exists in the very houses that he has to visit.   A. J. J.

International Clinics. A Quarterly of Illustrated Clinical Lectures and Especially Prepared Original Articles on Treatment, Medicine, Surgery, Neurology, Pediatrics, Obstetrics, Gynecology, Orthopedics, Pathology, Dermatology, Ophthalmology, Otology, Rhinology, Laryngology, Hygiene, and other topics of interest to students and practitioners.   By leading members of the medical profession throughout the world.   Edited by A. O. J. KELLY, M.D., Philadelphia, U.S.A., with the collaboration of Wm. Osler, M.D., Baltimore, U.S.A.; John H. Musser, M.D., Philadelphia; Jas. Stewart, M.D., Montreal; J. B. Murphy, M.D., Chicago; A. McPhedran, M.D., Toronto; Thos. M. Rotch, M.D., Boston; J. G. Clark, M.D., Philadelphia; Jas. J. Walsh, M.D., New York; J. W. Ballantyne, M.D., Edinburgh; John Harold, M.D., London; Edmund Landolt, M.D., Paris, and Richard Kretz, M.D., Vienna. With regular correspondents in Montreal. London, Paris, Berlin, Vienna, Leipsic, Brussels and Carlsbad.   Vols. I. and II.   Fourteenth Series.   1904.   Philadelphia: J. B. Lippincott Co.   Canadian agent: Chas. Roberts, Montreal.

Volumes I. and II. of the fourteenth series of " Clinics " are fully up to, and in some respects ahead of, some of their predecessors.   We are pleased to see that the name of Dr. Alex. McPhedran, of Toronto, has been added to the list of collaborators, and feel that such is a distinct acquisition and of additional value to the series.   Among the contributors to Volume II. appears the name of Dr. John McCrae, Lecturer in Pathology at McGill University.   One of the most valuable contributions to Volume I. is " The Progress of Medicine during 1903," by Drs. David L. Edsale, Joseph C. Bloodgood and A. A. Stevens.   The article covers over one hundred pages, and makes Volume I. worth purchasing, if for no other reason.   In it, Dr. Edsale covers Infectious Diseases, Parasitic Diseases, Diseases of Metabolism, of the Blood, of the Cardio-vascular, Respiratory and Gastro-intestinal Systems, and Diseases of the Liver and Kidneys.   Dr. Jos. C. Bloodgood takes up Surgery under the headings of Shock, Surgical Infections, Anesthesia, Blood Examinations, Blood Cultures, Burns and Scalds, Fractures, Tumors, and the Surgery of the

Stomach and Pancreas. Dr. A. A. Stevens deals with Treatment, viz., that of Infectious Diseases, Constitutional Diseases, Diseases of the Blood, Ductless Glands, Circulatory System, Diseases of the Kidney, Respiratory Tract, Stomach, Intestines and Liver.

Of Volume II., the first 128 pages are devoted to " Diseases of Warm Climates.'' Among those who contribute short articles to that department is Dr. John McCrae, who writes one of 22 pages on " Recent Progress in Tropical Medicine," a chapter well worth reading, and showing great scientific thought. Dr. C. Jarvis contributes 15 pages or so on " Sleeping Sickness," which is comparatively common in the Uganda country. A very interesting and instructive chapter, " Broncho-pneumonia in Children," is contributed by Dr. Isaac A. Abt, and one on " The Limitations of the Utility of Digitalis in Heart Disease," by Dr. Jas. M. French, is worthy of careful perusal.   W. A .Y.

Cap'n Eri. By JOSEPH C. LINCOLN. Toronto: William Briggs, Publisher.

The Cap'n is a man without a mate in the story-book line, excepting wonderful old David Harum. Eri lives, moves and has his being in and around Cape Cod; his quaintness has an. irresistible charm, and his love of comfort appeals to many a physician, especially those who have spent their earlier years in the country, and can remember being asked to step into the parlor and " set on the sofa "—to which invitation the Cap'n answers, " No, thanks; hair-cloth's all right to look at, but it's the slipperiest stuff that ever was, I cal'late. Every time I set on a hair-cloth sofa I feel's if I was draggin' anchor."   W. A. Y.

A Text-book of Alkaloidal Therapeutics. Being a condensed resume, of all available literature on the subject of the active principles, added to the personal experience of the authors. By W. J. WAUGH, M.D., and W. A. ABBOTT M.D., with the collaboration of E. M. EPSTEIN, M.D. Chicago: The Clinic Publishing Co. 1904.

This work covers a field that, up till now, has been largely ignored by the bulk of the profession. The tide, however, has been gradually turning till to-day physicians, who decried the system most vehemently, are now among its active supporters. There is little doubt that anything that is new, as a rule, is slowly taken up, and the headway made is discouraging. Alkaloidal medication is to-day receiving a good deal of attention, and the Waugh-Abbott text-book consists of 400 pages of literature, covering the 138 different alkaloidal preparations, their toxicology, physiological action, etc. As the authors say, " The mission of our book

8

is to get together from all sources all the facts obtainable concerning the alkaloids and active principles, and present them in a ' ready-to-use ' truly ' alkaloidal' form." The volume is well written and will prove, we feel sure, the means of adding many to the list of converts to this new, but, very often, indeed, successful method of medication.

A Manual of Practical Medical Electricity, the Rontgen Rays, Finsen Light, Radium and Its Radiations and High Frequency Current. By DAWSON TURNER, B.A., M.D., F.R.C.P. (Edin.), M.R.C.P. (Lond.), President Royal Scottish Society of Arts, Vice-President British Electro-Therapeutic Society, Fellow of the Physical Society, Lecturer on Experimental Physics, Surgeons' Hall, Edinburgh, etc. Fourth edition, revised and enlarged. University series. London: Bailliere, Tindall & Cox, 8 Henrietta Street, Covent Garden. 1904. Canadian agents: *J.* A. Carveth & Co., Toronto.

It is but two years or so since we had the satisfaction of reviewing the third edition of Dr. Turner's excellent work, and now we have before us the fourth edition still further enlarged. In his edition of 1902, the author devoted a good deal of space to a subject which was new then, viz., the treatment of disease by means of the ultra violet light, and since then it has been proved what rapid improvement can take place by this method in malignant cases. In the last edition, Dr. Turner has paid a good deal of attention to the use of sinusoidal currents in treatment, and also to the consideration of radium and its uses. He also goes into the therapeutics of high frequency currents. Quite a number of illustrations have been added.

The Clinical Study of Blood-Pressure. A Guide to the Use of the Sphygmomanometer in Medical, Surgical and Obstetrical Practice. With a Summary of the Experimental and Clinical Facts relating to the Blood-Pressure in Health and Disease. By THEODORE C. JANEWAY, M.D., Lecturer on Medical Diagnosis, University of Bellevue Hospital Medical College, New York City. With seventy-five illustrations in the text, many in colors. New York and London: D. Appleton & Co. 1904.

Instruments of precision for ascertaining blood-pressure have not been of much service in the past, but this author believes that, with modern instruments in the hands of those who understand their use, diagnosis, prognosis and therapeutics cannot but gain in efficiency through blood-pressure determinations at the bed-side and in the office.

The work is divided into three parts. Part I. deals with the purely physiological aspect of blood-pressure along the same lines that are followed by our leading text-books on physiology.

Part II. deals with the technical construction and application of various kinds and makes of instruments. The author favors the use of the modern instrument called the sphygmomanometer, several varieties of which are described, and attention is drawn to their several advantages and disadvantages.

The main interest centres in Part III., where the clinical aspects of the subject are discussed under such headings as, " The blood-pressure in disease in general," " In internal disease," " In nervous and mental diseases," " In surgical conditions," and " In obstetrical conditions."

Practical results have been obtained in nephritis, in perforation and hemorrhage complicating typhoid fever, in shock and collapse from various causes, and in a host of other conditions. During the administration of chloroform, any serious depression of the blood-pressure is at once indicated, and shows that the chloroform should be stopped and ether substituted.

In obstetrics, the greatest importance attaches to the arterial pressure as a means of foretelling, and, as a consequence, possibly forestalling, an eclamptic seizure. The author says, " To take the arterial tension is far easier than examining the urine, and the information thus obtained is no whit less valuable."

It is impossible, from a hasty perusal of the work, to determine the practical clinical value of obtaining blood-pressure as a routine practice in all cases. There can be no doubt, however, that the value of such tracings is very great in some, if not all, cases. I am sure that everyone who reads this work will be pleased with it. A. E.

Insanity in Every-day Practice. By E. G. YOUNGER, M.D. (Brux.), M.R.C.P. (Lond.), D.P.H., etc.; Senior Physician Finsbury Dispensary; Late Senior Assistant Medical Officer, London County Asylum, Hanwell; Formerly Assistant Medical Superintendent, Metropolitan District Asylum, Caterham. London: Bailliere, Tindall & Cox, 8 Henrietta Street, Covent Garden. 1904. Canadian agents: J. A. Carveth & Co., Toronto.

This little book is an excellent illustration of what may be accomplished by an intelligent and determined attempt at condensation. The usual experience of an author when undertaking to write on the subject of mental diseases is that so much important material presents itself to his mind that a large work is compiled before he can forgive himself for bringing it to a close. Dr. Younger, however, has contrived to present a comprehensive view of his subject within the compass of 106 octavo pages, and one reason why he has been able to successfully accomplish this surprising result may be found in the simple symptomatological classification which he has adopted. The wide divergence in the classification of various authors constitutes one of the discouraging difficulties to the professional mind in acquiring a knowledge of mental diseases, and Dr. Younger spares his readers by refraining from the introduction of a new terminology. He only refers to his monograph as an " outline chart," but certainly the masterly clearness and completeness with which he has sketched these outlines will cause every reader to hope that he may soon be induced to give the profession what he would regard as a more exhaustive treatise on mental diseases.   N. II. B.

Tuberculosis and Acute General Miliary Tuberculosis. By Dr. G. Cornet, of Berlin. Edited, with additions, by Walter B. James, M.D., Professor of the Practice of Medicine in the College of Physicians and Surgeons (Columbia University), New York. Handsome octavo volume of 806 pages. Philadelphia, New York, London: W. B. Saunders & Co. 1904. Canadian agents: J. A. Carveth & Co., 434 Yonge Street, Toronto. Cloth, $5.00 net; half morocco, $6.00 net.

This is the seventh volume to be issued in Saunders' American Edition of Nothnagel's Practice. Professor Cornet's exhaustive work appears at a time when the subject of tuberculosis has a peculiar claim upon the attention of mankind. Within a few years both professional and general public interest in the disease has made great advances. In almost every civilized community societies for the prevention of tuberculosis are being organized, and these are composed not only of physicians, but of laymen, while governments themselves are taking an active part in the movement. Under these circumstances, and at this time, the work is of interest to practitioners, for there is no other treatise which gives an equally clear and comprehensive view of this subject.

As to the relation of human to bovine tuberculosis, it is pointed out that while the bacilli of bovine tuberculosis are more virulent for cattle, and those of human tuberculosis for man, the two are, nevertheless, to some degree interchangeable, and we are, therefore, not justified in relaxing our efforts to prevent the use of milk and meat from tuberculous cattle.

However, the fact cannot be reiterated too often, that the great danger lies in dried tuberculous sputum. This is the great source of infection for human beings at all ages, from birth to old age. A second fact of equal importance is that bacilli die within a few hours if exposed to sunlight, and within a few days in diffused light. In the light of these facts, all that is required to prevent the spread of tuberculosis is cleanliness, light and fresh air.

The editor is to be congratulated on the excellence of the translation. His own additions, though few, are excellent, and materially add to the value of the work.   A. M'P.

The Practical Medicine Series of Year-Books. Comprising Ten Volumes on the Year's Progress in Medicine and Surgery. Issued monthly, under the general editorial charge of GUS-TAVUS P. HEAD, M.D., Professor of Laryngology and Rhinology, Chicago Post-Graduate Medical School. Vol. V., Obstetrics. Edited by Joseph B. DeLee, M.D., Professor of Obstetrics, Northwestern University Medical School. April, 1904. Price, $1.00. Vol. VI., General Medicine. Edited by Frank Billings, M.S., M.D., Head of the Medical Department and Dean of the Faculty of Rush Medical College, Chicago; and J. H. Salisbury, M.D., Professor of Medicine, Chicago Clinical School. May, 1904. Chicago: The Year-Book Publishers, 40 Dearborn Street. Price of series, $5.50; of this vol., $1.00.

These volumes are parts of a series of ten issued at monthly intervals and covering the entire field of medicine and surgery. Each volume is complete for the year prior to its publication on the subject of which it treats. These volumes are published primarily for the general practitioner, but being arranged in several volumes, those interested in special subjects may buy only the parts they desire.

Volume V., on Obstetrics, takes up Pregnancy, Labor, the Puerperium and Operative Obstetrics.

Volume VI., on General Medicine, treats of Typhoid Fever, Malaria, and Diseases of the Digestive Organs. General medicine, being a large subject, is divided into two volumes, viz., May and October. We are very much pleased with these volumes, and can recommend them to our friends.   W. J. W.

Epilepsy and Its Treatment. By WILLIAM P. SPRATLING, M.D., Superintendent of the Craig Colony for Epileptics at Sonyea, N.Y. Handsome octavo volume of 522 pages, illustrated. Philadelphia, New York, London: W. B. Saunders & Co. 1904. Canadian agents: J. A. Carveth & Co., Limited., 434 Yonge Street, Toronto. Cloth, $4.00 net.

If for no other reason than that it is now well over a quarter of a century since any work of any account on epilepsy has come from the press, Dr. Spratling's volume will be welcomed by the profession. The author has had the necessary experience as a neurologist to write the book, and, judging from what we have read of it, it is a volume that will interest, not only the specialist, but the general practitioner alike. In comparing the method of treatment adopted in epilepsy twenty years ago with that of the present day, one cannot but see what wondrous advance has been made, so that, for that reason, too, this volume should find a ready sale. The section that interested the reviewer most is that dealing with the medico-legal aspects of epilepsy, thirty pages full of thought, and yet conservative.

A Text-Book of Mechano-Therapy (Massage and Medical Gymnasties). For Medical Students, Trained Nurses and Medical Gymnasts. By AXEL V. GRAFSTROM, B.Sc., M.D., Attending Physician to the Gustavus Adolphus Orphanage, Jamestown, N.Y. Second edition, revised, enlarged and entirely reset. 12mo of 200 pages, fully illustrated. Philadelphia, New York, London: W. B. Saunders & Co. 1904. Canadian agents: J. A. Carveth & Co., Limited, 434 Yonge Street, Toronto. Cloth, $1.25 net.

Dr. Grafstrom considers in this small book Mechano-Therapy in 17 chapters, and takes up such in different departments and from different aspects; *e.g.,* Gymnastic Postures, Medical Gymnastics, Massage, A General Massage Treatment, Disease of the Respiratory Organs, Movements and Cardiac Diseases, Mechano-Therapy used in the Treatment of Rheumatism and Gout, Diseases of the Urinary Organs and their Treatment by Mechano-Therapy, Chronic Constipation and Diseases of the Liver, a short review of Mechano-Therapy in connection with Obstetrics, Mechano-Therapy as an Agent in the Treatment of Diseases of Children, Diseases of the Nervous System, Local Treatment, Massage of the Eye, Ear, Nose and Throat, and Pelvic Massage. The last two chapters are additions to Volume IL, and have not appeared before. The volume is not only of interest to medical gymnasts and nurses, but to medical practitioners as well.

Atlas and Epitome of Diseases of the Mouth, Pharynx and Nose. By DR. L. GRUNWALD, of Munich. From the second revised and enlarged German edition. Edited, with additions, by James E. Newcomb, M.D., Instructor in Laryngology, Cornell University Medical School; Attending Laryngologist to the Roosevelt Hospital, Out-Patient Department. With 102 illustrations on 42 colored lithographic plates, 41 text-cuts, and 219 pages of text. Philadelphia and London: W. B.

Saunders & Co. 1903. Canadian agents: J. A. Carveth & Co., Limited, Toronto. Cloth, $3.00 net.

In designing this atlas the author has kept constantly in mind the needs of both student and practitioner, and, as far as possible, typical cases of the various diseases have been selected. The illustrations are described in the text in exactly the same way as a practised examiner would demonstrate the objective findings to his class, the book thus serving as a substitute for actual clinical work. The illustrations themselves are numerous and exceedingly well executed, portraying the conditions so strikingly that their study is almost equal to examination of the actual specimens. The editor has incorporated his own valuable experience, and has also included extensive notes on the use of the active principle of the suprarenal bodies in the materia medica of rhinology and laryngology. The work, besides being an excellent atlas and epitome of the diseases of the mouth, pharynx and nose, serves also as a text-book on the anatomy and physiology of these organs. Indeed, we wonder how the author has encompassed so much within such a limited space. We heartily commend the work as one of the best we have seen.

Obstetric and Gynecologic Nursing. By EDWARD P. DAVIS, A.M., M.D., Professor of Obstetrics in the Jefferson Medical College and in the Philadelphia Polyclinic. 12mo volume of 402 pages, fully illustrated. Second edition, thoroughly revised. Philadelphia, New York, London: W. B. Saunders & Co. 1904. Canadian agents: J. A. Carveth & Co., Limited, 434 Yonge Street, Toronto. Polished buckram, $1.75 net.

Every practitioner sees daily the immense value of good nursing, the boon it is to the patient, and the manner in which it removes a large part of the burden from his own shoulders. A perusal of Dr. E. P. Davis' volume will still further assist the medical attendant and help him so as to systematize what his nurse ought to do so as to make his task all the lighter and more enjoyable. Apart from that, the book should be in the hands of every nurse who is anxious to be thorough and proficient in her life's work.

Fatigue. The Science Series. Edited by PROF. J. McKEEN CATTELL, M.A., Ph.D., and F. E. BEDDARD, M.A., F.R.S. Toronto: William Briggs.

This small volume is divided into 12 chapters, dealing respectively with The Migration of Birds, Carrier Pigeons, History of the Study of the Movements of Animals, Origin of the Energy of the Muscles and of the Brain, General and Special Characteristics of Fatigue, Substances Produced in Fatigue, Muscular Contracture and Rigidity, Law of Exhaustion, Attention and Its Physical Conditions, Intellectual Fatigue, Lectures and Examinations, Methods of Intellectual Work, and Overpressure.

Before "the dog days" cease to be for 1904 it would be a good thing to purchase from Wm. Briggs a copy of Prof. Cattell's unusual book, and, lying in a hammock when you think you are fatigued with a big day's work, peruse it and find how quickly that "tired feeling" will disappear.

W. A. Y.

Diseases of the Stomach and Their Surgical Treatment. By A. W. Mayo Robson, F.R.C.S., and B. G. A. Moynihan, M.S., London, F.R.C.S. Second edition. London: Bailliere, Tindall & Cox, 8 Henrietta Street, Covent Garden. 1904. Canadian agents: J. A. Carveth & Co., Toronto.

Less than a decade ago, it was considered out of the question to attempt to treat diseases of the stomach by surgical interference. During the past two or three years, however, opinion along this line has materially changed, and the surgery of the stomach is now a source of active discussion at any and every medical society meeting. The authors have a record of over 600 operations, the death-rate of which during the last year or two has been cut down to less than 5 per cent. Mr. Robson is strongly of the opinion that in cancer cases gastrectomy has advantages over gastro-enterostomy, and that, even as a palliative operation, partial gastrectomy can afford great relief. It may be said that the whole book has been rewritten, or nearly so, and the authors are deserving of congratulation for the literary character of the volume now before the profession.

The Canadian Journal of Medicine and Surgery

A JOURNAL PUBLISHED MONTHLY IN THE INTEREST OF
MEDICINE AND SURGERY

VOL. XVI.   TORONTO, OCTOBER, 1904.   NO. 4.

Original Contributions.

PRESIDENT'S ADDRESS.*

BY SIMON J. TUNSTALL, B.A., M.D., VANCOUVER, B.C.

Mr. Chairman and Gentlemen,—I feel that my first duty to-night is to offer you my very hearty thanks for the honor you have conferred upon me in electing me President of the Association for the ensuing year.

When I recall the names of those who have preceded me in this chair, I can only ask your indulgence for the deficiencies you may find in me, of which I am very conscious, and express the hope that under my presidency the interests of the Association may in no wise suffer nor its honor be in any way tarnished.

The present occasion is no ordinary one. In the appointment of a President from among the members of the Association whose home and work lie in this far distant portion of the Dominion, and in our meeting here to-day at the Doorway of the West, a new departure has been made.

I am far too modest to suppose for an instant that any particular merit of mine has induced the Association to make this departure; rather I conceive it to be due to a general recognition of the claims and standing of the western members as a whole, and of the growing importance of this fair Western Province.

I should be performing my duties but poorly did I not seize this opportunity to thank you on behalf of my western confreres, and on behalf of the people of this Province in general, and of this city in particular, for the compliment you have paid us in

---

* Delivered at meeting of Canadian Medical Association, Vancouver, B.C., August, 1904.
4

selecting this Province and this city as the place of meeting for this year, and I feel I am only expressing their wishes in tendering you a hearty western welcome to our midst, and their hopes that your brief stay among us will be both pleasant and profitable to you all.

To many of you, probably to most of you, the rapid progress and general development of this' young Province will come as a surprise. It does to most of our visitors from the older parts of the Dominion who know how recent has been the settlement of the West. And certainly, looking round one, it does seem scarcely realizable that the site of this rapidly expanding city, of which its citizens are so justly proud, and this very spot on which this building stands, surrounded by so many comforts and refinements of modern life, was, less than two decades ago, a wild and almost impenetrable virgin forest, the haunts of the bear, the deer and the primitive savage.

It is less than a score of years by two that the incorporation of this city took place, and yet to-day it will compare favorably with many cities of the older Provinces twice and thrice its age. From the medical standpoint it is reaching after a high ideal.

The incomparable water supply which is brought in closed steel conduits from the bosom of the mountains to the north of us; the sewerage system, with its septic tanks, that deliver their effluent into tidal waters;. the paved streets, with their array of cleaners; the cement sidewalks which are now throughout the city, rapidly replacing the earlier and cruder planking; the public and private hospitals; the General Hospital, which is now being built, and which, when finished, will be the peer of any hospital of its size, all make it clear that we are endeavoring to keep abreast of the times, as well in sanitary as in other matters.

It is no idle boast, then, if I say that in the West events move rapidly. Time is no sluggard here, and we see history fashioning itself before our eyes. The whole of this great Province was in indisputed possession of savage aborigines a half century ago. The closing years of the first half of the nineteenth century saw the first real settlement made on Vancouver Island at a place called Camosun in the native tongue, now Victoria, the capital of the Province.

A few years later, in 1858, an Act was passed in the Home Parliament to provide for the government of this new colony, thereafter to be known as British Columbia. From this date the real settlement of the Province begins. The discovery of gold in the Fraser and Cariboo soon made these districts as famous and as widely known as Sacramento or Ballarat, and a great inrush of population was the result. But a very few years later the conception of that colossal and momentous undertaking, the building of the Canadian Pacific Railway, began to shape itself in men's minds, and was finally carried out. You are all, doubtless, familiar with the history of this great undertaking and know the almost insuperable difficulties its earlier promoters had to contend with, and how in the end, in spite of political, natural and every other obstacle and hindrance, they successfully carried through the scheme and made possible the union of British Columbia and the great North-West with the rest of Canada, and gave us as a result that splendid heritage, that united land which stretches from ocean to ocean, from the rising of the sun to the going down thereof—a land of which all her sons and daughters are so proud—our beloved Canada.

It is gratifying to the profession to know that it has been ably and honorably represented among those history-makers in the persons of Drs. Helmcken and Tolmie, who were the first medical men to settle in the colony, about the middle of the last century. Both took prominent parts in the earlier events of the Province. The former still remains with us; the latter has gone to his rest. Prior to their advent the native Medicine-man had it all his own way.

There is a significance, not without interest to my mind, in the fact that this Association, representing as it does to-day in its various members the highest medical knowledge of this enlightened period of the world's history, should meet here in this new country, where Shamatism, or the cult of the savage Medicine-man, so recently prevailed, and does to some extent still prevail. The old and the new order of things are thus brought into suggestive contrast and juxtaposition, and we are led naturally to reflect upon the stages and steps we have passed since the days when all medical knowledge was comprised in the superstitious and rude practices of our savage prototypes; and in spite of our sometime failures and our lack of knowledge, still in certain directions the reflection on the whole is a pleasant and gratifying one, both to ourselves and humanity at large. It certainly would not be the least interesting of subjects were I to attempt on this occasion a general survey of the march and progress of medical science from the days and practices of the primitive Medicine-man as we find him even_in this Province, down to the times and discoveries of Lister, Pasteur, Virchow and their followers.

But it is not my intention to undertake such a task to-night, interesting and appropriate as it might under the circumstances be, although I cannot leave the subject without calling your attention briefly to a fact of which all of you may not be aware, and which gives pertinence to my reference to the old-time Shaman or Medicine-man. We are all familiar with hypnotism, but there are few of us, perhaps, aware that in the employment of hypnotism as a therapeutic agent we are returning to primitive methods, to the practice of our savage prototypes. Those who have made special study of the practices and customs of savage races inform us that the primitive doctor, or Medicine-man, was not that self-conscious fraud and humbug, knowingly duping his credulous patients, he is thought to have been, but a person who had a real belief in his own powers and cures; and that those powers and cures were, when genuine, generally, if not always, attributable to hypnotism, especially to that phase of it known as suggestion. A state of hypnosis was induced in his patient by the monotonous droning of his medicine song and the noise of his rattle, and when in this condition his attempt to extract the spirit of the disease from the patient's body, and his statement that he had presently accomplished it, acted suggestively upon the imagination of the patient and effected the cure. " Extremes meet," and " there is nothing new under the sun," we are told, and the school of Nancy, which is founded upon the suggestive phase of hypnotism, is not a new practice but an unconscious return, or rather I should say it is an unconscious modification and extension of these primitive methods which were in vogue among our savages here up to a few years ago, and may be to this day, for aught I know to the contrary.

But enough on this head. It is my intention rather to bespeak your consideration to-night of a point or two which I, in common with many of the members of the profession, have very much at heart, and which I deem of such importance as to merit our most careful consideration and endorsement.

I have reference, in particular, to: 1. The Canadian Medical Protective Association. 2. The Federal Health Bill. 3. The Dominion Medical Council. 4. The Treatment of Inebriates.

With regard to the first, The Canadian Medical · Protective Association, I would desire to urge upon members the strong claims this Association has upon the profession. I am among those who believe in the need of such an Association and that it may be made a valuable means of assisting and protecting members of our profession from wrongful actions-at-law, to which we are all of us at all times liable: actions brought by irresponsible persons for alleged malpractice, or by unscrupulous persons for the purpose of obtaining money under threats of injury to our professional character.

It is well known that a medical man's professional prospects depend to a very large extent, if not entirely, upon his professional reputation, and it is not difficult, therefore, for nuprincipled persons to attempt to levy blackmail upon him by threatening to bring action against him for malpractice or professional incapacity, which action, though wholly groundless and undeserved, may have the most disastrous effects upon his career and pocket.

During the past two years the Association has fought out several such cases successfully, and has amply demonstrated its usefulness and justified its existence. It is, therefore, a matter of wonderment to many of us that the Association has thus far received so little encouragement or support from the profession as a whole. Out of a possible 5,500, the total membership last year was only 252. This is altogether too small a number to make the aims and work of the Association effective or sustain it in a solvent condition, and I welcome this opportunity to invite your earnest co-operation in enlarging its membership and strengthening the hands of the Executive, and would to this end suggest that a special committee be struck during the Convention for the purpose of considering how best to enlist the sympathies and support of our brethren who are not yet members. I cannot but think that a large increase in the membership must inevitably result if the aims of the Association be once rightly understood.

The objects of the Association are such as all can subscribe to. It is not intended to defend or assist in defending unworthy members, or those who are actually guilty of malpractice, or who have brought discredit upon the profession. It aims rather to assist the worthy, those of its members who are wrongfully charged and whose character and reputation are placed at stake; and also to deter irresponsible and unscrupulous persons from bringing action against members of the profession for the purpose of spiting or injuring them, or of exacting a bribe for their silence; and it is only by uniting ourselves together in such a way as this Association offers that we can hope to secure the support of our brethren and become immune to many attacks which would otherwise be made upon us.

I feel, therefore, that we have but to devise some plan of arousing the interest of our brethren in the matter to ensure their support and co-operation.

And now a word or two as to the Federal Health Bill. Thanks to the energetic efforts of the special committee appointed to attend to this matter, considerable progress has been made towards the attainment of our desires in this behalf. The interest and sympathy of the Ministers of the Crown have been secured, and the Ministetr of Agriculture, the Hon. Mr. Fisher, under whose department the matter more directly falls, has taken the matter up most courteously and is thoroughly alive to its urgency and need. For the information of those not familiar with this subject, I would briefly say that the Association, at its meeting in Montreal in 1902, placed itself on record by resolution to the effect that it is expedient that a Department of Public Health be created by the Dominion Government and administered under the authority of one of the existing Ministers of the Crown, thus bringing all general questions relating to sanitary science and public health under one central authority, to be known as the Public Health Department. There is no need for me to dwell upon the importance or desirability of this step; it must commend itself to every member of the profession.

Thus far the Government has not seen its way to grant the desired measure. The work is not yet accomplished, and the need of pushing the matter still exists. I sincerely hope the meeting will not dissolve without first passing a strong resolution in favor of the measure, and thus encourage and strengthen the hands of the committee who have this work in hand.

And now I desire to touch upon my third point, which I regard as of the highest importance. I refer here to the Dominion of Canada Medical Act, which was assented to in the Federal House in 1902. We are under a deep debt of gratitude to the members of the special committee, and especially to Dr. T. G. Roddick, for his untiring efforts to get this measure placed upon the statutes of the country, and it is with great regret that I notice so much misapprehension as to the scope and powers of this Bill still exists in certain quarters. It has been thought that it would encroach upon the rights and privileges of the different Provincial Medical Boards and interfere with their autonomy, and I gladly hail this opportunity to say a few words which may help to remove this misapprehension. It was, and is, not in any way intended to interfere with existing provincial rights or intrench upon the prerogatives of Provincial Medical Boards. As an instance, in my own native Province, Quebec, our French-speaking brethren will have the right of examination in their own language.

Provincial registration and Provincial Boards will still continue to exist, and each Province will be at liberty to fix whatever standard it pleases for its own practitioners. They can, where they wish, continue as examining boards with power to grant provincial licenses, as they do now, and in any case in their hands will be left all matters relating to taxation and professional discipline.

The Bill is a purely permissive one, and though it has been placed upon the statutes of the country, it will be necessary, before it can become operative, to have the consent and co-operation of all the Provincial Medical Boards. Each Provincial Board will have to seek a slight amendment to its present Medical Act. This is all that is now required to make this most desirable measure effective, and I sincerely trust that this consent and co-operation will not be long wanting, for the aims and scope of this Act are such as should commend themselves to every member of the profession. Briefly, I would say that the main purpose of this Bill is to establish a Central Medical Council of Canada, with power to examine candidates and grant licenses, the possession of which shall ensure to the holders thereof such a medical status as will enable them to practice not only in all parts of the Dominion but in the United Kingdom as well, or, indeed, in any portion of His Majesty's Empire, in short, to do away with those mortifying disabilities under which a medical man trained in Canada now labors, and put him upon a footing of professional equality with his brethren in other parts of the Empire. This is assuredly a laudable and most desirable object, and one which, in my humble opinion, should call forth the best efforts of each one of us to bring about its accomplishment; and I sincerely trust that some concerted action will be taken in this matter before the meeting closes.

It is the least, I think, we can do to show our appreciation of the strenuous efforts exerted in securing the passage of so important a measure.

This brings me to my fourth and last point, " The Treatment of Inebriates." A conviction has been steadily growing in the minds of most medical men of late years that something should be done for the care and control of dipsomaniacs and inebriates in the form of founding establishments combining the main features of a hospital and an insane asylum, where drunkards could be legally confined under medical authority and treated in a systematic and enlightened manner. The practice, hitherto, of treating them as criminals subject to a fine or short periods of confinement in the common prisons of the country, has been shown to be wholly unsatisfactory and often productive of the greatest evil to themselves and those who may be dependent upon them.

There can be no doubt, I think, that the care and treatment of those unfortunate members of society is a question of the gravest and most vital importance, and should command the interest and attention of medical men as a subject, which, coming well within their province, affects so seriously the general commonwealth.

A movement towards this end has already been taken in Ontario, and a Bill drafted, the principles of which have received the endorsation of the Toronto Medical Society and also of our own Association; but what we want is a Dominion Act affecting the whole country; and it would be the source of the greatest satisfaction to me if this meeting would take this question up seriously and nominate a committee to draft a measure that could be submitted to the Federal authorities. This could be done either on the lines of the Ontario Bill or any others that might commend themselves.

Speaking personally, I may say that I shall be only too glad to help in drafting such a measure and giving any other assistance in my power, for I am convinced that the adoption and carrying out of the provisions of a bill of this kind will do much to diminish the volume of sickness, pauperism, vice and crime that now stains the annals of our country and restore to lives of usefulness and self-respect many of those poor unfortunates whom it is the design of such a measure to control and help.

Before closing my address, I wish to express to our visiting brethren my appreciation of the kindly feeling and interest which have actuated them in taking part in the deliberations of our National Association, and to hope that their stay may be fruitful of pleasant reminiscences.

And now, gentlemen, I must thank you for your kind reception of me as your President this year, and for the patient and courteous hearing you have given to my remarks, and trust that the suggestions I have ventured to offer may meet with your approval and receive your support.

THE SURGICAL TREATMENT OF COMPLETE DESCENT OF THE UTERUS.*

BY E. C. DUDLEY, M.D., CHICAGO.

COMPLETE descent of the uterus, descent to the third degree, which may be defined as that deviation in which a part or the whole of the uterus is outside of the vulva, is always associated with extensive injury to the pelvic fascia, the pelvic connective tissue, the muscles of the vaginal outlet, the perineum and the vaginal walls; in fact, these injuries of the pelvic floor constitute the essential lesion, the mal-location of the uterus being an incidental factor.

The uterus in its normal position lies across the pelvis, the fundus pointing in a slightly upward anterior direction, and the external is in a slightly downward posterior direction. The long axis of the uterus in this normal direction makes an acute angle with the long axis of the vagina, which extends from the vulva upwards and backwards in the direction of the hollow of the sacrum. Generally speaking, mobile anteversion with some degree of anteflexion is the normal position of the uterus; at any rate, the uterus in its normal range of movements does not deviate, unless temporarily, beyond the limits of a certain normal anteversion and anteflexion.

In the etiology and treatment of descent the practical significance of this acute angle between the axis of the uterus and vagina is very great, because the uterus in the act of prolapse must descend through the vaginal canal in the direction of that canal, that is, a coincidence of the two axes is a pre-requisite of descent. Now, if the essential condition of descent is a coincidence of the axes, it follows that one factor, at least, in the treatment of descent must be to restore the normal angle between the axes.

In labor the anterior wall of the vagina is depressed, stretched and shortened by the advancing child that during and after the second stage the anterior lip of the cervix uteri may be seen behind the urethra. This location of the cervix—so close to the anterior wall of the pelvis—necessarily involves great stretching of the utero-sacral supports which normally hold the cervix uteri, and together with it the upper extremity of the vagina close to the hollow of the sacrum. This function of the post-uterine ligaments having been temporarily impaired, the

* Read at meeting of Canadian Medical Association, Vancouver, B. C., August, 1904.

upper extremity of the vagina is displaced forward, so that the uterus, having sufficient space between itself and the sacrum, instead of maintaining its normal anterior position, may fall backward into retroversion and thereby bring its own axis into line with the direction of the vagina. Frequently the change in the direction of the vagina from the normal oblique to the abnormal vertical is still further increased by injury to the vaginal outlet; the perineum may be torn in any direction, and what is more serious, it may be torn away from its pubic attachments and in this way may be displaced backwards towards the tip of the coccyx; in fact, such displacement is so common, as the result of injuries to the perineum, as to suggest the propriety of a change in terminology from laceration to displacement of the perineum. The upper extremity of the vagina being displaced forward and the lower extremity backward, and the direction of the overstretched, dilated vagina now being vertical, the heavy uterus, having its long axis in the same vertical direction, has all the conditions favorable to progressive descent.

If the puerperium progress favorably with prompt involution of the pelvic organs, and if the relaxed vesico-vaginal wall and other parts of the pelvic floor, especially the utero-sacral supports and the broad and round ligaments, recover their normal tone, then the whole pelvic floor, including the uterus, resumes its normal relations. But if the enlarged heavy uterus remain in the long axis of the vagina, and especially if the fundus uteri be incarcerated under the promontory of the sacrum, with the sacral supports stretched so much and for so long a time that they cannot recover their contractile power; and if normal involution of the pelvic organs be arrested, then descent may not only persist, but may progress with constantly increasing cystocele and rectocele until the entire uterus has extruded through the vulva.

It is most important to remember that complete prolapse of the uterus is only an incident to prolapse of the pelvic floor. The whole mechanism is that of hernia, and the condition is hernia, for the extruded hernial mass drags after it a peritoneal sac which, hernia-like, contains small intestines. This sac forces its way to the pelvic outlet and extrudes through the vulva, having the inverted vagina for a covering.

The prolapsing uterus may be related to the vaginal walls in either one of two ways: the prolapsing vaginal walls may drag the uterus down after it, or the uterus itself may descend along the vaginal canal by force of its own weight and drag with it the reduplicated vaginal walls. Extreme prolapse of the uterus, the organ being covered thus by reflected vaginal walls, has given rise to considerable confusion in pathology, and by many standard authors wrongly has been called hypertrophic elongation of the cer-

vix uteri. In a given case, the possibility of infra-vaginal elongation may be settled easily by placing the patient in the knee-breast
position, when the uterus of its own weight will fall toward the
diaphragm and, the reduplicated vaginal walls will unfold and
utero-vaginal attachment will appear in the normal place instead
of being, as it seemed to be, high up on the walls of the uterus.
Those cases in which reduplication of the vaginal walls does not
almost entirely explain apparent great elongation of the cervix,
are rare exceptions. When formerly these mechanical conditions
were attributed to hypertrophic enlargement of the uterus itself,
and were regarded as adequate indications for the removal of
the cervix, the surgeon, in the attempt to remove what he supposed was the elongated cervix uteri, sometimes invaded the
bladder anteriorly and the rectus posteriorly.

Surgical Treatment.—In passing, it may be well to mention,
for the purpose of condemning it, an operation perhaps more frequently performed than any other for the cure of complete descent, namely, the operation which generally passes under the
name of Stoltz. This operation is designed to narrow the
vagina, and thus to maintain the uterus somewhere in the pelvis
above the constriction. Operations of this class usually consist
of the removal of an elliptical piece from the anterior or posterior
vaginal wall, or from both, and of closing the exposed surfaces by
means of a purse-string suture. No effort is made to destroy the
normal axis of the uterus and vagina. The whole purpose is to
make the vagina so narrow that the uterus cannot pass through it.
Such operations generally fail, because they leave the uterus and
vagina in the same axis, and because the restricted vagina cannot resist the downward force of the uterus, which almost invariably dilates the vagina a second time and forces its way through
with reproduction of the hernia. Moreover, the operation always
does permanent harm, because it shortens the vagina, thereby
making it draw the cervix away from the sacrum towards the
pubes, so that the body of the uterus may have room to fall backward to the position of incurable retroversion. We may, without discussion, perhaps, throw out all operations belonging to the
Stoltz group. The same may be said of all plastic operations in
which the vaginal surfaces are exposed by superficial denudation
and brought together by sutures.

After a prolonged trial of the principal surgical procedures
which have been made use of for the cure of complete descent,
I am prepared to lay down certain essential principles, as
follows: An efficient operation on the vaginal walls should have
for its object, not narrowing the vagina, but restoring the normal direction of it with a double purpose, so that (*a*) the upper
extremity, together with the cervix uteri, shall be in its normal

location within an inch of the second and third sacral vertebras, just where the utero-sacral ligaments would hold it if their normal tonicity and integrity could be restored, and so that (*b*) the lower extremity of the vagina shall be brought forward against the pubes.   The fulfilment of these two indications will restore the normal obliquity of the vagina, and will hold the cervix uteri so far back toward the sacrum that the corpus uteri must be directed forward in its normal anterior position of mobile equilibrium.   With these conditions, the uterus being at an acute angle with the vagina and having little space posteriorly, cannot retrovert and turn the necessary corner which would permit it to prolapse in the direction of the vaginal outlet.   In order to accomplish this, two things usually are necessary:

1. Excision of the Cystocele.

Anterior Colporrhaphy.—The plastic operations performed on the anterior and lateral walls of the vagina by Sims, Emmet, myself and others, which have consisted of superficial denudation and reefing of the anterior or lateral walls of the vagina, have been only partially successful, first, because they did not adequately force the cervix uteri into the hollow of the sacrum; second, because efficiency requires deeper work than superficial denudation can accomplish, and third, because these operations did not utilize the broad ligaments sufficiently for support.

The above principles, emphasized by Reynolds in a recent paper, have led me to modify my own operation materially. Complete prolapse, being hernia, should be treated according to the established principles of herniotomy by reducing it and then excising the sac in such a way as to expose strong fascial edges, which should be firmly united by sutures.   The absurdity of treating any other hernia by superficial denudation and reefing or tucking in the surfaces by sewing them together must be apparent to any one.   In order to indicate the part which the broad ligaments must have in a correct operation, it is only necessary to observe the fact that vaginal hysterectomy commonly results in holding up the pelvic floor and with it the rectum, vagina and bladder, because in this operation the broad ligaments are usually fixed to the vaginal wound.   But why should not the same result be aimed at by similar means, even though the uterus is not removed?   The operation which I would urge is performed as follows:

First Step.—To split the antero-vaginal wall—that is, the vaginal plate of the vesico-vaginal septum—by means of scissors, from the cervix uteri to the neck of the bladder, then to strip off the vaginal from the vesical layer of the vesico-vaginal wall and cut away the redundant part of the vaginal plate.

Second Step.—The redundant part of the vaginal wall having been removed to extend the incisions and remove the mucous and submucous structures to either side of the uterus, being sure to reach the fascial structures, which are in direct connection with the lower margins of the broad ligaments, or, what is better, to reach the ligaments themselves.

Third Step.—To introduce silk worm gut or chromic catgut sutures so that when tied they will draw the loose vaginal tissues and the broad ligament structures on either side of the cervix uteri in front of the cervix so as to force the cervix back into the hollow of the sacrum.

Fourth Step.—The sutures introduced in the third step having been tied, additional interrupted sutures are introduced to unite the vaginal wound from side to side; this suturing is continned to a point near the urethra, when most of the redundant vaginal wall will have been taken up; there will usually remain, however, the lower portion of the cystocele and perhaps some urethrocele, which cannot be disposed of by bringing the margins of the wound from side to side, but can be taken up by uniting the remaining part of the wound in a transverse direction.

Even at the risk of prolixity I repeat that it is essential to remove the entire thickness of the vaginal layer of the vesico-vaginal septum.

Contraindications to Elytrorrhaphy.—Elytrorrhaphy is usually unnecessary, and therefore contraindicated in descent of the first degree. The special province of the operation is in complete prolapse or procidentia when associated with cystocele. The operation further is contraindicated by tumors and adhesions which render replacement and retention impossible, and in diseases of the uterus or its appendages, which demand their removal. When such contraindications do not exist, elytrorrhaphy and perineorrhaphy in a majority of cases are quite as effective, and therefore to be preferred to the more dangerous and mutilating operations of hysterectomy.

2. Perineorrhaphy and Posterior Colporrhaphy.

As already stated, it is most important to appreciate the fact that in nearly every case of procidentia the lower extremity of the vagina is displaced backward. This is consequent upon subinvolution of the pelvic floor, and especially upon subinvolution or rupture of the perineum or of some other portion of the vaginal outlet. Unless, therefore, the posterior wall of the vagina and the perineum can be brought forward to their normal location under the pubes, so as to give support to the anterior vaginal wall, the latter will fall again, will drag the uterus after it, and the hernial protrusion (cystocele and prolapse) will be reproduced.

The treatment, therefore, of procidentia must always include an adequate operation on the perineum, or, more comprehensively speaking, upon the posterior wall of the vaginal outlet. The operation must be performed so that it will carry the lower extromity of the vagina forward to the normal location close under the pubes; then, if the anterior colporrhaphy has been adequate, and has carried the upper extremity backward, the whole vagina will have its normal oblique direction, and its long axis will make the necessary acute angle to the long axis of the uterus.

Hysterectomy, if indicated, should be performed by the vaginal route. As an operation for procidentia, hysterectomy is open to the following comments: Procidentia, as already shown, is hernial descent, not merely of the uterus, but also of the vagina, bladder and rectum. Complete prolapse often occurs after the menopause, when the uterus has become an insignificant rudimentary organ, and therefore may be removed easily. Cases are numerous in which, after vaginal hysterectomy, the pelvic floor, and with it the vaginal walls, have protruded again through the vulva—a result which may be expected unless the operation has included anchorage of the upper end of the vagina to its normal location by stitching the severed ends of the broad ligaments into the wound made by removal of the uterus. The indications for perineorrhaphy as a supplement to hysterectomy are the same as after anterior elytrorrhaphy.

As laid down in the foregoing paragraphs, the utilization of the broad ligaments is the essential factor in the treatment of complete procidentia. The operation of elytrorrhaphy, above described, unfortunately either may fail to bring the lower edges of the broad ligaments sufficiently in front of the uterus to enable them to hold up the uterus and vagina, or the ligaments having been stitched in front, the stitches may not hold. Consequently, in complete procidentia, elytrorrhaphy, even though well performed, may fail; at least, this has been my experience in a number of cases. Therefore, the completely prolapsed uterus may have to be removed in order to secure the entire outer ends of the broad ligaments to the upper part of the vagina, and thereby give absolute support. As before stated, the operation should include the treatment of the hernial factor in the lesion, that is, removal of the redundant portion of the anterior vaginal wall. Generally speaking, the indications are somewhat as follows:

1. Extreme cystocele, not associated with the most extreme procidentia, should be treated by anterior colporrhaphy and perineorrhaphy.

2. Cystocele associated with complete procidentia properly, may be treated by hysterectomy, anterior colporrhaphy and perineorrhaphy. Anterior colporrhaphy in all cases.

3. Conditions intermediate between the two conditions indicated above, and cases of very feeble or very aged women, will call for special judgment whether hysterectomy be omitted or performed. It is, however, a fortunate fact that the completely prolapsed uterus, even in aged women, is removed usually with ease and safety.

Other Operations of Questionable Value.—Other operations, designed to decrease the weight of the uterus by removel of it, are of questionable value. Amputation of the cervix to lighten the weight of the uterus has been practised much for the spurious hypertrophic elongation already described. Since this condition is rare, if not indeed unknown, it follows that it seldom will furnish an indication for amputation of the cervix uteri.

Alexander's operation and abdominal hysterorrhaphy belong to the surgical treatment of retroversion and retroflexion, not of procidentia. The object of these operations is to suspend the uterus from above. Hysterorrhaphy, which perhaps fulfils this indication better than shortening the round ligaments, may be indicated in cases of extreme relaxation of the uterine supports and greatly increased weight of the uterus. The results of it in complete procidentia, however, usually will not be permanent unless it is supplemented by adequate surgery to the vagina.

Proceedings of Societies.

THE GREAT WEST AND THE VANCOUVER MEETING OF THE CANADIAN MEDICAL ASSOCIATION.

IN a previous issue, through the kindness of a collaborator, a former resident of the North-West, we published a short, illustrated article on the beauty of the trip to the Coast, in order to try and infuse an added desire on the part of the members of the medical profession here to overstep all barriers and be among those present at this year's Canadian Medical Association meeting at Vancouver. As ever, *L'homme propose et Dieu dispose*, and many who had planned to go were detained: some were sick, others in England, and "some had friends who gave them pain," usually relations, and so the treat of a trip to the great West was missed. One more opportunity, however, of a similar character, presents itself, to take the trip, and even a further one, out to Portland, Oregon, to attend the American Medical Association convening there in July of next year. We here insert the remaining number of half-tones illustrative of the picturesque beauty of the tarrying spots along the way to Vancouver, which we hope ere long all the delinquent members of the C.M.A. of this year may view with delight. We physicians need more holidaying and surely more change of scene.

Perhaps the wonderful mountains are to the traveller the most inspiring sight of all.

Banff is the most famous pleasure resort of the Canadian Rockies. It enjoys a situation peculiarly advantageous for realizing the magnificence and charm of the mountain scenery. Not only are there mountains on every side with all the sublimity of snow-capped peaks and rocky steeps, but many valleys radiate from it, affording a delightful contrast. The Canadian Pacific Hotel stands at almost the point of the angle that the Bow River makes round the foot of Mt. Rundle, as its course changes from north-east to south-east. At the same point the Cascade River comes down from the north by the side of the mountain of the same name, and a considerable flat is formed—one of the most beautiful spots of the National Park, in the vast area of which it is included.

The course of the Bow River before its turn has been transverse to the run of the mountains. The heights are ranged in

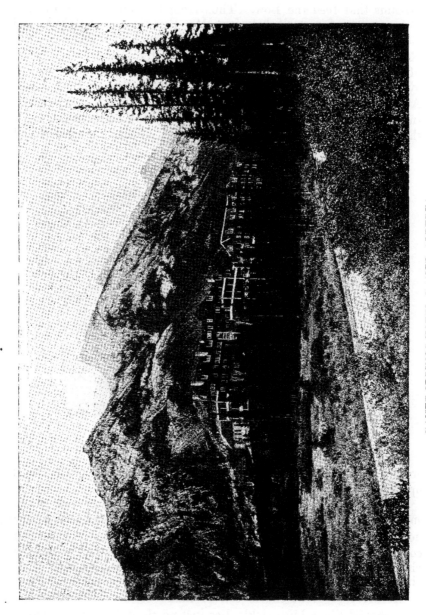

BANFF SPRINGS HOTEL, BANFF, ALBERTA.

almost parallel lines north and south, the valley of the Bow, when
it has resumed its southerly direction, being between Mt. Rundle
and the Fairholme Range.   Between the ranges come down small
streams that feed the Bow.   Thus from the south the Spray has
cut a valley for itself between Mts. Rundle and Sulphur, and
the Sundance Creek is between Mt. Sulphur and the Bourgeau
Range.   From the north, besides Cascade, the Bow receives Forty
Mile Creek, which flows between the Vermilion and Sawback
Ranges and then winds round the spurs of Stoney Squaw Mt.
An enlargement of the Bow forms the Vermilion Lakes, charming sheets of water, that with many meandering waterways occupy
the low ground of the valley and give the visitor unexpected and

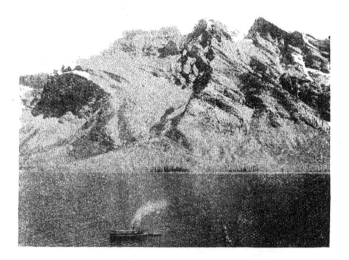

LAKE MINNEWANKA. NEAR BANFF ALBERTA.

lovely views of the giants that surround them and unsurpassed
opportunities for boating.

Banff Hotel stands on the south bank of the Bow, close to the
mouth of the Spray.   It has recently been enlarged, and now
accommodates three hundred people.   It is fitted up in the most
comfortable fashion, with rooms single and en suite, and may
challenge comparison with any other summer hotel on the continent.

A drive of great charm can be made to Lake Minnewanka
that, shaped like a huge sickle, lies just north of Mt. Inglismaldie.
It is eight miles from Banff, and the road leads up the valley of
the Cascade under the shadow of that glorious peak. The lake is
nearly ten miles long, and its waters are strangely diversified in
hue, deep blue and pale green giving way to yellow or grey, while

a streak of red appears here and there where some glacial stream debouches, and its peaceful surface reflects the ranges with absolute fidelity.

From the lake extends the valley of the Ghost River, one arm of which runs along under the shadow of the Devil's Head Mt., a peak that rises black and sombre to the north-east. The granite crags contain deep caves, the rivulets disappear to hidden reservoirs and the river runs along with mysterious, subterranean rumblings—a solitary, awesome region. The reasons of these uncanny manifestations were quite beyond the Indians, who for ages were the sole human beings to tread the valley, and it is not surprising that they saw in the great rocks, piled in majestic confusion, and the deep rumblings issuing from the bowels of the earth, the agency of powers supernatural and terrible. Even

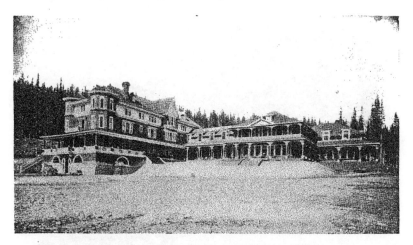

LAKE LOUISE CHALET, LAGGAN, ALBERTA.

now the visitor, fortified by all the knowledge of a scientific and rationalistic age, can, if he chooses, call up the feelings of the superstitious savage, and must be deeply impressed by the Valley of the Ghost.

The track from Banff to Laggan runs with thick groves on either side through a world of mountains. The observation car, attached to the trains, admirably fulfils the purpose for which it was designed, and gives uninterrupted views of the scenery all round; but the tourist may also travel between Banff and Laggan, if he so prefers, by special motor cars, built on the model of the open street railway car. They are driven by gasoline engines of twenty horsepower, and have a possible speed of twenty-five to thirty miles an hour. They are constructed with the sole idea of affording passengers the opportunity of enjoying the magnificent mountain vistas in the greatest comfort and at their leisure, and they have become a popular institution, as it is found they give a latitude the exigencies of the regular trains cannot allow.

After leaving Banff, the track runs through the tangled bottom, where sleep the Vermilion Lakes, a labyrinth of waterways, set off by grassy banks and thick woods.

Laggan is a station for a land of rare beauty. Within the mountains that overshadow it are enclosed the three lakes in the clouds, Paradise Valley, and the Valley of the Ten Peaks. The scenery differs from that which excited admiration at Banff, but it is of even greater charm, and those who pass by Laggan without halting have missed one of the most dainty bits ever carved by nature's deft fingers.

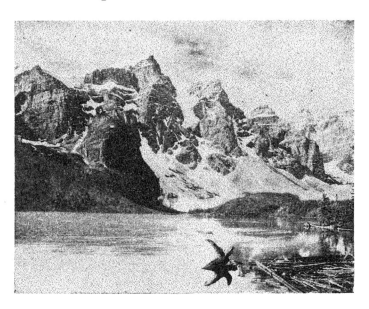

MORAINE LAKE, LAGGAN, ALBERTA.

The first sheet, Lake Louise, is reached from Laggan station by a drive of two and a half miles ever upward through a spruce forest. Here, on the very verge of the water, in the midst of the evergreen wood, the C.P.R. has built a lovely châlet, which has since been enlarged to a great hotel. It is open from June 1st to September 15th, and at it Swiss guides, horses and packers can be hired for excursions near or far.

As the name, Moraine, implies, the lake is situated at the foot of a moraine, as the mass of debris and rocks of every size and kind a glacier brings down is called. A great glacier has found its way down the heights at the head of the lake and has forced its course between and round the peaks. For a third of the distance from the lake to the summit the ice is entirely covered by a pic-

:turesque mass of rocks, piled in such disorder as chance directed the ice should leave them. It is a picturesque and awe-inspiring .sight. On either side the rocks rise sheer from the glacier, and as the sun lights up one precipice, gilding and bringing into relief every detail of pinnacle or crevice, while the other is left :in deepest shadow, the effect is magnificent in the extreme.

An interesting feature about this glacier is that it seems to be advancing. For some reason that cannot be explained, the .glaciers, not only in the Canadian mountains, but the world over, have of late years been receding, and the Moraine Lake ice-river is, therefore, an exception to the usual rule. Its force is tremendous, and it is most impressive to note how the woods have fallen before its resistless force.

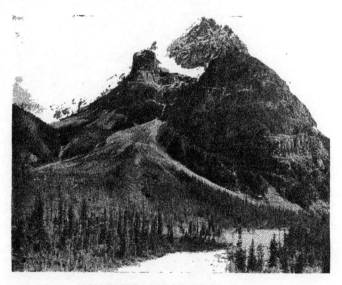

MOUNT STEPHEN, FIELD, B.C.

At Field the prospect widens, and the Kicking Horse River for a short distance flows across broad, level flats, that are only covered when the water is high. The place itself is a prosperous little village, but is dwarfed into insignificance by the splendid mountains that hem it in. On one side is Mt. Burgess, on the other Mt. Stephen, one of the grandest of all the Rockies.

Looking from the shoulder of Mt. Burgess or Mt. Stephen the valley seems narrow, the river a mere stream, and the dwellings in the villages dolls' houses. From below Mt. Stephen fills all the view; so rounded, so symmetrical that the spectator hardly realizes at first that he has before him a rock mass towering 10,000 feet above sea level and 6,500 feet above the valley. But as he gazes its majesty bears in on him and he is filled with a :sense of awe and wonder. One great shoulder is thrown forward,

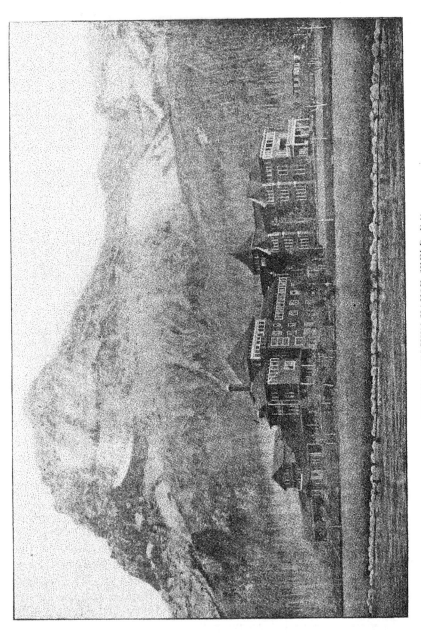

MOUNT STEPHEN HOUSE, FIELD, B.C.

a mountain in itself, and then the dome swells, gently, easily, till it reaches the clouds. Sometimes, indeed, the mist settles on it and obscures half its bulk; sometimes the sun lights up its crevices and touches its peak with gold; sometimes a cloud lies like a mantle across its face; but with it all it dominates everything and seems to defy man and nature. There is nothing broken or rugged in its outline, no suggestion of wildness or desolation; it impresses by its sheer bulk and massiveness and forces the admiration of the most careless.

To practised climbers the ascent of Mt. Stephen presents no insuperable difficulties, and indeed the trip to the summit and back from Mt. Stephen House has been made in eight hours. Swiss guides are stationed at the hotel, and will help the ambitions to accomplish the feat. The lower slopes of the mountain have one spot well worth visiting, the Fossil bed, where for 150 yards the side of the mountain for a height of 300 or 400 feet has slid forward and broken into a number of shaly, shelving limestone slabs. These fragments are easily split and reveal innumerable fossils, principally trilobites, a perpetual delight to geologists.

From the top of Mt. Stephen a magnificent view is obtained, that well repays the toil and difficulty of the ascent. The Van Horne range is seen beyond the Kicking Horse Valley to the west, the Emerald group occupies the north, while on the east the peaks that line the Yoho Valley, Mts. Habel, Collie, Gordon, Balfour, and many another are in full view. Across the river to the south, a number of fine mountains are in sight, Mts. Assiniboine, Goodsir, The Chancellor and Vaux. For miles and miles the tourist can see over valleys and peaks, and he realizes the immensity as well as the beauty, of the Rockies.

The summit of the Rogers Pass has an elevation of 4,300 feet, and from it a view is obtained of a splendid array of peaks stretching in all directions. Sir Donald, however, claims the chief attention, its position accentuating the impression its mere bulk creates. It stands at the end, at the climax of a line of heights, Mt. Avalanche, Eagle Peak and Uto Peak, and overlooks the Great Glacier of the Illecillewaet. Every inch of its 10,600 feet impresses the observer, and as it towers a mile and a quarter above the track, everything seems to sink into insignificance before its splendid presence, for it rises a sharp-pointed pyramid, bare and bold, from the valley below.

The dense forests creep up the low slopes, but fail long before they reach the base of the central height, and above is a glacier on which falls the snow that cannot lodge on the sheer crags of the soaring peak. A col, or ridge of rock, is thrown out towards the range, and at its foot lies another glacier, which feeds

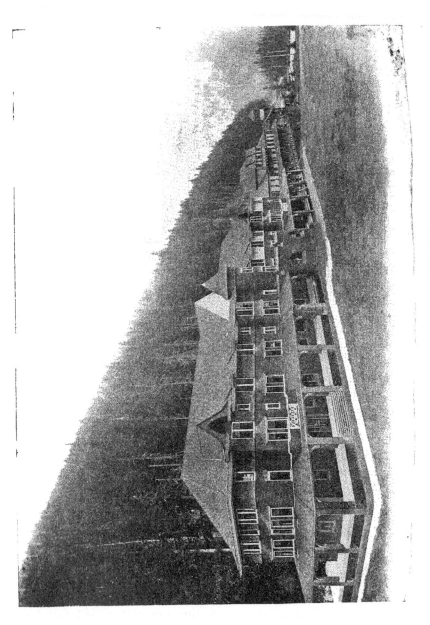

GLACIER HOUSE, GLACIER, B.C.

.a stream that finds its way down a deep-scarred gully to the vale below. It is this stream, perhaps, that brings out most clearly the magnificence of the mountain; the eye dwells on its course, follows its windings and ascends its bed for hundreds and thousands of feet to find there is still a tremendous pile of rock, above and beyond, that seems to pierce the very heavens. The verdure of the grass, the darker hues of the forest, the yellows and browns of the cliff, the blue of the glacier and the blinding, dazzling white of the snow, combine to make Sir Donald a mountain that artists love to paint. It is named after Sir Donald Smith, now Lord Strathcona, one of the chief builders of the Canadian Pacific Railway.

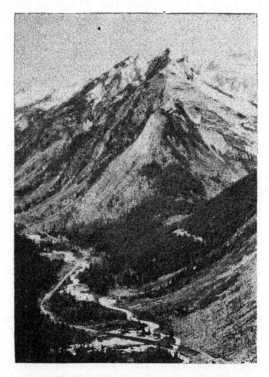

ILLECILLEWAET VALLEY, GLACIER, B.C.

Close by is Glacier House, the Canadian Pacific Railway hotel, enlarged to twice its original size for the second time last winter. Its popularity with tourists is growing steadily, and the Company purpose extensive additions before the end of the next year.

The Illecillewaet Glacier, like nearly every other observed glacier in the world, is receding. It is reckoned the sun drives it back thirty-five feet a year, and recovers this much from the bonds of ice. However, after the ice is gone, the moraine remains, and it will be many centuries before the great rocks carried down by the glacier are reduced to dust, and the land thus reclaimed supports renewed vegetation.

It is utterly impossible for us to even name more than one or two of the places which attracted most attention on the way across the continent, and space does not permit of our going into any further detail. We append what we trust our readers will find to be an interesting account of the meeting, and hope to report several of the papers read from month to month.

The Convention of the Canadian Medical Association, which opened in the O'Brien Hall at 9.30 o'clock on August 23rd, was a notable gathering even for a city so renowned for conventions as Vancouver. In the first place the delegates comprised some of the leading men in the profession from many of the foremost nations of the earth, and for a few days Vancouver possessed such a supply of grey matter as it had never known before.

The visitors began to arrive in small groups, but it was not until the day before that they came in any number. Among those who arrived early was Dr. Mayo Robson, of London, England, who reached Vancouver the Saturday evening previous. Dr. Mayo Robson came West principally on a hunting trip. He has an international reputation, and his address on surgery at the Convention on Wednesday was looked forward to with interest by the members of the Association. Among other notable arrivals were Dr. Ovialt, President of the Wisconsin Medical Association, and Dr. C. H. Mayo, of Rochester, Minn. These gentlemen are well known in the States for their successful surgical operations, and attended the Convention as visitors. Another eminent American physician is Dr. E. C. Dudley, of Chicago, who arrived on the Sunday night and contributed a paper on the following Wednesday evening.

Among the members of the Association on hand were Dr. H. Howard, Guelph; Drs. Chown and England, Winnipeg; Dr. H. G. McKid, Calgary; Dr. Wilson, Edmonton; Dr. T. W. Smith, Aylmer, Ont.; Dr. Mather, Tweed, Ont.; Dr. Boulet, Montreal; Dr. F. Martin, Dundalk; Dr. Pamiraud, Sherbrooke; Dr. Tierney, Prince Albert; Dr. L. G. De Veber, Lethbridge; Dr. Halder Kirby, Toronto; Dr. Geoffrey Bayfield, Portage la Prairie; Dr. A. A. Macdonald, Dr. B. E. McKenzie, Dr. G. Elliott, of Toronto, and lots of others.

Dr. Kirby was the guest of Mr. and Mrs. W. E. Burns, and Dr. Bayfield stayed with his brother, Mr. H. Bayfield, on Davie Street.

Some thirty-five or forty delegates arrived by the Pacific Express on the 22nd, but the bulk of the delegates materialized on the Imperial Limited the day of the opening, and still another batch the same evening. Among other arrivals was Dr. Small, of Ottawa, the General Treasurer of the Association. The rest were nearly all from Eastern cities, Montreal especially being strongly represented. Drs. Tunstall, Weld, Brydone-Jack, Monro and others of the Reception Committee had a busy time receiving and introducing the visitors. Though a little disappointed by the tardy arrival of the delegates, the Convention opened on time, and business was proceeded with in quite the regular order. The beauty of the mountain scenery was chiefly blamable for delayed arrivals, as delegates who had never seen the Rockies and Selkirks before could not be got to hurry through them.

O'Brien Hall, where the sessions were held, had been elaborately prepared for the Convention, and was well worth a visit. Tho stairway had been carpeted, and extra seats placed in the large hall to accommodate the visitors. The lesser hall had been converted into a hall of exhibits. A large space was occupied by Messrs. Chandler & Massey, of Toronto, with their display of surgical instruments and appliances. Enamelled operating tables occupied a prominent place, and on the side tables was a glittering display of surgical instruments of every kind. Gazing at the collection of catheters, forceps, probes and knives of every kind, one was very apt to realize that science has left very little undone towards the relief of human ills. Messrs. H. K. Wampole & Co. had a very neatly arranged display of their medicines, and Appleton's and Lippincott's both made a fine showing of medical books. Mr. J. H. Chapman, of Montreal, also had a large assortment of surgical instruments of French and English make on view. In the hallway there was a medicinal food exhibit, and just across from it the Deimel Mesh Underwear Co. displayed its goods. This portion was in charge of Dr. J. C. Cracknell, of Montreal.

All arrangements possible were made for the comfort and convenience of the delegates. A private writing room had been set off. At the head of the stairs on the second floor were placed the desks of the Secretary and Treasurer, and there was a post office box, a telephone, and a stenographer and typewriter; and to the rear of these a reading and smoking room. The arrangements reflected great credit on the local President, Dr. Tunstall, and the local Secretary, Dr. Brydone-Jack, and those who faithfully assisted them in their labors.

The head of the stairway in the O'Brien Hall was populous at an early hour with medical men assembled for the opening of the Convention. After an hour or more passed in signing the register and in informal chat, the President, Dr. Tunstall, of Vancouver, called the meeting to order in the large upper room.

Owing to the delayed arrival of the Imperial Limited, the

attendance at first was not as large as had been expected, but it was very representative, delegates being there from every part of the Dominion, as well as from several outside countries. On the platform were Dr. Tunstall, President; Dr. Geo. Elliott, of Toronto, General Secretary; and Dr. W. D. Brydone-Jack, Chairman of the Committee of Arrangements.

In opening the meeting, Dr. Tunstall stated that they had several distinguished guests among them, and he would be pleased to have their names introduced to the meeting.

The first one to be introduced was Dr. E. C. Dudley, of Chicago, a distinguished gynecologist, and author of " The Principles and Practice of Gynecology."

Dr. Dudley spoke of the pleasure it had given him to attend the meeting of the Provincial Medical Association of British Columbia three years ago, and said he felt sure that that pleasure would be more than repeated now.

Dr. C. H. Mayo was introduced by Dr. McKid, of Calgary. Dr. Mayo said he was pleased to be present at such a gathering, no matter where it might be held, as their profession recognized no international boundaries.

After the adoption of the minutes and the reading of the General Secretary's report, Dr. Small, of Ottawa, moved a resolution to introduce a new by-law into the constitution, empowering the Provincial Medical Associations each to appoint three members, who, with the President, should form an Executive Committee.

The resolution was adopted with very little discussion.

Dr. Brydone-Jack, Chairman of the Committee of Arrangements, then reported to the delegates on the provisions that had been made for their pleasure and comfort. He stated that they would hold occasional Masonic meetings for members of that fraternity. He also read a letter from the Secretary of the Lawn Tennis Club, offering the delegates the freedom of the grounds, and told of the entertainments and excursions which had been provided for the visitors.

Mayor McGuigan was received with applause on going forward to welcome the visitors. He said that he was sorry that the atmosphere was so murky that they could not see the beauties of the surrounding country, as we had here some of the finest scenery in the world. He hoped, however, that they would not blame it on the Council, who usually got blamed for everything unfavorable, bad weather included. He was pleased to offer them the freedom of the city, as he jocularly remarked that it was not always easy for the police to recognize a distinction in people. (Laughter.) He spoke of the value of the Convention in bringing to the Eastern part of the Dominion a knowledge of what the West really was. He told them there was a valuable organization in the city known as the Tourist Association, whose members would be glad to show them all that was to be seen.

He noticed that the American Medical Association was going to meet in Portland, Oregon, next year. He was sorry that the two bodies had not met on the Coast this year, but as it was he trusted they would both do much to dispel the false notions that prevailed in the East as to conditions in the West. He had just come from a trip to the East, and he knew there was a great deal of ignorance about the Coast. A prominent doctor in Montreal had asked him if they managed to get the *Daily Star* in Vancouver, evidently imagining that there were no daily papers here. He hoped that gentleman was out here now, and if he were he would see that we had as large a number of daily papers and as high a quality as any city of our size in the Dominion.

He spoke particularly of those physicians who were here from the Old Land, and of the tidings they would carry back with them, and it was in many ways a good thing for the medical profession and for the country that this meeting should take place here.

Speaking from a medical standpoint, he said that there was even a higher standard of professional ethics here than in the East, and instanced the entire absence of professional advertising. He stated that there was to his knowledge no illegal practitioner either in Vancouver or Victoria. In conclusion, he offered them the freedom of the city, and as Chairman of the Police Commission, he guaranteed that they would find the police and the city officials ready to give them all the information and assistance they might need. (Cheers.)

The following resolution was then moved by Dr. R. E. Mc-Kechnie, of Vancouver, and seconded by Dr. R. E. Walker, of New Westminster:

"*Whereas* tuberculosis has been positively proved to be an infectious disease;

"*Whereas* the patient is the focus of infection and is capable of infecting and does infect dwellings, clothing and private and public places generally. Statistics already available prove that compulsory notification with educational oversight of the patient and those under exposure to the contagion, together with disinfection of infected materials, has resulted in a diminution of the number of cases;

"*Whereas,* such action in the Dominion of Canada lies with the various Provincial Governments;

"*Therefore,* be it resolved, that the various Provincial authorities be and are hereby urged to at once take the necessary steps to bring these suggestions into effect, and that the Secretary be requested to forward copies of this resolution to the Secretaries of the various Provincial Boards of Health."

Dr. C. J. Fagan, of Victoria, Provincial Health Officer, spoke briefly in favor of the resolution. He said that some years ago he had brought up a similar resolution, but owing to the apathy with which it had been received by the medical men of the province, he had let the matter drop, until recently, when the urgent necessity for some measures had encouraged him to take up the matter again.

Owing to the non-arrival of some gentlemen who were down for addresses, Dr. Fagan was next called upon and read a paper on "Patent Medicines" which gave rise to a great deal of discussion. Whilst all seemed to agree with his views there was some difference of opinion as to how the evil should be treated. The thanks of the Association were moved by one member, who declared that the use of patent medicines was a growing evil and should be dealt with. He said that he understood that at the last session pressure was to have been brought upon Sir William Mulock to introduce some measures to check the spread of this evil by pamphlets sent through the mails, but nothing had been done. He was pleased, however, to notice that Dr. Sullivan had brought up a resolution in the Senate that the authorities should take this matter up and deal with it.

Another doctor suggested that it should be brought before the Minister of Inland Revenue that the sale of these medicines vastly exceeds that of alcoholic stimulants, from which the country derives a great revenue, and a greater revenue could be derived by taxing these proprietary medicines. In this way something might be done without infringing on the imaginary rights of people.

It was finally resolved that Dr. Fagan and such gentlemen as he wishes to associate with him, should be appointed a committee to draft a resolution on this question of patent medicines.

At the conclusion of the discussion on Dr. Fagan's paper, the Convention adjourned to meet again at 2.30 p.m.

At the opening of the afternoon session, Dr. Tunstall read the following telegram:

NEW YORK, AUGUST 23RD.

S. J. TUNSTALL, M.D.,

Thanks for kind invitation. I greatly regret cannot attend meeting. The press here, medical and lay, refers triumphantly to Osler's appointment as Regius Professor of Medicine at Oxford. King Edward approved it. Osler has accepted for next year. God bless dear old Canada, McGill and Osler.

Yours faithfully,

WILFRID NELSON.

Dr. Davie, of Victoria, Vice-President of the College of Physicians and Surgeons of British Columbia, then came forward to welcome the visitors to the Province.

Dr. Davie said that in the absence of the President of the College of Physicians and Surgeons it gave him much pleasure to welcome the visitors. He said that this was the first meeting of the kind in the Province, but they had the same interests and studies in common, and it gave him much pleasure to bid them heartily welcome.

Dr. R. E. McKechnie then gave an "Address on Medicine," which contained a very interesting sketch of the progress of medical science from the earliest ages. The address will be found under our original articles in next month's issue of the JOURNAL. He also gave an interesting account of his experiences with a rival "medicine man" among the Indians on the Coast. The concluding part of the address dealt with the progress of medicine in recent years. At the conclusion of the address a vote of thanks to Dr. McKechnie was moved by Dr. Lafferty, of Calgary, and seconded by Dr. England, of Montreal. Before putting the motion the President explained that the address redounded the more to the credit of Dr. McKechnie because less than two weeks ago he had stepped into the place of a gentleman who had been set down for it, but was unable to attend. The vote of thanks was then heartily carried.

As several gentlemen who were down for addresses had not arrived, an exhibition of "The new color test apparatus" was given by Dr. Glen Campbell. Mr. Mansfield, Fleet Surgeon on H.M.S. *Grafton,* had been billed for this, but as his ship had been called away to Honolulu, Dr. Glen Campbell had kindly consented to read the paper he had prepared and to work the color test.

The machine in question is shaped something like a camera, with two knobs and different eyeholes in frout, but is closed up behind, and is meant for testing the eyesight of candidates for the Army and Navy.

That the members of the Association might better observe this instrument, the meeting was adjourned for fifteen minutes.

When the meeting was again called to order, a paper on "Movable Kidney" was read by Dr. Kenneth McKenzie of Portland, Oregon.

Dr. Robert H. Craig, of Montreal, followed with a paper on "Case Reports."

Dr. Hackett and Dr. Irvine, both of Montreal, spoke briefly on Dr. Craig's paper, both congratulating him on the success of his operations.

The Convention then adjourned till 9.30 next morning.

The conversazione given by the Association at the Hotel Vancouver in the evening was a brilliant social affair. By ten o'clock there must have been fully 500 people in the large dining room of the hotel, and the hum of many voices in conversation almost drowned the strains of Harpur's orchestra, which was playing at the further end of the room. Among the many guests were the wives and daughters of the visiting medicos, and the members of the Committee on Arrangements, conspicuous by their bright badges, had a busy time making introductions. Among the many guests from the city were the Mayor and several members of the City Council, and many of the city officials. There were also several representatives of the city clergy, and the legal profession was present in large numbers. That those present enjoyed themselves was shown by the cordiality and freedom from restraint with which conversation was carried on.

Up to the evening of the first day, 157 members and visitors had registered on the books of the Association, but this was augmented to well on towards 300 by the following night's arrivals.

Speaking of the departure of a number of London people to Vancouver to attend the meeting of the Canadian Medical Association, the *Free Press,* London, says: " A large party of medical men and their wives left the city on Monday night for a pleasant transcontinental trip, in the course of which they will attend the convention of the Dominion Medical Association to be held in Vancouver, B.C. Among those who left—all travelling by the C.P.R.—were Dr. and Mrs. Drake, Miss J. Moore and Dr. Norman Henderson, of this city, and Dr. and Mrs. McCallum, Miss McCallum and Dr. and Mrs. Bell, of the Asylum.

" Dr. and Mrs. Eccles and Dr. and Mrs. Meek also left, but were members of a special party that was made up, in addition, of the following: Dr. Wardlaw and wife, Galt; Dr. Hobbs and wife, Guelph; Dr. Rooney and wife, Shelburne; Dr. Ross, Dundas; the Misses Bain, Dundas; Dr. Secord, Brantford; Miss Howell, Brantford; Dr. Holmes, Chatham; Dr. Savage, Guelph; the Drs. Thompson, Strathroy; Dr. McCullough, wife and daughter, Alliston; Dr. Gilchrist, wife and daughter, Orillia; Dr. Stewart, Milton. This latter party went to Owen Sound, and thence by C.P.R. steamer *Alberta* to Fort William, where they took a special car on which they travelled to the Coast."

It may be interesting to know that the handsome badge worn by so many of the Medical Association, was designed by the worthy President, Dr. Tunstall. It is a neat heart-shaped button, surmounted by the miniature arms of Vancouver (the Sunset Gateway of the Dominion) as a crest. Through the centre runs the golden staff of Mercury, and round the edge is inscribed

" Canadian Medical Association, 1904." The button was neatly finished off in alternate stripes of white and blue, and is a credit both to the designer and the maker.

That the Medical Association is growing was abundantly proved both by the report of the General Secretary and the large number of names proposed for membership.

Among the other arrivals on the Pacific Express the second evening was Senator Sullivan, of Kingston, Ont.,

Dr. Moorehouse, one of the Nova Scotia delegates, was unfortunately taken ill while en route to the Coast. The ambulance was in attendance on the arrival of the Imperial Limited, and conveyed him to the Vancouver General Hospital, where he speedily recovered.

A pleasing feature of the first day's proceedings was the attention with which everyone present listened to the various papers, very few leaving the room before adjournment.

A notable exhibit was an X-ray outfit by Heinz & Co., of Boston, Mass. The expert who had charge of this machine gave several exhibitions before the Association. Mr. J. J. Dougan also installed an exhibit of the many valuable medical works for which he is agent.

The smoothness with which the Convention was conducted is largely due to the following gentlemen, constituting the Committee of Arrangements: Vancouver—W. D. Brydone-Jack, Chairman; F. McPhillips, Secretary. Victoria—Dr. Fraser, Chairman; H. M. Robertson, Secretary. Finance—J. M. Lefevre, Chairman; J. M. Pearson, Secretary. Printing—F. T. Underhill, Chairman; G. P. Young, Secretary. Reception— O. Weld, Chairman; J. S. Conklin, Secretary. Exhibit—A. S. Monro, Chairman; X. McPhillips, Secretary.

In honor of the visitors the streets were illuminated till a late hour in the evening.

On Thursday evening a meeting in the interests of Dr. C. J. Fagan's plan for the proposed tuberculosis sanitarium was held in the O'Brien Hall at 7.45 o'clock. The Mayor presided and Dr. Mayo Robson, the celebrated English surgeon, delivered an address.

Second Day's Session.

There was a considerable increase in the number of members attending the second day's session of the Canadian Medical Association and O'Brien Hall was well filled. Many new members were placed on the roll. Dr. Brydone-Jack, Chairman of the Committee of Arrangements, made several welcome announcements of entertainments and outings provided for the visitors. He stated that cheap rates had been obtained for those wishing to visit New Westminster, and for those who did not

6

wish to go, the steamer *Kestrel* had been retained, and they could explore the beauties of the Inlet. He also announced that all guests of the Association were to receive free tickets to the dinner at the Hotel Vancouver that evening. He further stated that on Wednesday evening there would be a special Masonic meeting, at which members of the fraternity visiting the city would be made especially welcome. For the ladies accompanying the visitors, carriages would be at the Hotel Vancouver at 2.30 to take them around the Park.

The first paper read was doubtless one of the most notable addresses of the Convention. It was that of Mr. Mayo Robson, of London, Eng., on "Surgery." Mr. Mayo Robson's address, *which we hope to reproduce next month,* was vividly illustrated by a superb series of lantern slides, showing the formation of the internal organs, and was listened to with the keenest interest throughout the whole hour that it occupied, and was received with loud applause.

At the conclusion a hearty vote of thanks to Mr. Mayo Robson was tendered by the audience.

Dr. F. J. Shepherd, of Montreal, then read a paper on "Hernia of the Bladder, Complicating Inguinal Hernia." The paper was followed by short discussions by Dr. A. A. Macdonald; Dr. Meek, London, Ont.; Dr. Secord, Brantford; and Dr. Eagleson, Seattle.

A paper on "Movable Kidney" was then read by Dr. K. McKenzie, of Portland, Oregon. Those taking part in the discussion were Dr. R. C. Coffey, Portland, and Dr. Eccles, London, Ont.

Dr. S. R. Jenkins, of Charlottetown, P.E.I., then read a short paper on "Report of Hypertrophy of the Breasts."

Before adjournment, Dr. Brydone-Jack announced that those who wished it might go with Dr. Underhill to inspect the septic tanks—that was if they preferred that to the lunch in the Pender Hall. There were also bowling and croquet games and lawn tennis at the Lawn Tennis Club grounds.

The Convention then adjourned for luncheon.

The first business to come up in the afternoon was the election of the Nominating Committee. Drs. Brydone-Jack and Shepherd were appointed tellers, and a ballot was taken on the following:

Prince Edward Island—Dr. McLaren and Dr. Houston.

Nova Scotia—Dr. James Ross, Dr. J. B. Black.

New Brunswick—Dr. Morehouse, Dr. T. Walker.

Quebec—Dr. Shepherd, Dr. R. Craig, and Dr. Boulet.

Ontario—Dr. Meek, Dr. Howitt and Dr. A. A. Macdonald.

Manitoba—Dr. McArthur, Dr. Smith and Dr. Chown.

North-West Territories—Dr. De Veber and Dr. Stewart.

British Columbia—Dr. Davie, Victoria; Dr. R. E. McKechnie, Vancouver.

There are only two candidates elected for each Province, so that only the results in Ontario, Quebec and Manitoba remain to be known.

Dr. McGillivray, of Edinburgh, and Dr. Sinclair, of Manchester, Eng., were introduced to the Association and welcomed by the President.

A paper on " Diseases of the Eye " was then read by Dr. J. W. Stirling, of Montreal.

Dr. D. Cruikshanks, of Windsor, Ont., followed with a paper on " Therapeutic Hints from Bacteriology," giving many interesting descriptions of the actions of bacteria on animals. He was of opinon that too much medicine was used in bacterial diseases as a general rule, and thought that the twentieth century would witness a radical change in treatment.

At 4 o'clock the meeting adjourned, most of the members going to the Pender Hall, where a reception was held, while others went for a drive round Stanley Park. The reception was quite a brilliant affair. It was attended by several hundred people, and Mrs. Tunstall and the wives of other local doctors who constituted the Reception Committee, had a busy time receiving their guests. The hall was decorated in a manner that reflected the greatest credit on Mr. O'Callaghan and those who had assisted him in the work. The windows were treated with a dark green dressing, which admitted a softened light. The roof was done in terra-cotta, and the electric lights were festooned with orange shades and ivy. Undoubtedly the beautiful setting of the scene did much to enhance the success of the gathering.

There was a large attendance at the evening session, and the Presidential address of Dr. Tunstall was listened to with great interest. Before commencing his address, Dr. Tunstall asked Dr. Powell, of Ottawa, to take the chair.

In doing so, Dr. Powell referred to the pleasure he felt at being at a meeting of the Association presided over by his old friend, Dr. Tunstall.

Dr. Tunstall then delivered his masterly address, which will be·found among our original contributions in this issue of the JOURNAL.

The Hon. Senator Sullivan, in quite a lengthy speech. proposed a vote of thanks to Dr. Tunstall for his very able address. He spoke of the gratitude due to this young province for entertaining in its midst this cultured and enlightened gathering. He spoke of the history of the Canadian Medical Association, which had been first established thirty-eight years ago. He congratu-

lated Vancouver on securing so many visiting doctors from the
neighboring States, and said that if Canada was invaded it would
not be by way of Tacoma. (Laughter.) He said he intended to
have given them a little of the wisdom of the hoary East, but Vancouver was so much West that she was neither East nor West.
He spoke with approval of the suggestions made by Dr. Tunstall, and said he hoped they would travel East and be taken up
with enthusiasm by the profession as they went till they covered
the whole Dominion. He again moved a vote of thanks to the
President for the very able and practical paper he had given them.
Dr. Sullivan's speech was replete with witty points and flashes
of rhetoric, and was received with great applause.

The vote of thanks was seconded by Dr. Eccles, of London,
Ont., and carried with enthusiasm.

Dr. E. C. Dudley, of Chicago, then gave an address on
" Gynecology," illustrated by a series of fine lantern slides. It
was listened to with close attention, and at the close Dr. Dudley
received a hearty vote of thanks from the audience. (Dr. Dudley's
address will be found on pages 237 to 243 of this issue.)

A number of pictures of the new Vancouver Hospital building were then thrown upon the screen, and were explained to the
meeting by Mr. G. W. Grant, of the firm of Messrs. Grant & Henderson, the architects of the building.

As the hour was late, the Convention adjourned to meet again
in the O'Brien Hall at 9 o'clock next morning.

During the course of the evening session, the following announcement was made by Dr. Brydone-Jack, Chairman of the
Committee of Arrangements:

The excursion tickets were quite free to all their guests, and
the Committee hoped that every member present would take advantage of them and take their wives and daughters with them.

He announced that transportation to Victoria would be free
to all members from the East, and if any had not tickets, all that
was necessary was to apply to Mr. Coyle, Passenger Agent of the
C.P.R., and they would receive them. As they wished to estimate
the number going to Victoria, he asked all who intended going to
stand up, and nearly everyone in the room rose, whereupon Dr.
Fraser, of Victoria, said he hoped that everyone would go, as there
was much to show them.

Dr. Brydone-Jack apologized for not being able that afternoon to carry out their arrangements to visit the septic tanks,
but he said provision had been made that that morning at 10.30
Dr. Underhill and Colonel Tracy would be at the disposal of
any members who wished to view the tanks.

He also announced that the Maritime Provinces Association
meeting would be held sharp at 12 o'clock, when the members

here would present an address of welcome to the visitors from their old home.

During the previous day's session, the following announcements were made:

A meeting of the members of the Canadian Medical Association, who hail from the Maritime Provinces, is called at 12 o'clock. The meeting will be held in the smoking-room of the O'Brien Hall, and is called for the purpose of meeting the local members of the Maritime Provinces Association. It was understood that the members of the latter Association intended to extend a formal welcome to the visiting " Blue Noses," and also present the visitors with an address.

A cordial invitation was also extended by the Art and Historical Association to the visiting members of the Canadian Medical Association to visit the Carnegie Library, at the corner of Westminster Avenue and Hastings Street, on the upper floor of which is the Society's museum, which is open for the inspection of the visiting doctors. The interesting collection on view there is well worthy of a visit.

A meeting of the Executive Committee of the Association was called for 2.30 p.m.

Those who wished to get tickets for the New Westminster excursion were requested to apply at the Secretary's desk in the O'Brien Hall, and meet at the tram office at 1.30 p.m. Special cars were provided and run half-hourly during the morning.

THIRD DAY'S SESSION.

At the opening of the third day's session of the Canadian Medical Association, the attendance was smaller than before, as many had chosen to go out to the septic tanks, and different outside attractions had taken away others.

Many new members were proposed and elected, and Dr. Brydone-Jack announced that the Government steamer *Kestrel* would be ready at the C.P.R. wharf at 2.30 to take out any that had not gone to New Westminster.

The first paper read was that of Dr. C. H. Mayo, of Rochester, Minn., on " Tubercular Peritonitis." The fact that the Mayos have an almost international reputation for the treatment of tubercular diseases, lent additional weight to his words, and his paper was followed with close attention.

A vote of thanks was moved by Dr. Macdonald, Brandon, and seconded by Dr. McKid, Calgary.

Dr. Davie, Victoria, discussed the paper at some length, complimenting Dr. Mayo on opening up new theories of treatment for these troublesome diseases, and praised the ingenuity of the American physicians in the methods they had adopted.

Dr. Holmes, of Chatham, Ont., also spoke a few words expressive of the pleasure he had derived from listening to Dr. Mayo's paper.

Dr. Howitt, of Guelph, Ont., read a paper on "Meckel's Diverticulum, Report of Cases." During the reading of his paper, Dr. Howitt had several photographs of diverticula he had treated handed round for inspection.

Dr. Mayo discussed the paper at some length. He said that in these physical freaks it often took a gravestone to teach them anything. He also said that while the lungs would stand a great deal of operation, a small intestine would stand very little.

Dr. C. W. Wilson, of Montreal, read a paper on "Results (after one year) of the Lorenz Operation for Congenital Dislocation of the Hip," illustrated by a number of radiographs. He showed that of cases treated there had been about 10 per cent. of perfect replacements, and perhaps 50 per cent. of good results.

The paper was discussed by Dr. B. E. McKenzie, of Toronto, who cited many cases of dislocated hip which had come under his own observation.

Dr. E. R. Secord, of Brantford, Ont., gave an address on "Operative Treatment of Spina Bifida," which was the last paper read before the Association, as one or two others whose names were on the programme had failed to appear. Dr. Secord's paper was well received, and at the conclusion he was made the recipient of a vote of thanks.

The Convention then adjourned till 9 o'clock next morning, when a business meeting was held and officers elected for the ensuing year and reports of committees handed in.

After the adjournment of the morning session, a number of the officers and members of the Maritime Provinces Association met in the lesser O'Brien Hall to present an address to the visiting doctors from their home land. Several ladies were present, and before opening Miss Burpee very tastefully played a selection on the piano. When the visitors had gathered together, Mr. John Johnstone, President of the Maritime Provinces Association, presented them with the following address:

To the Maritime Provinces Members of the Canadian Medical Association—

The Maritime Provinces Association of Vancouver desires to extend to you a very hearty welcome to the Pacific Coast and especially to the Lion's Gateway, our fair city of Vancouver.

Our Association, now numbering over one thousand, resident in or near Vancouver, was formed for the purpose of bringing together natives of Nova Scotia, New Brunswick and Prince Edward Island in friendly and social intercourse, and of keeping in mind the varied and romantic history of the provinces by the sea, and the many distinguished men whose memories should never be allowed to fade.

We regret that your stay in Vancouver is so limited, and that your time is too fully occupied to permit us to meet with you publicly. Our members would gladly embrace the opportunity to mingle with you and renew old acquaintances.

We can assure you that we have not forgotten the homes of our childhood, whether these were on the rugged shores of Nova Scotia or in its beautiful valleys; or by the peaceful Cape Breton lakes; in the garden of the Gulf, the fruitful Island of Prince Edward, or in forest-clad New Brunswick, with her wealth of beautiful lakes and glistening streams.

Your visit brings these old scenes back to us, and mitigates, to some extent, the three thousand miles intervening between us and " home."

We trust you will carry away with you pleasant memories of your visit among us, and of this great Province in which you are sojourning, which is so vast in area, so rich in resources and endowed so beautifully in scenery and climate.

Here in Vancouver the grass remains green all winter, roses and other flowers bloom in the gardens in January and February, and the balmy breezes of the Pacific breathe perpetual summer.

With renewed expression of our interest in your visit, and trusting that British Columbia will appeal to you in all its varied beauty, we ask you to convey our salutations to old friends at " home," and assure them that while loyal to the land´ of our adoption, our pulse yet beats true to the Maritime Provinces, and that we ever follow with warm interest their continued prosperity and development.

Signed on behalf of the Maritime Provinces Association of Vancouver, this 25th day of August, A.D. 1904.

> EDWYN S. W. PENTREATH,
> Archdeacon of Columbia,
> > *Honorary President.*
> JOHN JOHNSTONE,
> > *President.*
> T. B. CROSBY,
> > *Honorary Secretary.*

Dr. J. Ross, of Halifax, then read the following address in reply:

To the Maritime Provinces Association of Vancouver—

The Maritime Provinces members of the Canadian Medical Association are deeply grateful to you for the hearty welcome and words of cheer extended to us.

That such an Association as yours exists, with its large number of members, and showing strong evidence of a healthy growth, pictures that spirit of true fellowship that should fill the hearts of all those who have not forgotten their nativity.

Since we arrived in your city we have been received with the greatest hospitality and particularly from those whose "homes" are so intimately associated with our own in the far East.

We will carry away glad memories of our visit, and particularly the knowledge that your hearts will ever beat true at fond memories of Home, Sweet, Home.

(Signed)　　S. R. JENKINS, Charlottetown.
　　　　　　JAMES ROSS, Halifax.
　　　　　　F. S. YORSTON, Truro.
　　　　　　GEO. M. CAMPBELL, Halifax.
　　　　　　J. B. BLACK, Windsor.
　　　　　　C. I. MARGESON, Hantsport.

Vancouver, August 25th, 1904.

At the conclusion Dr. Ross called upon Dr. Black, of Windsor, N.S., the senior member of the delegation, for a few words.

Dr. Black said he had been delighted with this country and the reception that had been given them by the people here. He wanted to say that no man could ride from Halifax to Vancouver and not be a bigger man mentally when he arrived in Vancouver. He believed he would be a more loyal man, more of a Canadian and less of a colonist, and it would give him a more abiding faith in Canada and her institutions. Whilst he was not here as a politician in any sense of the word, but simply as a physician attending the Convention, he believed that, as full-grown, self-respecting men, we feel, or ought to feel, that this Canada of ours should be wholly governed by ourselves. He was not a secessionist, and had not the least desire to break any of the links with the Old Land, but he thought they should be part of a British federation entirely controlling their own affairs. They had their own hopes and ambitions and aspirations, which could not be shared by England, Ireland, Scotland, or any other part of the British Empire. The artisans of the cities of these countries were the men who elected the men that sent them their Governors-General. He believed, however, that the people of Canada had ability and courage enough to choose for themselves. "Time turns the old days to derision," Swinburne told them, and he believed that it was rapidly turning the old days of colonialism to derision, and teaching them that they must look to themselves. In conclusion, he said he was glad to see that their people here had not forgotten the best part of the Dominion down by the sounding sea.

Archdeacon Pentreath said he was only sorry that circumstances had prevented them giving the physicians a large public reception, as they would like to have done. He spoke with regret of the late ex-Lieutenant-Governor McInnes, who, with others, was a prime mover in founding the Association. They had now on the books nearly a thousand members, which showed that there was a strong and excellent element building up Vancouver and British Columbia. He spoke of the growing national spirit in Canada, and said it was something they should do all in their power to foster.

Before the visitors dispersed all were presented with beautiful bouquets by the ladies present.

About two hundred doctors, with their wives and daughters, went over to New Westminster in the special cars provided for them the same afternoon. After having made a short inspection of the Royal City, they embarked on two steamers and were taken down the river past Ladner to Steveston. There the medicos were duly initiated into the mysteries of salmon canning, the different canneries being thrown open for their inspection. They were also taken on a tour through Chinatown, where they caught a glimpse of life in China as it is transplanted in the far West. Afterwards Mr. Coyle, Assistant General Passenger Agent of the C.P.R., met them at the depot and saw them safely installed in the special train he had provided, and about 6 o'clock they returned to Vancouver, quite refreshed by their outing.

In the morning between twenty and thirty of the doctors drove round with Dr. Underhill, Medical Health Officer, and Colonel Tracy, City Engineer, and inspected the septic tanks.

In the afternoon several delegates, who did not visit New Westminster, were taken for a cruise on the Inlet on the *Kestrel*.

The dinner of the Canadian Medical Association, given at the Hotel Vancouver that night, was a distinguished and successful affair. There were about two hundred medical men present, nearly all of whom were visitors to the city, and who were attending the Convention of the Association. Many of the visitors who came on Sunday had gone either to Victoria or Seattle, consequently there were fewer of the members present than were anticipated. As it was, however, the event was a highly pleasant one. Dr. Tunstall, the President of the Association, occupied the seat of honor at the table, and on the right hand was Mr. Mayo Robson, whose address at the Convention was so instructive and interesting; Prof. Dudley, of Chicago University; His Worship the Mayor, Dr. McGuigan; Dr. Sullivan, Senator, who wittily replied to the address of the President on Wednesday evening. On the left of the President were Dr. Shepherd, of Montreal; Dr. Powell, President of the Canadian Medical Protective Association; Mr. R. Marpole, General Superintendent of the Pacific Division of the C.P.R.

The spacious and well-appointed dining-room was well fitted to accommodate the large assembly. The brilliancy of the electric light was augmented by the glint of lighted tapers, and High-

field's orchestra provided music in such a style as to elicit applause
from time to time.

After the repast, the toast list was announced by the President, Dr. Tunstall. First, "The King," responded to enthusiastically by the entire assembly singing "God Save the King." "The President of the United States" was also drunk heartily when "The Star-spangled Banner" was the air. "Canada," proposed by Dr. Brydone-Jack, Secretary of the British Columbia Provincial Association, called for the hearty singing of "The Maple Leaf."

This toast was coupled with the names of Dr. Sullivan, of Kingston, and Dr. McGuigan. Dr. Sullivan's reply opened very wittily, his remarks beginning really when he told of how proud we should be that we were residents of the Dominion, and particularly of Vancouver, the best in Canada. He was glad to see so many from the United States on such an occasion. Dr. Sullivan told of whom he represented from Ontario, and waxed warm and witty over their grand attributes. He humorously objected in the strongest terms to having been pounced upon to reply to a toast without having had any notification, his remarks causing laughter throughout.

Mayor McGuigan reminded the members that in the holding of the Convention in Vancouver, the Association had completed the extent of Canada from Prince Edward Island to British Columbia. The members would go down to Victoria on Friday, and that would complete the trip to the Pacific Coast. Touching upon Vancouver, he informed his hearers that when he first came to the city the spot on which dinner had been eaten was forest, where grouse could have been obtained in season. Since then the city had grown into one of the best in Canada, with all the up-to-date appurtenances of a modern city. He hoped the members of the Association would carry back kind remembrances of their visit to the Pacific Coast. (Applause.)

A song by Dr. Powell was a pleasant interpolation. The selection, entitled "Where'er St. George's Banner Waves," was rendered in fine voice.

Dr. Chown, Winnipeg, in proposing the toast of "The Canadian Medical Association," said his first opportunity of seeing Vancouver was when the Association held its Convention at Banff fifteen years ago. Since then the city had been greatly developed, and the early day anticipations had been fulfilled. Now, with continental railway development it was an easy matter to traverse the Dominion and hold a convention here. It was due to Eastern members in the larger cities that the Association was maintained in active organization, and the present session was remarkable for its large attendance and success. With his toast he coupled the names of Dr. Shepherd and Dr. Good.

Dr. Shepherd, of McGill University, Montreal, after an in-troductory remark that he recognized some of his old pupils, among them the Mayor, said that the first President, Sir Charles Tupper, was still alive, which was worthy of note. The cause of its inception had been to get a Medical Bill passed, but this was ineffectual. The earlier efforts had been surpassed by the great meetings of later days. He had come to Vancouver, too, when the Convention had been held at Banff, but the same smoke seemed to still hang over Vancouver. (Laughtor.) He hoped, when he came West again, that there would be an opportunity to confirm the report that there was scenery here. (Laughter.)

Dr. Good, of Winnipeg, who had been referred to by Dr. Shepherd as the silver-tongued orator, turned the remark in a very pleasant way, and spoke of the benefits of the Convention, referring humorously to the length of the papers read. One of the objects of the Association was to bring men together, which had proved beneficial. In his reference to Vancouver, he said it was pleasing to note that a member of the profession occupied the Mayor's chair, and if a judgment could be made from adiposity, Dr. McGuigan was certainly an excellent Mayor. (Laughter.) Dr. Good said he had come from the County of Bruce (cries of " Hear, hear ") and had sat at the feet of the President, Dr. Tunstall, and from that school teacher had imbibed many of the noble ideas from which he now suffered. (Laughter.) Dr. Good upheld the reputation ascribed to him, and was interesting and humorous in his remarks, which were greeted with applause.

Dr. Brydone-Jack read two telegrams which had been received by Dr. Tunstall. One was from J. B. Eagleson, whicsh contained the following: " Yankee doctors on their way home give three cheers for the Convention and the Entertainment Committee." The other was from Hon. Richard McBride, and read: " Kind invitation just received. Regret impossible to be present."

Mr. R. G. Macpherson, M.P., wrote: " Through unavoidable circumstances I am unable to be present at your dinner to the Canadian Medical Association to-night. Will you please express my sincere regrets that I am unable to attend, and at the same time trusting that joy will reign supreme round your festive board, and that the members of your noble profession will carry away the most pleasant remembrances of their visit to Vancouver."

Dr. Weld proposed the toast of " Our Guests." He said that the success of the present Convention was due to the presence of distinguished doctors from other countries. Among these were Mr. Mayo Robson, from London; Dr. McGillivray, from London; Dr. Dudley, from Chicago, and others, whose papers had been of great profit. When they came again he hoped that Vancouver would have a hospital where operations could be carried on with less inconvenience than on the present occasion. This called forth an enthusiastic " For They Are Jolly Good Fellows," followed by hearty cheers. With this toast were coupled the names of Mr. Mayo Robson, Dr. McGillivray, Dr. Dudley, Dr. Mackenzie, of Portland, and Dr. Manning, Everett.

Mr. Mayo Robson said Canada was a great country, not only in its details, but in its grandeur. Entering Belle Isle Straits he thought he was near Quebec, but after he had travelled a day and saw the extent of that province, he wondered how great Canada was. When he had crossed the continent, his expectations were realized. When he went back he would know that England was smaller than ever and that Britain was greater than ever. (Applause.) All that was needed was the federation which was now coming about. What was required was to have more Englishmen come to Canada for them to become followers of Mr. Chamberlain. Now the narrow policies of the Georges were replaced by those of a king with a wide knowledge and broad understanding, and the future would be guided by the policy Mr. Chamberlain was now inaugurating. This was a day of aggregation, not segregation. As a medical man he should not have any politics. He had not seen a more enthusiastic gathering. It was a great pleasure to see four hundred or five hundred men together at the extreme west side of the continent. He complimented the resident doctors upon the prospect of a new hospital, and upon the equipment of the present institution. There was no want of learning nor of care among the medical men of this part of Canada.

Dr. E. C. Dudley's first information of Canada was when he was a barefoot boy, and he had formed many opinions of Canada at that time. Since then these good opinions had increased. Proceeding, he said the lack of preparation had left him only one resource, to tell the truth. Before doing so (loud laughter) he said he would like to remark on the different periods in the feeling between the United States and Canada, the latest of which was the period of brotherly love, which was here to remain. Earlier in the evening the President had proposed the toast of the President of the United States. In the United States the toast of the King of England was never proposed. He had been present at many affairs of this kind in his own country, and the toast was " The King," and everyone knew. (Applause.) British stock and American stock was common stock, and this was preferred stock. (Cheers.) Dr. Dudley touched upon the Russo-Japanese War, and said that while he was in favor of the Japs, as a cosmopolitan he hesitated about being in favor of a Japanese victory, as it might be a menace. He closed with a reference to the unanimity of Canada and the United States.

Dr. McGillivray, Edinburgh, said he had learned since coming to the Dominion what true hospitality meant, and said if he remained here he would know what it was to be killed by kindness. The memory of his stay in Canada would remain with him long after he returned to his native country. (Applause.)

Dr. Mackenzie, Portland, Ore., extended hearty thanks for the generous hospitality extended to the delegation form Oregon. It had distinctly a western flavor, which was to him a rare exotic. Since he had made Oregon his adopted home, twenty or thirty years ago, he had found that the people of that side of the line were much the same as they were in Canada. He was proud to belong to the great Anglo-Saxon race, which would ultimately win in the racial struggle now going on. Practically Canada and the United States were one, only a line, delimited by some engineers, separating them. Next July the American Medical Association would convene in Portland, and as Chairman of Arrangements he extended an invitation to be present. (Cries of " We'll be there.")

Dr. Manning, Everett, made a pleasing reference to the similarity of peoples, and said that it would be difficult to find a mistake in the actions of the Canadian Medical Association. Upon the question of mistakes he spoke eloquently and humorously, dwelling upon the mistakes of the profession. In closing he thanked the Canadian Medical Association for the loyal manner in which they had entertained their guests. Dr. Manning was greeted with applause.

Dr. A. A. Macdonald, who was called upon for a Scotch song, said he thought when he came here he was so far from his native heath that he would never be called upon for a speech or a song. Had it not been for the Convention of the Canadian Medical Association, he did not think it probable that he would have visited the West. He was always a Canadian, but he never appreciated the extent of this great country. This was the preface to a very catchy song with a nasal chorus in which all joined, accompanied with much laughter and absence of harmonious tune.

Dr. Lafferty, Calgary, proposed the toast of " The Learned Professions." He deprecated his ability to perform the task, but succeeded admirably. This toast was responded to by Mr. W. R. White, K.C., barrister, of Pembroke, and Prof. Sinclair, of Manchester, England.

Mr. White said he was at a loss to express his feeling at being present at such a gathering of ability and learning from all parts of America and Britain. He found very appropriate words, however, and his remarks were able and entertaining. He spoke at some length upon the subject, and was followed with considerable applause.

Prof. Sinclair declared that this was the first time in his life he had had the pleasure of responding to this toast.

Dr. Powell, Ottawa, said he felt it a high honor to propose a toast to the President, Dr. Tunstall. He had known the President for many years, and his appreciation of him was sincere.

When those present had sung heartily " He's a Jolly Good Fellow," Dr. Tunstall thanked the proposer for his high encomium. When he had received the appointment as President of the Association, he began to think in what way he could carry on the labors of those who had preceded him. If he had succeeded in making this Convention a successful one, much was also due to those who had assisted him, and to those also who had come thousands of miles to give their help. If he had done as well as was said, he was satisfied. (Applause.)

The healths of the Treasurer and Secretary, Dr. Small and Dr. Elliott, were also drunk, to which suitable responses were made. Dr. Small, Ottawa, recalled the fact that this was the third largest Convention in the history of the Association. The number of visitors from Great Britain and the United States has also been larger than heretofore, and he hoped to see greater co-operation between those of the medical profession in the two countries.

Dr. Elliott, Toronto, who for three years had been General Secretary of the Association, affirmed that he had not served with greater satisfaction under any President than under Dr. Tunstall, of Vancouver.

The toast to the health of the local Secretary, Dr. Brydone-Jack, was proposed by Dr. Shepherd.

Dr. Brydone-Jack said the success of the Convention was not due so much to the Secretary, as to the united efforts of the medical men generally.

The banquet closed with the singing of Auld Lang Syne and God Save the King.

Fourth Day's Session.

Probably owing to the lateness of the banquet the night before, combined with preparations for departure, the attendance at the final meeting of the Canadian Medical Association was much smaller than it had been before. The principal business was the receiving of the reports of committees, and election of officers.

The Nominating Committee sent in the following names as officers for the ensuing year, and they were duly elected:

President—Dr. John Stewart, Halifax.

Vice-Presidents—Prince Edward Island, Dr. McLaren, Montague Bridge; Nova Scotia, Dr. J. B. Black, Windsor; New Brunswick, Dr. A. B. Atherton, Fredericton; Quebec, Dr. James E. Dube, Montreal; Ontario, Dr. H. Meek, London; North-West Territories, Dr. W. S. England, Winnipeg; British Columbia, Dr. R. E. Walker, New Westminster.

Local Secretaries—Prince Edward Island, Dr. H. D. Johnson, Charlottetown; Nova Scotia, Dr. G. C. Jones, Halifax; New Brunswick, Dr. T. D. Walker, St. John; Quebec, Dr. J. D. Cameron, Montreal; Ontario, Dr. Stuart, Palmerston; North-West Territories, Dr. Hewittson, Pincher Creek; Manitoba, Dr. Popham, Winnipeg; British Columbia, Dr. A. S. Monro, Vancouver.

General Secretary—Dr. Geo. Elliott, Toronto.

Treasurer—Dr. H. B. Small, Ottawa.

Executive Council—Drs. G. M. Campbell, J. Ross, C. D. Murray, Halifax.

Upon motion, the President cast the ballot for the above-named candidates, and they were declared elected.

It was also decided that the next annual meeting of the Association should be held in Halifax.

Dr. Powell, of Ottawa, presented a report of the Committee on a Federal Health Department. He said that in accordance with a resolution passed in London last year, the committee had interviewed the Government, and he was sorry to report that it could not give them any assurance that the resolution in the matter would be practically considered. He said there seemed to be a general fear lest such a department should interfere with the autonomy of the Provincial Boards, but he had pointed out that there was no fear of that, as many matters would come up for consideration that could not be touched by the Provincial authorities. He instanced the medical treatment of Indians, which was under the supervision of the Minister of the Interior, and the Quarantine Department, under the control of Dr. Montizambert. There were such matters, besides, as sickness on trains and in camps, which could be dealt with by a Federal Department, and he did not see that there was the least need that it should in any way interfere with the Provincial Departments.

Dr. Fagan said he quite agreed with Dr. Powell's remarks, because, as a Provincial Medical Health Officer, he had often been faced with the very same difficulties of which he had spoken. Cases were brought to his notice that were not within the range of the Provincial Department, and when he applied to Ottawa he was told that they could not deal with them there.

The following resolution was then carried unanimously: " That the Canadian Medical Association regrets that the Canadian Government has not seen fit to carry out the resolution of this Association in favor of the creation of a Federal Health Department, and be it further resolved that the Association continue to press this matter before the Government, and that the Special Committee in charge of the same be re-appointed and requested to continue its efforts to this end, and that copies of this resolution be sent to the Prime Minister, the Minister of Agriculture and the Secretary of State."

Dr. Fagan then brought in the following resolution on "Patent Medicines": "That in view of the large amount of patent medicines which are now on the market containing alcohol and various drugs which, being taken, lead to the formation of evil habits, and are dangerous to the health, and in special view of the false statements concerning these remedies made through the press and by other means, some means should be adopted to control and restrict the sale of such medicines and to prevent fallacious statements advertising the same. Further, that a memorial to the Government be sent to the proper department concerning the matter."

Dr. Shepherd, of Montreal, thought the resolution might have been a little more specific. There was a complaint, but no remedy suggested. He thought that, considering the amount of alcohol used in these preparations, the manufacturers should be compelled to print a table of the ingredients, as was done in Germany.

Dr. Fagan said the committee had considered that it would be better first to bring the matter before the authorities in a general way, and let them take what action they might think fit. He scarcely thought it would be courteous to tell them what to do.

Dr. Lafferty said that he agreed with Dr. Fagan in this matter, though, if the Government seemed willing to take the matter up, they might make some suggestion to them next year.

The resolution was then passed unanimously.

The Hon. Dr. Sullivan then brought up a resolution urging energetic legislation in connection with the correct registration of medical practitioners.

Dr. Powell said there had been a great deal of prejudice in the Province of Quebec against the change proposed, and the Association must try to remove this misunderstanding on which that prejudice was founded.

Dr. Tunstall said that the great obstacle in Quebec was that the people did not understand our language, but he thought that once this matter was placed clearly before them the difficulties would vanish. The resolution in no way interfered with local practitioners in the Province—all that is required is that anyone wishing to be placed on a par with physicians all over the British Empire must undergo a Dominion examination.

Dr. Lafferty thought that a memorial should be sent to the Dominion Government in this matter, and that it should be propagated in the press.

The resolution was then carried.

The Auditor's report showed the handsome balance of $602 on the books.

It was also resolved that the usual honorarium be granted to the Secretary.

Dr. Black, of Windsor, N.S., moved, and Dr. Lafferty

seconded, a vote of thanks to the ladies of Vancouver for their efforts in making their stay so pleasant.

Dr. Shepherd moved that a vote of thanks be given to the Canadian Pacific Railway Company for the kind way in which they had treated them on their journey.

Dr. Brydone-Jack moved a vote of thanks to the press for their kindness during the Convention. They had been very good in carrying out the instructions given them, as well as in making announcements from time to time. He also included in the motion a vote of thanks to Mrs. McLagan of the *World* for her generous donation of papers to the members.

It was resolved also that an acknowledgment should be sent to the British Medical Association for their appointment of Dr. Roddick as representative of the Canadian Medical Association.

A hearty vote of thanks was passed to Dr. Tunstall for the able manner in which he had presided over the Association, and this brought this most successful Convention to a close.

Most of the delegates then commenced to say " Good-bye " to Vancouver. A large number of them went down to Victoria on the *Princess Victoria,* a programme having been arranged for their entertainment at the Capital City, including drives and steamboat excursions and a reception in the Parliament Buildings.

Directly after the close of the meeting of the Canadian Medical Association, a meeting of the Canadian Medical Protective Association was held.

Dr. Powell, the President, said that when this Association was first started they had hoped that 75 or 80 per cent. of the Medical Association might join them. He thought some alteration was necessary in the constitution to bring this question home to members in distant provinces. He thought there ought to be some one in each province to keep alive the interest in this Association.

Dr. Powell then read his annual report, which dealt strongly with the necessity of more increased activity in soliciting membership, though full of faith for the ultimate success of the organization.

Dr. Tunstall said he quite agreed with Dr. Powell as to paucity of membership in the Association, and would suggest a few changes in the constitution. In the first place he thought they should combine the offices of Secretary and Treasurer, and place more clerical help at the disposal of the President. In consequence of the need of this, there had been a great deal of irritation among members about having no acknowledgment for the receipt of dues and other matters. He also proposed the appointment of a small Executive in each province whose duty it should be to pass upon all cases occurring within the province and to solicit membership. He moved a resolution to that effect, the Executives for this year to be nominated by the President.

7

Dr. Powell said he had found himself under great difficulties for want of assistance in the provinces in this way. When a case of malpractice occurred, he had to communicate directly with the person, instead of with some disinterested party who was on hand and understood the matter. He regretted to say that a very unfortunate circumstance had occurred in this very city, owing to that position of affairs, whereby the good name of the Association had been smirched in the minds of the profession in British Columbia. He found that the person in charge occupied a very high position in British Columbia, and somebody pretending to act on behalf of this Association published a false telegram in the Vancouver press, the object of which was to show that this person did not occupy in the profession the same place as in the Police Court reports. When he found it out, he had at once telegraphed to Vancouver to say that the telegram was false. Had he had a local Executive to assist him it would have never allowed the good name of the Association to be dragged in the mud in this way. He wished to explain that he had an exact copy of the telegram he had sent, which was to the effect that they were to send a sworn statement from the accused that he was innocent, and another from his lawyer to the same effect, together with his receipt, and if the Executive thought it was a case to defend they would do so, but not otherwise. They were willing to defend those whom they thought to be wrongfully accused, but the Association would never defend any doctor for wrong-doing.

Dr. Fagan wanted to know whether they were going to pursue any inquiry as to the origin of the false telegram. He said that as a result of it a Victoria paper had published an editorial attacking the profession and the methods they pursued.

Dr. Powell said that until he had consulted with the solicitor of the Association he could take no further steps in the matter. Several telegrams had been sent to him asking for aid in the case, and one of these was signed " P. H. Weld," which was manifestly a forgery. He said he thought the position of the Association was quite plain. He had been a good deal attacked since coming here for acting on such slight information, and he was glad to have this opportunity to clear matters up. The Association always investigated a case before dealing with it. Some cases they refused to handle, others they advised to settle out of court, and some cases they defended. In no case would they defend wilful wrong-doing —they simply could not do so.

The matter was then dropped without further discussion.

Dr. Powell was re-elected as President of the Association, and Dr. James A. Grant, jr., also of Ottawa, was chosen as its first Secretary-Treasurer, and the Association adjourned to meet in Halifax next year.

The Canadian
Journal of Medicine and Surgery

J. J. CASSIDY, M.D.,
EDITOR,
43 BLOOR STREET EAST, TORONTO.

Surgery—BRUCE L. RIORDAN, M D ,C M., McGill Univer sity; M D University of Toronto, Surgeon Toronto General Hospital ; Surgeon Grand Trunk R R ; Consulting Surgeon Toronto Home for Incurables , Pension Examiner United States Government : and F. N. G. STARR, M B., Toronto, Associate Professor of Clinical Surgery, Toronto University , Surgeon to the Out-Door Department Toronto General Hospital and Hospital for Sick Children.

Clinical Surgery—ALEX. PRIMROSE, M B , C.M Edinburgh University ; Professor of Anatomy and Director of the Anatomical Department, Toronto University ; Associate Professor of Clinical Surgery, Toronto University; Secretary Medical Faculty, Toronto University

Orthopedic Surgery—B. E MCKENZIE, B A., M D , Toronto, Surgeon to the Toronto Orthopedic Hospital ; Surgeon to the Out-Patient Department, Toronto General Hospital ; Assistant Professor of Clinical Surgery, Ontario Medical College for Women ; Member of the American Orthopedic Association, and H. P. H. GALLOWAY, M D., Toronto, Surgeon to the Toronto Orthopedic Hospital ; Orthopedic Surgeon, Toronto Western Hospital ; Member of the American Orthopedic Association.

Oral Surgery—E H. ADAMS, M.D , D.D S., Toronto.

Surgical Pathology—T. H MANLEY. M D., New York, Visiting Surgeon to Harlem Hospital, Professor of Surgery, New York School of Clinical Medicine, New York, etc , etc

Gynecology and Obstetrics—GEO T MCKEOUGH, M.D., M.R C S Eng , Chatham, Ont ; and J. H LOWE, M.D., Newmarket, Ont

Medical Jurisprudence and Toxicology—ARTHUR JUKES JOHNSON, M.B , M R C S Eng , Coroner for the City of Toronto ; Surgeon Toronto Railway Co., Toronto , W. A YOUNG, M D., L.R C.P Lond ; Assoc ate Coroner, City of Toronto.

Pharmacology and Therapeutics—A. J HARRINGTON M D , M R C S.Eng , Toronto

W. A. YOUNG, M.D., L.R.C.P.Lond.,
MANAGING EDITOR,
145 COLLEGE STREET, TORONTO.

Medicine—J J. CASSIDY, M D , Toronto, Member Ontario Provincial Board of Health , Consulting Surgeon, Toronto General Hospital ; and W. J WILSON, M D. Toronto, Physician Toronto Western Hospital

Clinical Medicine—ALEXANDER MCPHEDRAN, M D., Professor of Medicine and Clinical Medicine Toronto University ; Physician Toronto General Hospital, St Michael's Hospital, and Victoria Hospital for Sick Children.

Mental and Nervous Diseases—N. H. BEEMER, M.D , Mimico Insane Asylum ; CAMPBELL MEYERS, M D., M R C S L.R.C.P (L ndon, Eng), Private Hospital, Deer Park, Toronto , and EZRA H. STAFFORD, M.D.

Public Health and Hygiene—J. J CASSIDY, M D , Toronto, Member Ontario Provincial Board of Health ; Consulting Surgeon Toronto General Hospital , and E. H. ADAMS, M D , Toronto.

Physiology—A. B EADIE, M D., Toronto, Professor of Physiology Woman s Medical College, Toronto.

Pediatrics—AUGUSTA STOWE GULLEN, M D., Toronto, Professor of Diseases of Children Woman's Medical College, Toronto ; A R GORDON, M D., Toronto.

Pathology—W H PEPLER, M D., C.M., Trinity University; Pathologist Hospital for Sick Children, Toronto ; Associate Demonstrator of Pathology Toronto University; Physician to Outdoor Department Toronto General Hospital , Surgeon Canadian Pacific R R , Toronto ; and J J MACKENZIE, B A , M B., Professor of Pathology and Bacteriology Toronto University Medical Faculty.

Ophthalmology and Otology—J. M MACCALLUM, M D , Toronto, Professor of Materia Medica Toronto University ; Assistant Physician Toronto General Hospital , Oculist and Aurist Victoria Hospital for Sick Children, Toronto

Laryngology and Rhinology—J D THORBURN, M D , Toronto, Laryngologist and Rhinologist, Toronto General Hospital

Address all Communications, Correspondence, Books, Matter Regarding Advertising, and make all Cheques, Drafts and Post-office Orders payable to "The Canadian Journal of Medicine and Surgery," 145 College St., Toronto, Canada.

Doctors will confer a favor by sending news, reports and papers of interest from any section of the country. Individual experience and theories are also solicited Contributors must kindly remember that all papers, reports, correspondence, etc., *must be* in our hands by the fifteenth of the month previous to publication.

Advertisements, to insure insertion in the issue of any month, should be sent not later than the tenth of the preceding month. London, Eng Representative, W. Hamilton Miln, 8 Bouverie Street, E. C. Agents for Germany Saarbach's News Exchange, Mainz, Germany.

VOL. XVI.   TORONTO, OCTOBER, 1904.   NO. 4.

Editorials.

AMERICAN SURGERY SEEN THROUGH FRENCH EYES.

DR. J. L. FAURE, of Paris, gives his impressions of American surgery in an article published in *La Presse Médicale,* July 27th, 1904. Premising, he recognizes that the general doctrines of scientific surgery are the same in both countries. He thinks that the operating room of the Mount Sinai Hospital, New York, is the handsomest he has ever seen. It is an extraordinary room, remarkable in that the walls and even the ceiling are covered with immense single sheets of white marble; but such decorative opulence, instead of capturing his admiration, gives him rather the sensation of prodigality run to riot.

The washing stands, with their taps worked by hand or foot, are similar to those used in France, and just like them, the mixing taps sometimes give the user of a basin a burst of hot water, and at other times pure cold water. He observes that the American sterilizing machines, particularly the autoclaves, which are of large size and placed in a horizontal position, are generally superior to the French ones, though he cannot pronounce authoritatively on their internal value.

He remarks that, during operations, American surgeons are covered from head to foot in sterilized garments; the nurses also wear caps, so as to conceal the hair. Almost all the operators and their assistants wear rubber gloves. On the other hand, he thought that the toilet of the anesthetized patient's skin was done less carefully and with less 'asepsis than in French hospitals. He thinks that the number of assistants at operations is excessive—two, three or four assistants to touch the patient and the instruments, while two or three nurses are busy with the compresses, passing them from hand to hand. This is, of course, contrary to the practice of French surgeons, whose ideal is to operate with only one assistant.

No operating table which he has seen in America is, in his opinion, equal to Mathieu's. The table most generally used is, however, a good one, being made of sheets of plate glass, which are easily taken apart, although it is defective in not allowing a sufficient inclination, so as to execute easily all the manoeuvres required in pelvic surgery.

He pronounces American surgical instruments vastly inferior to those made in France, the instruments used in gynecology and general surgery being heavy, coarse and primitive in make. This inferiority in surgical ware rather surprised him, but he explains it by the superiority of hand-made to machine-made goods, especially when the former are produced by artists, who put heart and brain into their work. To do first-class work in manufacturing surgical instruments, a long training, tradition and a direction met with only in Europe, and especially in France, are absolutely requisite.

The French nurse (*infirmiére*) is not in the same class as the American hospital nurse, and her work is not of equal value. The American nurse often belongs to a good family, and her general education is superior to that which falls to the lot of the French nurse. France cannot begin to compare with America in this respect, and Dr. Faure candidly admits that, while everywhere in American hospitals one sees well-educated young ladies acting as hospital nurses, a similar class of women is unknown in France. He describes how the trained nurse in America makes out clinical reports for each patient, noting such particulars as the temperature, pulse, excretions, sleep, nourishment, medicines, accidents, etc., details which in the French hospitals are noted by the externs, and not so scrupulously or carefully as in American hospitals.

With regard to the method of selecting surgeons for hospital positions, he thinks that the French method (*concours*) cannot be surpassed. In America, social influence and political wire-pulling are the mainsprings of success in many hospital appointments, and the instability of rival political parties sometimes occasions the premature disappearance of very able men.

Dr. Faure was favorably impressed with the surgical work done at a hospital in Rochester, a small town in Minnesota, by two brothers named Mayo. This hospital has accommodation for over a hundred patients, and has two small operating rooms. Patients go there from Canada and all parts of the United States. Each person's disease is diagnosed by one of a corps of eleven specialists, and if the case be suitable for a surgical operation, it is attended to by the brothers. Every morning, Sundays excepted, they do on an average about ten operations (three thousand per annum). On the day Dr. Faure was present at Rochester, he saw an operation for uterine polypus, an enucleation of tubercular glands of the neck, two prostatectomies, an abdominal hysterectomy for fibroma, a gastro-duodenostomy for pyloric stenosis, a gastro-enterostomy for cancer, a cholecystotomy, and a cholecystectomy for lithiasis of the gall-bladder.

American hospitality comes in for a good word: "They opened their operating rooms to me and welcomed me to their hearths."

Speaking of the relative merits of the surgeons of both coun-

tries, he says: " If the surgery of America is great, and if American surgeons are aware of their own greatness, we French surgeons have also the right to know our own value, and the right to
speak of it."

He advises French surgeons to travel, learning from foreigners
what they can, and imparting to others in return from the storehouse of their own knowledge.   Altogether a clever article, and
one which will do much good by removing misconceptions, showing Frenchmen that surgery in America has not been backward,
but that it is living up to the best traditions of European schools,
and, in some respects, is far ahead of the best of them.

J. J. C.

THE IMPERIAL CANCER RESEARCH FUND.

FROM the report of the Secretary of the Imperial Cancer Research Fund (*B. M. J.*, July 16th, 1904), we learn that this
English society, which is devoted to the study of cancer, has
established friendly relations with several institutions of learning in Europe and America.   Among individuals specially mentioned in this connection we notice the names of Professor Welch,
of Harvard University; Professor Adami, of McGill University,
and Professor J. J. Mackenzie, of the University of Toronto.

The report of the General Superintendent, Dr. E. F. Bashford, contained several noteworthy statements.   In opposition to
the view that vertebrates in a state of nature are not afflicted with
cancer, he said: " Altogether upwards of two thousand specimens have been examined during the year, and, wherever possible,
they have been studied not from the histological point of view
alone, but from the biological point of view as well.   The general
results may be thus summarized: Cancer has been discovered to
pervade the whole vertebrate kingdom and to present constant
fundamental characters.   External agencies, such as food, habitat,
and conditions of life generally have no causative influence.
The histological characters, methods of growth and absence
of specific symptomatology lead to the conclusion that it is not
permissible to seek for the causative factors of cancer outside of
the life processes of the cells."

With regard to the diagnosis and treatment of cancer, Dr.
Bashford stated: " No specific constitutional symptom of the

presence of a new growth has been observed, and the conclusion is drawn that cancer qua cancer in man and animals is without a specific symptomatology. Artificially transplanted tumors (cancerous) also afford the most favorable means of testing the claims made on behalf of various reputed empirical, therapeutic methods. Amongst these the action of radium bromide has been tested. Its investigation is not yet complete, but there is no ground at present for predicting the curative effect of radium upon deep-seated primary tumors.

In reference to hospital statistics, it appears that a plan whereby most of the great London hospitals place at the disposal of the Cancer Research Fund succinct accounts of all the cases of cancer which have been subjected to microscopic examination, has been at work for nine months.

An immediate practical result of compiling these hospital statistics is the proof afforded of the absence of specific clinical symptoms, hence the necessity of an early operation in a case which may not at the time appear to be malignant. It is also pointed out that in spite of the proportion of cases simulating new growths which appear in the tables, the surgeon should treat all suspicious growths as if he knew they were malignant, any delay in operative treatment in the hope that some means will be found to replace surgical interference being totally unwarranted."

The idea that cancer is a disease practically limited to civilized races is disproved, specimens of undoubted malignant new growths having been obtained from regions where intercourse with civilized man is at its minimum.

The low cancer death rate of Ireland is ascribed to the infrequency of necropsies and the neglect of microscopic examination of diseased specimens in that country. If it were otherwise, a cancer death rate proportionately higher than that of England would be found, in accordance with the higher age constitution of the Irish population.

Respecting the reputed increase in the prevalence of cancer, Dr. Bashford points out that cancer has now been discovered in animals formerly considered to be free from it, and that it has been shown to be relatively more frequent than hitherto recorded among uncivilized races. He concludes by stating that "there is nothing in the statistical investigations which points to an actual increase in the number of deaths due to cancer."

From an editorial in the August number of the *Montreal Medical Journal*, we gather that 275 cases of malignant new growths, reported from the Montreal and Royal Victoria hospitals, were included in the report of the Imperial Cancer Research Fund. Of these 275 cases, 212 were of carcinoma and 63 of sarcoma. In the carcinoma cases, the frequency of occurrence in the alimentary tract is striking: 60 per cent. of all the cases are in that situation, contrasted with 35 per cent. in the London series, but agreeing closely with the figure of 57 per cent. yielded by the Hamburg reports. Of all the cancers occurring below the age of 35, 63 per cent. were in the alimentary tract; of all the cancers of the alimentary tract, 62 per cent. occurred in the stomach. And again: "Of carcinoma in the male, 40 per cent. were situated in the stomach; in the female, 32 per cent. were in the stomach, 16 per cent. in the breast, 13 per cent. in the uterus."

One conclusion to be drawn from the Montreal cancer statistics is quite different from that of the Imperial Cancer Research Fund report. The latter confidently states that external agencies, such as food, habitat and conditions of life, generally have no causative influence in causing cancer; the latter makes it clear that "of all the cancers of the alimentary tract, 62 per cent. occurred in the stomach."

Now it may or may not be true that gormandizing is responsible for the large percentage of cancer of the stomach in the Montreal series of cases; but if that external agency was in no way responsible, then the fact that 62 per cent. of the 275 Montreal cases of cancer were located in the stomach must be regarded as a very strange coincidence indeed.   J. J. C.

THE VANCOUVER MEETING OF THE CANADIAN MEDICAL ASSOCIATION.

THE promise of a meeting beyond the Rockies, affording an opportunity not only to view the unrivalled mountain scenery of our West, but also to visit many friends who have gone into Manitoba and have located upon the fertile prairies, and the privilege of returning by way of United States cities, and espe-

cially by way of St. Louis, called out many from their daily toil
and grind to profit by a very genuine holiday. To travel from
the older portions of Canada by way of the C.P.R. palatial
steamers; to enter Winnipeg, the gateway of the West; to view
the grain fields of Manitoba; to inspect the train loads of cattle
moving eastward, fatted for market without corn, solely upon the
rich prairie grass; to visit many rapidly growing cities, such as
Brandon, Calgary and Edmonton; to talk with enthusiastic
immigrants, and thus to gain a knowledge from personal observation of the newer Canada, is, in itself, a liberal education.

The medical men of Vancouver had spared neither effort nor
money in arrangements tending to insure success. The late date
fixed by the Executive, however, for leaving the East, was responsible for the late arrival of many members at Vancouver,
causing disturbance in carrying out the programme, and detract-
ing much from the success of the scientific part of the convention.

Great interest was manifested in the papers presented by
our distinguished visitors, and the uniform appreciation of the
attention shown them won the golden opinions of the members.
Mr. Mayo Robson, of England; Dr. C. H. Mayo, of Rochester,
Minn.; Dr. Dudley, of Chicago, and Dr. Kenneth McKenzie, of
Portland, Oregon, contributed papers which added greatly to
the strength and interest of the programme.

Dr. McGuigan, Mayor of Vancouver, gave a cordial address
of welcome, granting to all the freedom of the city.

Many of the papers presented were of a high order, but lack
of time for discussion was felt to be a serious drawback. Greater
punctuality in opening the sessions and a feeling of personal
responsibility on the part of those who have allowed their names
to appear upon the programme, the recognition of an obligation
to carry out the promise made at the time appointed, would add
much to the enjoyment and value of the meeting.

No one was disappointed in finding that the social side of
the meeting had received much attention and was carried out
with marked success. Notable among the social features were
the visit to the canneries at Steveston, the conversazione at the
Hotel Vancouver, the annual dinner, and the visit to Victoria.

The Vancouver meeting was one of the most largely attended
yet held by the National Association, and fairly justifies the

plan of convening in distant parts of Canada. It is hoped that
a still further increase of interest will be manifested in the meeting to be held next year in Halifax. The number of those who
look forward to this annual gathering as an opportunity to
broaden their outlook, to cultivate the acquaintance of fellow-
practitioners, and to make the personal acquaintance of distinguished visitors, is increasing. Canadian loyalty should stimulate
the profession everywhere to give a generous and intelligent
support to the Canadian Medical Association, that it may in all
its departments be worthy of the great, rich and growing country
whose sons we are.   B. E. M'K.

EDITORIAL NOTES.

Protecting Masks and Jackets for Combatants.—During the
present Russo-Japanese war, many wounds have been caused,
especially during naval engagements, by shells, which, after bursting, are dispersed in a radiating manner. As one might expect,
such wounds are lacerated and much larger than bullet wounds.
Dr. Suzuki, chief surgeon of Admiral Togo's flagship, insists
(*British Medical Journal,* August 13th, 1904) on the need of
larger first-aid packages for such cases. In the same communication he also suggests the advisability of combatants putting on
clean clothes just before an action, as the fragments of a shell may
carry into the body of a wounded man pieces of his clothing, which
cannot be as sterile as shell fragments or rifle bullets. This
sounds a little naive, if one reflects that the naval surgeon
wears a sterilized gown when dressing a shell wound, while the
recipient of the wound may not have a change of clothes, or may
have slept in his clothes and has not equal laundry advantages
with the ship's surgeon. The Japanese sailors are fond of bathing their bodies, but probably do not spend the necessary time in
laundering their inner and outer clothing. Hence Dr. Suzuki's
advice to the fighting sailor, to put on clean clothes before an
action, is well taken. Referring to the protection from shell fragments afforded by knives, pocketbooks, etc., Dr. Suzuki thinks it
probable that in time all combatants will wear protecting masks
and jackets. It does seem reasonable to think that the body of
the modern combatant on sea or land should be protected against

shell wounds just as the bodies of the men-at-arms of the days of chivalry were shielded from thrust of lance or blow of sword. But if the masks and jackets are not flexible and of light weight, they will be thrown aside by naval gunners just at the time when they are working hard to silence an enemy's fire. Besides, in reference to soldiers, a coat of mail, while protecting an infantryman against wounds from bursting shells, would add a few more pounds to the already heavy load which he carries into action.

The Drug Habit.—The following is quoted from the *Analyst* of the State Board of Health of Massachusetts for the information of those who have acquired the self-dosing habit. Each article mentioned contains the percentage by vol. of alcohol indicated by the following figures: Lydia Pinkham's Vegetable Compound, 20.6; Paine's Celery Compound, 21; Holden's Liquid Beef Tonic, " recommended for treatment of alcohol habit," 26.5; Ayer's Sarsaparilla, 26.2; Hood's Sarsaparilla, 18.8; Dana's Sarsaparilla, 13.5; Peruna, 28.5; Hoofland's German Tonic, 29.3; Hove's Arabian Tonic, " Not a rum drink." 13.2; Mensman's Peptonized Beef Tonic, 16.5; Schenck's Seaweed Tonic, " entirely harmless," 19.5; Boker's Stomach Bitters, 42.6; Burdock Blood Bitters, 25.2; Hoofland's German Bitters, " entirely vegetable," 25.6; Hop Bitters, 12; Hostetter's Stomach Bitters, 44.3; Richardson's Concentrated Sherry Wine Bitters, 47.5; Warner's Safe Tonic Bitters, 35.7. Beer contains 2 to 5 per cent. of alcohol. Some of the above contain ten times as much, making them stronger than whiskey, far stronger than sherry or port, with claret and champagne far behind.

A Renunciation of Prudery.—We are all familiar with the story of the prudish dame who put pantalets on the legs of her piano; but a refreshing instance of prudery in the rural New England of three generations ago is noted by Dr. Norman Bridge, of Los Angeles, California, in an address delivered at the commencement exercises of the Training School for Nurses of the Pasadena Hospital, May 26th, 1904. In this instance the prudishness of the New England ladies took another direction, for they objected to the wearing of drawers by women to protect the lower extremities. This garment, it seems, had never been worn before by any woman of that country, and the innovation was a shock.

In a year or two the fashion had very properly spread to nearly
·every household in the community. The women came to their
senses. This episode shows in a grotesque way how foolish the
human genus may be when it acts without thinking. The woman
who first wore drawers in a New England village was taunted
with not only wearing the garments of men, but with having
designs on the vocations of men as well, and with being immodest.
There appears to be a certain amount of truth in the criticism
launched at this innovating lady, for the women of to-day not
only wear the garments of men (beneath their skirts, of course),
but have made serious inroads into the vocations of men, though
no unprejudiced man will say that the women of to-day are immodest. The latest census in Britain shows that women are continuing to encroach on fields of industry formerly reserved for
men. The returns, by occupations, show that there are 80 women
auctioneers, 6 architects, 39 bailiffs, 316 blacksmiths, 3,071 brick-
makers, 3,850 butchers,, 54 chimney-sweeps, 1 dock laborer,
5,170 goldsmiths, 9,693 printers, 745 railway porters, 117,640
tailors. and 3 veterinary surgeons.

Effects of Boric Acid and Borax upon General Health.—The
United States Department of Agriculture, Bureau of Chemistry,
H. W. Wiley, Chief, has issued Circular 15, giving the plan of
work and conclusions as to the effects of boric acid and borax on
digestion and health. The interest of these experiments turns
largely on the fact that borax is used in the preservation of butter
and meats. The report shows that those who habitually eat
butter and meat preserved with borax might be consuming half
a gram, or a little more. of boric acid per diem. Would the in-
gestion of this amount be injurious to an otherwise healthy man?
The report says: "The administration of borax and boric acid
to the extent of one-half gram per diem yielded results markedly
different from those obtained with larger quantities of the preservatives. This experiment, conducted as it was for a period
of fifty days, was a rather severe test, and it appeared that in
some instances a somewhat unfavorable result attended its use.
On the whole, the results show that one-half gram per diem is
too much for the normal man to receive regularly. On the other
hand, it is evident that the normal man can receive one-half gram
per diem of boric acid, or of borax expressed in terms of boric acid,

for a limited period of time without much danger of impairment of health." The report shows that the therapeutic value which these agents possess in certain diseases, does not have any relation to their use in the healthy organism, except when prescribed as prophylactics. The final conclusion of this report is: " It appears, therefore, that both boric acid and borax, when continuously ad-- ministered in small doses for a long period, or when given in large quantities for a short period, create disturbances of appe- tite, of digestion and of health."

Should Elastic Stockings be Worn by Persons who have Varicose Veins of the Inferior Extremities ?—Dr. Lucas-Cham- pioniére (*Academie de Medecine,* 26 Juillet, 1904) is strongly in favor of active movements of the lower extremities by persons who have varicose veins. He quotes with approval the opinions of Dr. Dragon, who shows that phlebitis should be treated by methodical movements, followed by a mild, regular and progres- sive massage of the limbs. Except in the cases of persons who are in a state of acute infection, or who have a high temperature, there is no danger from embolism. All of which goes to show that varicose veins are governed by the same vital laws as other living tissues, and that, in spite of their deformity, movement is useful to them. Dr. Lucas-Championiére also approves of Dr. Marchais' treatment. It consists in carefully massaging the varicose veins and in making the patient walk. Dr. Marchais re- calls an old saying to the effect that omnibus conductors suffer from their varicose veins, while rural postmen afflicted with the same complaint endure it very well, and walk long distances in spite of it. Dr. Marchais advises persons who have varicose veins to avoid standing in a motionless attitude. He forbids the use of elastic stockings. For two weeks he has the limbs massaged to lessen their sensitiveness, as well as to give tone to the muscles. He then makes the patient practise rapid walking. The walking must be done at a minimum rate of one hundred steps a minute. After some practice his patients can walk at this rate for from one to two or more hours. As substitutes for rapid walking, Dr. Lucas-Championiére recommends the bicycle or tricycle. Modern experience, he says, shows that exercise of the lower limbs does not induce phlebitis or embolism in people with varicose veins, and it will relieve them of the inconvenience and expense of elastic stockings.

The Chicago Drainage Channel.—In the Bulletin of the Health Department of Chicago for the week ending August 20th, 1904, Arthur R. Reynolds, M.D., Commissioner of Health, the pleasing statement is made that "no such healthful summer appears on record in the history of the city as this of 1904. . . . Lower and fairly equable temperature, an improving milk supply and absolutely pure water are the principal factors contributing to this result." As explanatory of the pure water supply of Chicago, the Bulletin states: "There is no obvious or plausible reason for this but the continuous operation of the Drainage Channel. This is the fifth year that an average of more than 300,000 cubic feet per minute, night and day, has been flowing from the lake, down the Desplaines and Illinois valleys, and during this time there has been the reduction in deaths from the impure water diseases, shown in the following table, the dividing line being January, 1900, date of opening the Channel:

Deaths from:	Four years 1896-1899.	Four years 1900-1903.
Acute Intestinal Diseases	8,119	8,898
Rate per 1000 of population	16.41	12.44
Typhoid fever	2,266	2,235
Rate per 1000 of population	3.68	3.10

If the rate of the four years, 1896-1899, before the opening of the Drainage Channel, had obtained during the last four years, there would have been 11,724 deaths from the acute intestinal diseases, and 2,629 from typhoid fever, or 2,826 more from the former and 394 more from the latter (a total of 3,220) than did actually occur."

Public Baths for Toronto.—Dr. Harrison, chairman of the Toronto local Board of Health, reports that in Buffalo, Boston and other cities of the United States, public baths are used, and in New York State the law requires them in every city of 50,000 inhabitants or over. In Buffalo the baths are free, soap and towels being furnished, and there is a laundry in which people can wash their under clothing or upper clothing, place them in a hot-air drier, and have them ready to put on again when they return from the bath. All the baths are sprays, there being no plunge or swimming baths, and each is in a room by itself. There is accommodation for one hundred men and one hundred women. The laundry is the unique feature in the Buffalo baths. The bathers do their own washing, but no charge is made for the use of the laundry. At the Boston baths a charge is made, a cent for a towel and a cent for soap. It will be remembered that a little while ago, Dr. Sheard, M.H.O., recommended to the Board of Education of Toronto the establishment of baths in some of the city schools, but no reply was sent to his letter. When an increased supply of water for general and fire purposes is considered by the Toronto Council, we hope that an item for a public bath will also be added to the estimates. Toronto has great facilities for a pure and abundant water supply, so that public bath would not be expensive. Baths are needed in cold weather as well as during hot weather, and a free use of the bath would add very much to the health, bodily comfort and cheerfulness of the citizens.   J. J. C.

University Senate Elections.—The usual elections for membership in the University Senate take place within a day or two now, and the results, so far, at least, as the four representatives in Medicine are concerned, are looked forward to with interest. Those whose names have been mentioned up till the date of going to press, who are desirous of representing the graduates in Medicine, are Dr. Adam Wright, Mr. Irving H. Cameron, Dr. W. H. B. Aikins, Dr. J. M. MacCallum, Dr. J. A. Temple and Dr. G. A. Bingham, the two latter to represent the Trinity element. Dr. J. A. Temple and Dr. G. A. Bingham have never run before for Senatorial honors, and, we understand, have been pressed into the fight by their friends. Though "comparisons are odious," yet, in looking into this subject recently, we find that there should be little difficulty in the matter of choosing the men most worthy of the honor of holding a seat in Toronto University Senate. In order to fulfil the duties properly, every occupant of the position must be prepared to give up a certain amount of his time to the work, and those who in the past have been delinquent in this respect cannot expect any support, and should be left " at home " when it comes to the signing of the ballot paper. We find from a report issued by Mr. James Brebner, Registrar of the University, that during the last term there were in all forty-eight meetings of the Senate. Of these, Prof. Cameron has attended twenty-nine; Dr. A. H. Wright, six; Dr. W. H. B. Aikins, seven, and Dr. J. M. MacCallum but three. Dr. Mac-

Callum, therefore, cannot expect further support, and we think that the best ticket would consist of Prof. Cameron, Dr. A. H. Wright (who has had more experience in this work than Dr. Aikins and is " in the inner ring "), and in order to give Trinity equal representation, Dr. J. A. Temple and Dr. Geo. Bingham, who, we feel sure, would represent in an efficient manner the medical graduates.   W. A. Y.

PERSONAL.

Dr. J. M. MacCallum, with Mrs. MacCallum and baby, spent the latter part of September around the Georgian Bay.

DR. J. J. CASSIDY has almost recovered from his recent accident. The doctor spent part of August at Preston Springs.

DR. B. R. O'REILLY has been appointed surgeon on the Canadian Pacific steamship *Tartar* and left the city on the 14th ultimo for Vancouver.

WE are glad to announce that Dr. H. A. Bruce, of 64 Bloor Street East, has almost entirely recovered from his recent attack of appendicitis.

DR. AND MRS. FRANKLIN DAWSON have returned home after spending a delightful four months touring through England, Scotland and France.

AMONG the city practitioners who will be removing soon into their new homes on Bloor Street are Drs. R. A. Reeve, Allen Baines and Clarence Starr.

PROFESSOR J. J. MACKENZIE, of Toronto University, and Mrs. Mackenzie, who have been spending the summer in England, arrived home ten days ago.

DR. LUSK has resumed practice, and may be found at his residence, 99 Bloor Street West. Office hours, 11 a.m. to 1, and 6 to 8 p.m. Telephone, North 2274.

AMONG the Toronto delegation to the Canadian Medical Association at Vancouver, B.C., were Dr. A. A. Macdonald, Dr. J. H. Watson, Dr. B. E. McKenzie and Dr. Geo. Elliott.

Dr. S. KITCHEN, St. George, and Dr. R. P. Boucher, Peterboro', have been appointed to represent the Provincial Board of Health at the Congress on Tuberculosis at St. Louis on the 3rd, 4th and 5th of October.

THE marriage of Dr. F. N. G. Starr of College Street, to Miss Annie Callender Mackay, of Hillshead, New Glasgow, N.S., took place at that place on September 14th. After a wedding trip of two weeks, spent amid the resorts of the St. Lawrence, Dr. and Mrs. Starr reached Toronto on the 1st inst.

SIR LAUDER and Lady Brunton, of London, Eng., were recently visiting Dr. McPhedran, of 151 Bloor Street. Sir Lauder is one of the most eminent consulting physicians and scientists of London. He is on his way to St. Louis to attend the Science Congress. This is his second visit to Toronto. He was here some years ago, and made many friends.

DR. C. K. CLARKE, Medical Superintendent of Rockwood Hospital, has been appointed co-editor of the *American Journal of Insanity,* the official organ of the American Medico-Psychological Association. This well-known quarterly is edited by a board of four editors, and is published by the Johns Hopkins Press of Baltimore. Dr. Clarke succeeds Dr. Henry Hind, the eminent Medical Superintendent of Johns Hopkins Hospital, in editorial work, although Dr. Hind will still act as consultant in the management of the affairs of the *Journal.* We heartily congratulate Dr. Clarke on the recognition of his advanced work in the medico-psychological field, and the medical profession certainly thoroughly appreciate the compliment paid to a Canadian. Dr. Clarke's editorial duties will in no way clash with his work at Rockwood Hospital.

❧ *Items of Interest.* ❧

Will of Dr. N. S. Davis.—The will of the late Dr. N. S. Davis, father of the American Medical Association, disposes of an estate valued at $39,000, of which $25,000 is real estate. The homestead is bequeathed to his widow, his library to his son, and a perpetual scholarship in Northwestern University to his grandson, Frank H. Davis.—*Med. News.*

Fourth Pan-American Medical Congress.—President Amador of the Republic of Panama has appointed the following officers of the Fourth Pan-American Medical Congress, to be held in Panama the first week in January, 1905: Dr. Julio Ycaza, President; Dr. Manuel Coroalles, Vice-President; Dr. Jose E. Calvo, Secretary; Dr. Pedro de Obarrio, Treasurer; Dr. J. W. Ross, Dr. J. Tomaselli, Dr. M. Gasteazoro, Committeemen. There will be but four sections, Surgery, Medicine, Hygiene and the Specialties, to which the following officers were appointed: Surgical Section—Major Louis LaGarde, President; Dr. E. B. Barrick, Secretary. Medical Section—Dr. Moritz Stern, President: Dr. Daniel R. Oduber, Secretary. Section on Hygiene—Colonel W. C. Gorgas, President; Dr. Henry E. Carter, Secretary. Section on Specialties—Dr. W· Spratling. President; Dr. Charles A. Cooke, Secretary.

The Emergency Hospital at the World's Fair, St. Louis.—This hospital is located near the parade entrance, where it can be easily and promptly reached from both the outside and inside of the grounds. The building is 103 x 109 feet, erected at a cost of $16,000, and has been operated since January 5. 1904. This institution, which is under the charge of the medical director of the Fair, Dr. L. H. Laidley, is thoroughly equipped in every detail, for handling all classes of injuries and illness. A special sunstroke ward, fitted with bath tubs, shower baths, ice boxes and wicker couches, occupies a well-ventilated room on the first floor. The leading medical magazines will be found on file in the library. Dr. Laidley has at present a staff of six physicians, besides nurses, ambulance drivers, clerks and orderlies. About six thousand cases have been treated in the hospital thus far. The entire equipment of the hospital was furnished by the Blees-Moore Instrument Co., of St. Louis.—*Med. Herald.*

The Physician's Library.

BOOK REVIEWS.

Diseases of the Intestines and Peritoneum. By DR. HERMANN
NOTHNAGEL, of Vienna. The entire volume edited, with
additions, by HUMPHREY D. ROLLESTON, M.D., F.R.C.P.,
Physician to St. George's Hospital, London, England. Octavo
volume of 1,032 pages, fully illustrated. Philadelphia, New
York, London: W. B. Saunders & Co. 1904. Canadian
agents: J. A. Carveth & Co., Limited, 434 Yonge St., Toronto.
Cloth, $5.00 net; half morocco, $6.00 net.

This is the eighth volume of " Nothnagel's Practice," and has
been issued almost simultaneously with the preceding one on
" Tuberculosis." It is written by Nothnagel himself, and is very
full. It is edited by Dr. Humphrey D. Rolleston, of London,
who has added very largely to the work, greatly increasing its
value. Besides short paragraphs throughout the work, he has
written short sections on Intestine Sand, Sprue, Ulcerative Colitis
and Idiopathic Dilatation of the Colon. The section on Intus-
susception has received large and valuable additions by D'Arcy
Power, of London, who has written so much on this subject.
Where all is so well edited it is invidious to select any for special
commendation. The section on the Urine in Diseases of the
Intestines is worthy of note.

The article on Appendicitis is long, and shows that little of
the voluminous literature published on that subject in recent
years has been overlooked. The conclusions of the author are
conservative, and not in agreement with the opinion so prevalent
in America that every case of appendicitis should be operated
on as soon as diagnosis is made, but rather that each case should
be treated on its own merits, a conclusion that will be approved
by the sanest of the profession in all parts of the world. The
editor quotes Dieulafoy and Osler to the effect that there is no
medical treatment of appendicitis; the latter transfers all his
hospital cases at once to the surgical side to be operated on if
necessary. If by medicinal treatment is meant curative treatment, is not the statement equally true of many other diseases,
both operable and non-operable, such as pleurisy, gastric ulcer,
nephritis, etc. ? The great majority of cases of these diseases

recover with care, and so do the majority of cases of appendicitis. It is only in the minority that operation is required, and the physician should know, as well as the surgeon, when an operation in any given case is advisable, and should be quite as alert in seizing the proper time for operation.

The translation on the whole is well done. The two words that occur in so many of the preceding volumes and are so much the stock-in-trade of United States speakers and writers, "factor" and "formulate," are much less in evidence. In some pages, however, "factor" occurs in every few lines, and in many cases without any reference to its true meaning. One sentence will suffice to show the absurdity of the use of the word "formulate": "Dunin has recently formulated the rule that habitual constipation is merely a symptom of neurasthenia," meaning simply that he has stated that as his belief. One is rather surprised to see the recommendation of ergot in intestinal hemorrhage passed over without comment by the editor. These defects are not of material·consequence, and it is a real pleasure to recommend the book to all physicians as being not alone interesting, but of great value to everyone engaged in practice.   A. M'P.

Modern Ophthalmology.   A Practical Treatise on the Anatomy, Physiology and Diseases of the Eye. By JAMES MOORES BALL, M.D., Professor of Ophthalmology in the St. Louis College of Physicians and Surgeons. With 417 illustrations in the text and numerous figures on 21 colored plates, nearly all original. 820 pages, extra large royal octavo.   Price, extra cloth, $7.00, net; half-morocco, $8.50, net. F. A. Davis Company, publishers, 1914-16 Cherry Street, Philadelphia.

The many diagrams, excellent illustrations and colored plates of external and of fundus diseases are what first attract attention.   Closer examination reveals the fact that these are not the stock illustrations found in most works on the eye. Quite a number are original; others are from sources of authority and are credited to them. The print and the paper is excellent, the one objection to be offered being the large size of the book, extra large octavo, which makes it clumsy to handle, and keeps one in dread lest the back shall split.

The first three chapters are devoted to a consideration of the embryology, anatomy and physiology of the eye. The examination of the eye is dealt with much more fully than usual, and will be found much more satisfactory. A departure has been made in handing over the dermatologic aspect of diseases of the eyelid to the care of Ohman-Dumesnil, the St. Louis dermatologist. A great deal of space is given to the various·blepharoplastic operations, which so often prove troublesome.   •

The diseases of the tear passages, so often cursorily treated in text-books, receive the greater space demanded by their frequency and their refusal to respond to treatment. This chapter, and those on the diseases of the conjunctiva, cornea and iris, in which the general practitioner is always interested, will be found complete and reliable. A short chapter is devoted to the hygiene of the eye. The rest of the volume is taken up with those diseases which more particularly concern the ophthalmologist.

One lays the book down, having formed a most favorable opinion of it. J. M. M'C.

The Doctor's Recreation Series. CHAS. WELLS MOULTON, General Editor. Vol. III.—"In the Year 1800," Being the Relation of Sundry Events Occurring in the Life of Doctor Jonathan Brush During that Year, by Samuel Walter Kelley, M.D. Akron, O., Chicago and New York: The Saalfield Publishing Co. 1904. Canadian Depot: Chandler & Massey Limited, Toronto, Montreal and Winnipeg.

We have taken occasion in two previous issues of the JOURNAL to state the fact that a series such as this would, we felt, meet with the support of the medical profession as a body. We understand that this prognostication has been fulfilled and that Charles Wells Moulton's volumes have " caught on." The reading is light and quite interesting, and will be the means of passing many a pleasant hour during the approaching winter months to all of us who become at times tired of the stereotyped medical works. Vol. III. is as good as, if not rather better than, its predecessors, and gives a most interesting account of events in the life of Dr. Brush over a century ago. W. A. Y.

Graves' Disease, With and Without Exophthalmic Goitre. By WILLIAM HANNA THOMPSON, M.D., LL.D., Physician to the Roosevelt Hospital; Consulting Physician to the Manhattan State Hospitals for the Insane, East and West; formerly Professor of the Practice of Medicine, New York University Medical College; Physician to Bellevue Hospital, etc. Pp. 143. New York: William Wood & Co. 1904.

The object the author had in view in writing the monograph on Graves' disease was to emphasize the fact that the constitutional and general derangements which are characteristic of Graves' disease, constitute the disease, and not the condition of the thyroid gland or of its accessories." This contention can hardly be said to be new, nor perhaps is it quite claimed by the author to be so, as he gives certain quotations from the works of others who have made somewhat similar observations.

The writer of this treatise has, however, given us ample evidence of the correctness of his contention, as set forth in the clinical histories of twenty-eight patients who at no time showed any sign of exophthalmic goitre and, for comparison, that of forty-two patients who had goitre as an accompanying symptom.

Whilst the fact may thus be established that goitre may not exist in a typical case of Graves' disease, still we have as yet no proof that in such cases the thyroid function is normal. It is quite possible that derangement of thyroid function may exist in the absence of gross pathological lesion of the gland. It is a well-known clinical phenomenon that many of the characteristic symptoms of Graves' disease may precede thyroid enlargement, the goitre developing late.

The monograph will be read with interest by all students of clinical medicine. It contains quite a wealth of material in recording the clinical features which presented themselves in a large number of cases under the observation of the author of the work.

A. P.

A Practical Treatise on Genito-Urinary and Venereal Diseases and Syphilis. By ROBERT W. TAYLOR, A.M., M.D., Clinical Professor of Genito-Urinary Diseases at the College of Physicians and Surgeons (Columbia University), New York; Consulting Genito-Urinary Surgeon to Bellevue Hospital and to City Charity Hospital, New York. Third edition, thoroughly revised, with 163 illustrations and 39 plates in colors and monochrome. New York and Philadelphia: Lea Brothers & Co.

Dr. Taylor's "Genito-Urinary and Venereal Diseases" is really a magnificent work, which does credit to the author and his country. It is not, therefore, a matter of wonder that an Italian translation of the second edition of this work has been issued by the Union Tipografico Editrice of Tprin.

Dr. Taylor has had thirty years of experience and large opportunities of studying genito-urinary and venereal diseases in hospital and private practice. He is also the possessor of a felicitous style of writing, combining the merits of the writer and clinical teacher, so that the reader is never left in doubt as to the author's meaning.

Any physician of experience in the diagnosis and treatment of these diseases will be pleased with the perusal of Dr. Taylor's book, which gives evidence of modesty and good sense, directing to a useful purpose the data of clinical experience. Dr. Taylor believes firmly in the efficiency of nitrate of silver in gonorrhea, and he expresses but a poor opinion of argentamine, protargol, *et hoc genus omne.* In this respect he does not quite live up to the modified proverb which he quotes, " De novis nil nisi bonum."

In selected cases of syphilis he favors the hypodermic use of the perchloride of mercury, preferring it to any other salt of that base.

The influence of syphilis on the different organs and tissues of the body, particularly in the tertiary stage, is very fully considered, data being given of the tertiary affections of the viscera. A full description is given of the syphilitic affections of the nervous system.

Artistic illustration is a feature of the book. It is by far the handsomest book of the kind we have seen, and, as a standard authority, deserves a place in every practitioner's library. The book is beautifully printed and well bound.   J. J. C.

The Seaboard Magazine. Devoted to the Industrial and Agricultural Development of the South. Published monthly by the Industrial Department of the Seaboard Air Line Railroad, Portsmouth, Va.

To any and all who are interested in the South and its development, we say " Send for a copy or two of *The Seaboard Magazine.*" It is most interesting, and freely illustrated in half-tone. The issues we have had the privilege of looking over contain some articles on " The Land of the Manatee, the Land of Flowers," and goes to prove how rapidly this, up till recently unknown part of the South, has developed. The magazine also gives information as to Palmetto, where coffee and pineapples are cultivated to perfection; Sarasota, the winter and summer resort on the South-west Coast; Braidentown, the largest town in the Manatee section, and Pinehurst, " The City of the Ideal." Any physician will receive a copy of *The Seaboard Magazine* on presenting or mailing his card to the Industrial Department of the Seaboard Air Line Railroad, Portsmouth, Va.

The firm of H. K. Lewis, 136 Gower St., London, W.C., Eng., is too well known to require more than passing mention. Mr. Lewis has been a medical book publisher for many years now, and from his printing presses have come a large number of the best known English medical works. Their names are too numerous to mention; suffice it to say that a few of the most recent ones are:

" Diseases of the Skin: Their Description, Pathology, Diagnosis and Treatment." With Special Reference to the Skin Eruptions of Children, and an Analysis of Fifteen Thousand Cases of Skin Disease. By H. Radcliffe-Crocker, M.D. (Lond.); F.R.C.P., Physician for Diseases of the Skin in University College Hospital, London. Thoroughly revised and enlarged, with 4 plates (2 being colored) and 112 illustrations. 2 vols., large 8vo, 28s. net. " This is by far the most exhaustive work upon diseases of the skin which has as yet appeared. . . . The practising dermatologist cannot afford to be without it."— *Therapeutic Gazette.*

" Diseases of Women. A Practical Text-book." By A. H. N. Lewers, M.D. (Lond.), F.R.C.P. (Lond.), Senior Obstetric Physician to the London Hospital, and Lecturer on Midwifery in the London Hospital Medical School; Examiner in Obstetric Medicine to the University of London; Examiner in Midwifery and Diseases of Women at the Conjoint Board of the Royal College of Physicians of London and of the Royal College of Surgeons of England, etc. Just published, thoroughly revised, with 4 plates and 166 illustrations, crown 8vo, 10s. 6d. " This neat, bright and well-written volume. . . . It has what is much more valuable than the most correct photographs, a number of good diagrams. This book must recommend itself to every student and practitioner, for in it he will find the gist of the whole subject."—*Canadian Journal of Medicine and Surgery.*

" Handbook of Diseases of the Eye and Their Treatment." By Henry A. Swanzy, A.M., M.B., F.R.C.S.I., Surgeon to the Royal Victoria Eye and Ear Hospital, and Ophthalmic Surgeon to the Adelaide Hospital, Dublin. Just published, with 167 illustrations, post 8vo, 12s. 6d. " This favorite hand-book . . . Its popularity with students is as great as ever. It is received with growing favor by practitioners who have once perused it, because of its readability and the soundness of its teaching."— *Canadian Journal of Medicine and Surgery.*

" Hygiene and Public Health." By Louis C. Parkes, M.D., D.P.H., Lond. Univ. Lecturer on Public Health at St. George's Hospital School, etc., and Henry R. Kenwood, M.B., D.P.H., F.C.S., Professor of Hygiene and Public Health at University College, etc. Now ready, with 88 illustrations, pp. 763, crown 8vo, 12s. " As a general text-book covering the whole range of hygiene and public health the practitioner and student will find it thoroughly satisfactory."—*Lancet.* (English.)

A postal card to H. K. Lewis at above address will bring a catalogue by return mail.

Reference to page xcix. of this issue will reveal the advertisement of Mr. H. J. Glaisher, medical book publisher, 57 Wigmore St., London, W., England. His annual complete catalogue of Publishers' Remainders in all branches of literature, including medical, will be sent post free to any physician on receipt of calling card. Mr. Glaisher's prices are greatly reduced, so that it will repay any of our subscribers to communicate with the address as given.

The Canadian
Journal of Medicine and Surgery

A JOURNAL PUBLISHED MONTHLY IN THE INTEREST OF
MEDICINE AND SURGERY

VOL. XVI.   TORONTO, NOVEMBER, 1904.   NO. 5.

Original Contributions.

ADDRESS IN MEDICINE.*

BY R. E. McKECHNIE, M.D., VANCOUVER, B.C.

Mr. Chairman and Gentlemen,—In asking a member of the profession residing in the far West to deliver the address in medicine, I feel that a compliment has been paid, not so much to myself, as to the West. To demand that we, living so far away from the centres of learning, from the great teaching institutions of the East, should nevertheless be expected to keep ourselves abreast of the times and in touch with the latest discoveries, is surely expecting a great deal; and then to expect that one, living under such barren influences, should be able to give you an address equal to this occasion, containing some food for thought and pointing out the pathway of duty and practice, is to look still farther for a miraculous manifestation. But the genus of the West is ever equal to all occasions. It has grown accustomed to the knowledge that the best wheat in the world grows in our North-West: that our forests can supply the hugest sticks of timber known to commerce; that our fisheries can supply the world with illimitable quantities of salmon, halibut and other delicacies; always the best, the hugest, and the illimitable, ever the superlative. So it is not strange that a strong egotism has developed out here, sufficient even to accept this task, and hoping, but with misgivings, that its self-sufficiency may not suffer in the attempt. Personally, I feel that a great honor has been conferred on me, and I most sincerely thank the Association for its

* Read at meeting of Canadian Medical Association, Vancouver, B.C., August, 1904.

4

kindness and trust that its confidence may not have been misplaced.

As to-day we seek to adapt treatment according to the cause of disease, so, looking back to the remotest ages, we find the human instinct groping along the same pathway. But in the early ages of the race science was unknown, and miracle was seen in every unexplainable phenomenon. Hence disease was attributable to the wrath of a good being or the malice of an evil one, and treated accordingly. Among the ruder tribes the Medicine-man has ever held sway; but even in higher civilization we find that in Egypt the priests of Osiris and Isis claimed powers over disease; in Assyria, the priests of Gibil; in Greece, the priests of Aesculapius; in Judea, the priests of Jehovah. While these have ceased to exist with the decay of their respective religious systems, the ruder primitive tribes have persisted. They are found among the aboriginal tribes of Africa to-day, as also on this side of the Atlantic. Parkman, in discussing the customs of the Hurons, says: " A great knowledge of simples for the cure of disease is popularly ascribed to the Indian. Here, however, as elsewhere, his knowledge is in fact scanty. He rarely reasons from cause to effect, or from effect to cause. Disease, in his belief, is the result of sorcery, the agency of spirits or supernatural influences, undefined and indefinable. The Indian doctor was a conjurer, and his remedies were to the last degree preposterous, ridiculous or revolting.'

Among the Coast Indians in British Columbia the practice is still kept up, and it may interest you to hear me relate what I saw not forty miles from here only three years ago. In the Indian villages are to be found huge barnlike structures called rancheries, each consisting of one immense room and capable of accommodating twenty or thirty families. Living close to nature, the floor, of course, is mother earth. Rough stalls, arranged along the walls, separated by screens of rush matting, and open towards the centre, form the none too private retreats of the individual families. Each lights its own fire on the earthen floor opposite, whereon their rude cooking is done. The smoke escapes through the shingles, as there is no chimney, and in the absence of windows the light comes in through the cracks in the wooden walls. I went down one evening to such a place to see a sick Indian woman. It was dusk, and the waves of the sea were lapping the beach close at hand, while dusky children flitted by in the twilight, engrossed in some pastime. On entering the only door in the rancherie, I found it in utter darkness, excepting for a small fire burning at the extreme end of the building. Here was presented a study in light and shade to have suited a Rembrandt. Around the fire was arranged a circle of Indian women (it is always the women who are closest to the mysteries of nature), while at one side was the patient, too weak to sit up, but supported by a couple of sympathizers. Facing her was the Indian Medicine-man trying to cure her disorder by directing his energies to overcome the supposed cause of her disease. My diagnosis was tubercular pleurisy with effusion, but my Indian confrere had diagnosed possession by an evil spirit, and as he was in charge of the case, I could only look on. Each woman, with a stick in either hand, was beating on a piece of wood before her, making as much noise as possible, and adding blood-curdling explosives to the incantations of the Medicine-man, in a vain endeavor to drive out, to scare out, the possessing spirit. But unfortunately this kind comes not forth by such rude wooing. And so, from the gray dawn of time, down to what we imagine is the mid-day splendor of to-day, such forms of practice have persisted through all the ages.

But let us not imagine the air clear yet; the fog is only getting thinner. In other times the sun has attempted to shine through. Five hundred years before Christ, Hippocrates broke away from the old traditions of healing, the supernatural methods, and laid the foundations of medical science on experience, observation and reasoning. Later his teaching influenced the school of Alexandria, where positive knowledge was developed by the adoption of anatomic studies; and centuries later under Moslem patronage, the medical sciences reached their highest development in the Middle Ages. But Europe was less fortunate under Christian influences. There was a return to the belief in the supernatural origin of disease, and in the practice of supernatural methods to combat it. Retrogression prevailed over progression. Still believing in demoniacal possession, the various phases of exorcism were practiced, even combined with such practical methods as the following: " To disgust the demon with the body he was tormenting, the patient was made to swallow or apply to himself unspeakable ordures, with such medicines as the livers of toads, the blood of frogs and rats, fibres of the hangman's rope, and ointment made from the body of gibbeted criminals." For myself I would prefer the simpler methods of the British Columbia Medicine-man. Cures effected by relics, by pilgrimages and sacred observances obscured the horizon, while even the Divine Right of Kings gave the world the blessings of the Royal Touch for King's Evil. All these practices were injurious to the development of medical science, for " why should men seek to build up scientific medicine and surgery when relics, pilgrimages and sacred observances, according to an overwhelming mass of concurrent testimony, had cured hosts of sick folk in all parts of Europe?" But finally the tide turns. The discoveries of

Galileo, Kepler and Newton had their reflex on the sister science of medicine, and investigators made bold to pry into the secrets of life and learn her vital processes, to seek the true causes of disease and endeavor to find the cure. Relapses have occurred. As fanatics opposed the introduction of the fanning-mill because it infringed on the divine prerogative, which furnished the wind to winnow the wheat from the chaff, similarly opposition arose to the introduction of inoculation, vaccination and the use of anesthetics. And as supernatural agencies were invoked to cure diseases supposed to be of supernatural origin, so to-day we have the various sects of faith-healers, magnetic healers and what not.

But, as Carlyle says, " Only what is true will persist. Out of the merciless fire of modern criticism truth, like asbestos, will come forth purified; but vain theories, gaseous, will be dissipated among the waste winds forever."

But where do we stand to-day? Have the fogs all lifted and do we now see clearly? Unfortunately not. Investigators to-day are not numbered by tens but by hundreds, pursuing many diverse threads of thought, and giving to the world their conclusions, fully formed or immature, probable or fantastic, relevant or irrelevant.

The search for the causes of disease still continues as actively as ever, but disappointments are far more numerous than successes. Concerning sarcomata, Stimson, in this month's *Annals of Surgery*, says: " We are absolutely in the dark as to etiology, and no farther advanced in prognosis and treatment than were our colleagues a quarter of a century ago."

Dr. Snow, Chief of the London Cancer Research Committee, has come to almost identical conclusions regarding carcinoma. As regards these two classes of disease, we are, therefore, forced to be content, at present, with increased ability to diagnose them, and have to thank the surgeon largely for the groundwork of this advance.

In 1882 Koch proved tuberculosis to be due to a specific bacillus, and in 1890 startled the world with the announcement of a cure. We all remember the reaction, the tremendous disappointment felt not only by the laity but even more keenly by ourselves, when slowly, unwillingly, we were forced to admit that our expectations were not realized. Early in 1903, Behring delivered a lecture before the Vienna Medical Society, detailing his experiments on animals with his own special serum, and speaking very hopefully as to the future. Perhaps he, who with Roux, discovered in diphtheritic antitoxin the greatest remedial agent of recent times, will unravel the puzzle.

More recently. Marmorek, of Paris, has staked his great reputation by giving to the world the results of his labors in a new serum, and we can only trust that time will prove that it possesses some definite value. Later still, that our professionally agnostic brethren may not starve for want of food, an Italian professor has enunciated that Koch's tubercle bacillus is not the cause of phthisis, but rather an uncouth octopoid micro-organism of his own finding. Well may the general practitioner raise his hands in despair and wonder what he can believe.

But experience has shown that in tuberculosis, as in other things, prevention is better and surer than cure. Statistics are piling up year by year, adding proof where now none is needed, that, recognizing tuberculosis as an infectious disease and treating it accordingly, a definite gain can be recorded. Education of the public has already advanced so far that more positive steps should be enforced. Compulsory notification, as in other infectious diseases, proper disposal of infected excreta, disinfection of infected dwellings, etc., should be rigidly carried out, and the same positive results would be attained throughout the country at large as already obtain in the few places far advanced enough to follow this self-evident line of action. A resolution should be passed by the present meeting, urging the various Provincial Governments to introduce the necessary legislation, and I venture to affirm that, coming from so influential a body of scientists, the suggestion would be adopted. And, if adopted, as I have already said, the educated sentiment of the public would not obstruct, but rather would uphold the action of the authorities. Perhaps this body has already taken such action, but until the various authorities have adopted the suggestions, I consider it the duty of this Association to yearly reiterate the advice. Then finally will begin an era of diminution, until, as some of our more optimistic brethren affirm, fifty years will see the extinction of the Great White Plague.

Councilman's pronouncement as to the causative agent of variola still remains unchallenged; while more recently Mallory, of Boston, has described a protozoan which he has named cyclaster scarlatinalis, and which he believes has a causal relation to scarlet fever. In the winter of 1902-3, Mosher, of the Kinderspital in Vienna, announced the discovery of an anti-scarlatinal serum prepared from a coccus constantly found in the throats of subjects of that disease. His statistics, covering several hundreds of cases, both mild and severe, were, as such statistics usually are, certainly favorable; but he failed to prove his coccus as the cause of the disease, and the consensus of opinion inclines to believe that the favorable results were due to the combatting of the influences of a mixed infection. The same favorable results can also be obtained by the use of anti-streptococcic serum, which reagent, in other forms of infection, has not the wide use among the profession that its virtues demand.

To turn to another field, where surgery and medicine meet, we find that some definite progress has been made. Numerous operations on the stomach have shown that ulceration is more common there than formerly suspected. The physician of to-day must not expect to find all the classical symptoms, for we can have ulceration without pain as we also can have it without hemorrhage. Brilliant results have been obtained in most inveterate cases, by operative methods, results such as medicine has not afforded. Under these circumstances we have the added responsibility of advising some of our patients to submit to the risks of an operation, a responsibility which will often tax our courage to the utmost, but which we, as true men, should not shirk when the occasion arises.

In diseases of the biliary tract, surgery has also disclosed many new features. The post-operative biliary fistula, in cases of obstruction of the common duct, affords a positive means of correctly estimating the quantity and qualities of the bile. The use of cholagogues has an established place in our practice, but now our faith is rudely shaken. Although the term cholagogue has been in use for more than two thousand years, and is apparently as firmly seated as the everlasting hills, recent investigations have caused it to tremble, and it may eventually disappear as did many a mountain in some prehistoric cataclysm. Mayo Robson, in estimating the effects of certain so-called cholagogues, found that the old reliable calomel caused a diminution instead of an increase in the flow of bile. Enonynim gave the same result, while rhubarb and podophyllin, turpentine and benzoate of soda gave negative results. His conclusion is: " The supposed cholagogues investigated seem to rather diminish than increase the amount of bile excreted." Perhaps the most of us feel like saying as the fox to the grapes, " We did not think they were much good, anyway."

As regards cholelithiasis we have also learned a great deal, and have had to revise our views as to etiology, and must consider the typhoid bacillus and the bacillus coli the primal cause for the majority of the cases. The French school go so far as to affirm that, without infection at some stage of the disease, we will not have cholelithiasis. Legars says: " The infectious origin of biliary lithiasis is proved, for the following reasons: If we have shown that gall-stones do not depend on general and obscure humoral conditions but on a local infectious process, the disorder becomes for the most part also a local matter and as such accessible to direct local means. If the calculi are once formed, they increase and multiply, and we can still be sure that they are due to a single attack of lithogenous infection. At a given moment, microbian invasion of the gall-bladder took place. and these microbian invasions, of intestinal origin, depend on various causes and may occur in the course of different acute disorders; at any rate the calculous disorder comes from this primordial lithogenous cholecystitis.   Once more, it is a complaint of the gall-bladder and ducts, not of the bile, and lithogenous chole-cystitis is comparable to many other localized infections, such as appendicitis, for instance.   By removing the calculi, or the gall-bladder, recovery may be complete and final.   Finally, we find infection not only at the origin of lithiasis, but also at all stages of the disorder; it is the leading factor of the various complica-tions as well as of the prognosis of the complaint."

Deaver says: " It can be emphatically stated that gall-stones are always the result of precipitated salts and tissue debris, fol-lowing in the wake of bacterial infection, mild or severe in degree. Furthermore, the complications of chronic gall-stone disease, adhesions, ulceration, fistulæ, liver and pancreatic disease, are also due to infection."   He also says: " The treatment of chronic gall-stone disease, its complications and sequelæ, can only be surgical.   Gall-stones are formed through the aid of infection, and therefore the disease is local and requires local treatment, that is, operation, and not solvents or cholagogues to relieve a condition resulting from faulty metabolism."

Therefore, the same application can be made here as was made in reference to gastric ulceration.   We should realize the impotence of medicines.   Solvents do not dissolve, and the old treatment was merely that of temporizing, with the hope that Dame Nature would aid our misguided efforts by expelling the offending bodies through the natural passages.   Such expectancy is often dangerous.   Surgery holds out a positive cure in a large proportion of cases, but too many of us fear the responsibility of advising such radical treatment, and our patients suffer from our timidity.

Let us now return to a consideration of the work being done by our great army of investigators.   In reviewing their work, not only that of the past year, but of recent years, we see labor mul-tiplied, mountains heaped on mountains in the attempt to scale the heights of the unknown, until, considering the results attained, we might be forgiven for inquiring, " What avails so Titanic a struggle?"   The causes of disease are so intricate that they are reached only after ages of scientific labor.   Yet a few successes have made us impatient of the coming of complete victory.   Some successes have proved to be stars of the first magnitude, others but the smallest flint sparks to illuminate the truth, whilst many so-called discoveries have given no more light than when wax is struck on wax. idle theories, thoughts written on the brain, and now, let us hope, rubbed out forever.   Looking at the workers as constituting an army, one searches in vain for a controlling spirit, one which will concentrate the tremendous and apparently never-tiring energies of this mass of workers into a well-directed assault on some stronghold of the unknown. Modern investigators are, to quote a phrase of Carlyle's, "like a hapless servant gone masterless, unfit for self-guidance." To give an idea of the varied subjects being studied, let me quote the titles of a few of the papers published during the year in but one publication, *The Journal of Medical Research*: "On the Appearance and Significance of Certain Granules in the Erythrocytes of Man," "The Influence of Certain Bacteria in the Coagulation of the Blood," "The Relation of Specific Gravity and Osmotic Pressure to Hemolysis," "The Bacteriolytic Complement Content of Blood Serum," "The Agglutination of the Pneumococcus with Certain Normal and Immune Sera," "Cat's Blood: Differential Counts of the Leucocytes," "A Study of the Agglutinating Hemolytic and Endothelialitic Action of Blood Serum in Variola," and so on. I do not wish to speak slightingly of the labors which these titles of so diversified investigations portray, but I do affirm, that if the workers of some one strong school were under one sole control, their campaign planned against one enemy, and their work properly correlated, more progress would be made in a given time than by the independent, uncorrelated work of all the schools combined.

Such a view is perhaps too Utopian. The world will "gang its ain gait," and our workers will continue to work as before. Truths will gradually be unfolded and science will be developed in the medical field as in the other realms of science. As Marconi did not have to wade through all the drudgery of elaborating the data he needed, but utilized the work of others in perfecting his discovery; as Roentgen needed to win but a single step in advance of others in the race to gain the palm, so, too, can we confidently look forward to the appearance of a master from among our members, one who, building with the bricks made by others, will erect the edifice of truth containing the key which will unlock the secrets of nature and give us command over our most illusive foes. We all feel that that day is near at hand, and when it dawns we will join unselfishly, without a trace of jealousy, in crowning that master with the everlasting laurel.

In conclusion, Mr. Chairman and gentlemen, I thank you for the patience with which you have listened to this address, and wish you every success in your labors in the Section of Medicine.

CHEST EXAMINATIONS: A SYSTEM OF RECORDING OBSERVATIONS.*

BY J. H. ELLIOTT, M.B.,

Physician-in-Charge, Muskoka Cottage Sanatorium, Gravenhurst, Ont.

IT is scarcely necessary for me to preface my communication by any remarks as to the great value to the physician, and through him to his patient, and even to the profession at large, of carefully kept records of cases examined and under treatment. And though the value of such records is recognized, how few general practitioners make any attempt to properly record their findings upon examination of patients. Much valuable material is thus lost, and when at a later period he may be desirous of making some report on a case, there is only the memory, the prescription book and the cash book to be referred to by the physician for data.

The well-written, extensive history of the patient, his symptoms and the findings on physical examination, are of inestimable value to the student and young practitioner in teaching the importance of thoroughly going into details, and to train all the faculties of observation to the highest degree of perfection, and it is to be hoped with the constant extension of the curriculum of our schools, that nothing will ever interfere with our teachers in clinical medicine and surgery insisting upon proper case taking, with attention to the minutest details.

The busy physician feels the need of some short method of recording notes where many patients have to be seen daily. In my own work, with a large number of pulmonary cases under close supervision, with examinations at frequent intervals, I have found it necessary, in order that other work might not suffer, to adopt a graphic method of charting the auscultatory and other phenomena found upon chest examination. At first adopted purely to save time, I have found it of immense value not only in saving time in recording my findings at the time of examination, but also in comparing previous examinations and noting at once any changes.

A momentary glance at such a pictorial record gives one a clear comprehension of the conditions present, which if written *in extenso* would require several minutes to clearly picture to the mind the area involved and physical signs there present. Several lines of written matter cannot convey to one the picture given by a diagram of the chest on which is superimposed a few

---

*Read at meeting of the Ontario Medical Association, June, 1904.

simple symbols showing area over which abnormal physical signs are to be found, and the nature of the same.

For the method of graphic charting which is presented to you to-day, I cannot claim originality. I began the use of symbols on the suggestion of Dr. E. C. Ashton. It has grown with several years' experience, and I have incorporated what I have considered the best points of systems in use elsewhere. Those of Wyllie, of Edinburgh, and Sahli, of Bern, have been modified by various writers, but none of these have I been able to find satisfactory. To Dr. McPhedran and others I have been indebted for valuable suggestions.

Le Bureau central contre la Tuberculose was to consider two weeks ago in Paris the adoption of an international system of symbols. Their report is not available, and probably will not be final for another year or two. When adopted, I shall be pleased to report it to this Society.

In the meantime I present the system which I have found invaluable, which I trust will be of service in stimulating more accurate records of physical signs, as well as being useful in the saving of much time.

The underlying principles are:

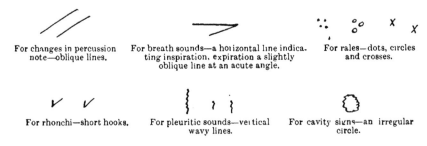

For changes in percussion note—oblique lines.

For breath sounds—a horizontal line indicating inspiration. expiration a slightly oblique line at an acute angle.

For rales—dots, circles and crosses.

For rhonchi—short hooks.

For pleuritic sounds—vertical wavy lines.

For cavity signs—an irregular circle.

The *length* of a line indicates the comparative length of the sound. The *thickness* of a line indicates the comparative density of the sound. A *dot placed above or below* indicates the pitch. For other physical signs, abbreviations are used.

PERC.: PERCUSSION.

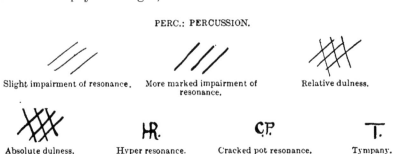

Slight impairment of resonance.

More marked impairment of resonance.

Relative dulness.

Absolute dulness.

Hyper resonance.

Cracked pot resonance.

Tympany.

As an alternative method of indicating percussion changes, shading the area with blue pencil may be used, superimposing on this the symbols indicating changes found by auscultation, etc.

B. S. : BREATH SOUNDS.

N. V.

Normal vesicular—if no note is made it is granted that B.S. are normal.

Inspiration slightly roughened. Expiration not prolonged.

Inspiration slightly roughened. Expiration prolonged.

Inspiration harsh. Expiration somewhat so and prolonged.

Bronchial breathing.

Rough, low-pitched inspiration with high-pitched expiration.

Harsh, wavy inspiration (cogwheel). Expiration not prolonged.

Both inspiration and expiration roughened and wavy. Expiration prolonged.

ADVENTITIOUS SOUNDS.

Crepitant rales.

Dry rales. (If these terms be used.) Moist rales.

Small, medium and large crackling rales.

Sibilant rales.

Rhonchi.

ADVENTITIOUS SOUNDS WHICH SEEM PLEURAL IN ORIGIN.

Pleuritic crackles.

Pleuritic rub.

Signs of cavity formation.

For conditions noted upon inspection and palpation, abbreviations which explain themselves are used. Many others than those shown here readily suggest themselves; *e.g.*,

Em.   Chest emaciated.
Clav. Prom.   Clavicles prominent.
Exp. Lim.   Expansion limited—

to which may be added notes showing comparison of the two sides.

Clav. Prom. Rt. +   Indicating that though both are prominent, the right is more so.
Exp. Lim. Rt. — — —   Expansion is limited, the left having very little movement.
V.F. + ⊣   = Vocal fremitus much increased.
V.R. —   = Vocal resonance diminished.

V.R. o   = Vocal resonance absent.
W.P.   = Whispered pectoriloquy.
W.V.   = Whispered voice.
Cond.   Written under any symbol indicates
                  that the sign is conducted.
Succ.   − Succussion splash.
Coin.   = Coin sound.
                  Placed over second left interspace near ster-
+   num would indicate that the pulmonary
−   second sound was increased or decreased
                  in intensity.
                To indicate impulse.

The use of the plus and minus signs saves a great deal of
writing, indicating whether the deviation from normal is slight
(+) (−): moderate (+ +) (− −); or marked (+ + +)
(− − −).

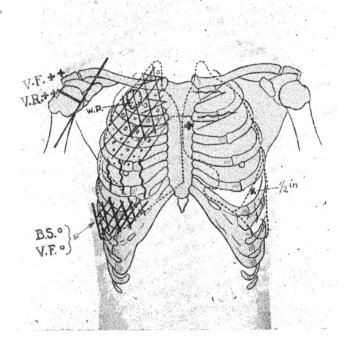

Em. Little Moot Rt.
Both clav. prom. Rt. + +

For example, this chart would tell one at a glance: Patient
emaciated. Both clavicles prominent. Rt. much more marked.
Fair expansion of the left chest. Movements of right much
restricted. Almost absolute dulness apex to third rib with vocal
fremitus much increased and bronchial breathing present. Area
full of moist rales with softening in progress and one well-marked
excavation. Comparative dulness for some distance below this
with small moist rales, then a friction rub well-marked, and below

this to the costal margin absolute dulness with absence of vocal fremitus and breath sounds. Harsh, wavy breathing left apex with no rales, probably compensatory. Apex beat displaced outward half an inch beyond nipple line. Pulmonary second sound accentuated. A few pleuritic crackles at left base.

It is of great assistance in using this or a similar system, to have a chest diagram of fair size; the average one placed on the market in the way of gummed diagram or rubber stamp is rather too small. After a long search for a suitable one, I have adopted that of Musser,* adding the outline of the lobes of the lung and of the pleura. The plate was prepared from a drawing made by Mr. Kelly, of the Toronto Lithographing Co., and should any member of this Association require such a diagram, I would be much pleased to have it used. I believe it is already in use in the Hospital for Sick Children in Toronto. In my own work I have the front and back of the chest printed on either side of a card of standard size, using it as a part of a card index system of recording cases, a system which I put into use on the advice of Dr. N. A. Powell, to whom I am also indebted for much help in the completion of the details of the same.

---

* John H. Musser, "A Practical Treatise on Medical Diagnosis." 3rd Edition.

THE ARID CLIMATES.*

BY J. FRANK McCONNELL, M D., LAS CRUCES, MEXICO.

CLIMATE is relied upon to a greater extent for the arrest of pulmonary tuberculosis than for any other disease.

If this be true, and it would be rash to gainsay it, a brief consideration of the so-called arid belt will serve to demonstrate the peculiar features of a region which has produced more permanent arrests of tubercular involvements than any locality extant.

For the purpose of this monograph it will be sufficient to refer to but Colorado, New Mexico, and Arizona, since those adjacent parts, which are politically in other States, are geographically of those named. For example, El Paso is politically in Texas, while topographically it is part of Southern New Mexico; similarly with portions of Wyoming, Utah and California.

Any consideration of this' region must of necessity be both general and particular, since all of the country tributary to the Rocky Mountains, from Canada to Mexico, and the desert to the west of them, presents features which are possessed in common, and at the same time, it is equally true that the various localities exemplify great variations of these characteristics, that are of deep interest to the student of climatotherapy.

The general features may be reviewed under the captions of altitude, purity of atmosphere, sunlight or sunshine, humidity and soil.

Altitudes may be arbitrarily classified as high, intermediate or moderate, and low.

High.—Localities situated more than 4,500 feet above sea level belong to this sub-division. The majority of the resorts in Colorado, Northern New Mexico and Northern Arizona, enjoy this distinction:

ILLUSTRATIVE POINTS :—   ALTITUDE.
Santa Fe, New Mexico 6,939
Las Vegas, New Mexico...................... 6,398
Colorado Springs, Colorado.................. 6,000
Denver, Colorado 5,294
Prescot, Arizona........................... 5,300
Oracle, Arizona........ 4,800

Adaptations.—Favorable: Incident or moderately advanced cases of the ulcerative type in subjects under forty-five years of age, who have no further lesions, and whose alimentation is favorably influenced by cold. Unfavorable: Far advanced cases; those in whom emphysema and marked fibroid changes co-exist;

* Read at meeting of the Ontario Medical Association, Toronto, June, 1904.

those in whom the circulation is feeble; those subject to catarrhs, to whom rapid variations in temperature are a serious menace. Hemoptysis is not a contra-indication.

Intermediate or Moderate.—Localities which are between 2,500 and 4,500 feet above sea level:

Illustrative points :—	Altitude.
Las Cruces, New Mexico	3,873
El Paso, Texas	3,600

Adaptations.—Favorable: Incipient and moderately advanced cases in subjects of all ages; those in whom the circulation is inclined to be feeble, especially the catarrhal types; laryngeal complication. Unfavorable: Cases with emphysema, progressive fibroid change, kidney and heart lesions.

Low.—Localities which are less than 2,500 feet above sea level:

Illustrative points :—	Altitude.
Tucson, Arizona	2,400
Phœnix, Arizona	1,100
Yuma, Arizona	140

Adaptations.—Favorable: Advanced cases in subjects of all ages, particularly in those who are menaced by marked variations in temperature; laryngeal complications, cases exhibiting lesions of other organs, especially of the genito-urinary tract; and those in whom there is accentuation of the pulmonary second sound. Unfavorable: Young adults of good physique; especially those whose appetite is mal-influenced by heat. It is but meet that at this point mention should be made of Indio, a locality situated in the California desert, some hundred feet below sea level. The writer has seen several far advanced cases that had not improved in various altitudes go on to a considerable degree of improvement in this region.

Purity of the Atmosphere.—Owing to the mountainous and desert character of the various localities comprised in the arid belt, the comparative paucity of those essentials conducive to the support of a large population, there is no lack of an abundance of pure air. Again, the practical absence of any opportunity for decaying vegetable matter precludes the possibility of organic combustion arising from chemical, physiologic or zymotic agencies, which are favorable to the development of the tubercle bacillus, and other pathogenic micro-organisms. The aseptic feature of the atmosphere is of the greatest moment, however, in preventing favorable opportunity for converting a tubercular focus into one of mixed infection, *since the most untoward accident which may befall a tubercular individual is that he should become consumptive.*

Sunshine or Sunlight.—That there is a direct and intimate relationship between sunlight and dryness cannot be successfully denied, but in the writer's opinion the real feature of value is summed up in the term brightness. Nowhere is sunlight more brilliant and of greater duration than in the arid regions, where it may be truthfully stated that there is sunshine on almost every day of the year.

Solar heat increases all the functions of animal as well as vegetable life; *peripheral circulation* is more active, to the advantage of internal organs, which thus free themselves from stagnant blood charged with excrementitious principles. Light, also, as seen in vegetation, plays a most important part through its active rays. " It reddens the blood, it cures chlorosis, in the same manner as it restores the color to plants bleached in darkness."

Humidity.—It is to this part of our subject that we would most particularly invite your attention, since it is the consensus of opinion among the practicians of this region (of New Mexico at least) that the low relative humidity or atmospheric dryness which the south-west possesses, plays a role in the therapy of pulmonary diseases which is deserving of a better recognition than that of being classified as a mere " useful adjunct."

The relation between temperature and humidity is an intimate one. The amount of water that can exist in the gaseous state depends on the temperature. The higher the temperature the greater the possible humidity; the lower the temperature the lower the possible humidity. Water exists in the gaseous state at all observed temperatures.

The amount of moisture in the atmosphere in any given locality will be governed, firstly, by the temperature of the region; secondly, by the nature of the evaporating surface of the place; thirdly, by the rate at which the humidity is carried away; and, finally, by the rate at which humidity is brought to the region by the prevailing winds. As the temperature declines with altitude, it is evident that the humidity possibilities of elevation must decline; though in relation to the last statement it must be recollected that during certain seasons and on mountain slopes upon which the clouds gather the humidity is increased. *The dryness of the atmosphere in the arid belt is a primary requisite for the early arrest of the tubercular process.*

  Soil.—Whether the soil belongs to the gravel, sand or adobe types it possesses the special characteristic of dryness. It is an unfortunate feature that many of the towns have been built in old river bottoms, where the adobe clay becomes pulverized and makes itself noticeable whenever there is wind or much traffic.

It is worth mentioning that among the alfalfa meadows there

	Elevation	Latitude	Soil	Normal Air-Pressure	Temperature			Humidity				No. of Cloudy Days	Mean Monthly Wind Movement
					Annual	December	August	Relative	Absolute	Dew Points	Rain-fall		
Santa Fe, N.M	7,000	33.34	Sand and Adobe..	24.50	51	32	71	50	1.90	30	16.1	52	5451
Colorado Springs, Colo.	6,000	38.51	Gravel.	24.03	47	28	70	51	1.84	29	15.2	58	6565
Denver, Colo.	5,280	38.76	Gravel and Sand.	24.18	49	29	76	50	1.86	30	14.1	63	4898
Flagstaff, Ariz.	6,300	34.26	Gravel and Sand.	......	53	33	74	51	2.18	38	16.0	51	5150
fa, Ariz.	4,650	32.50	Gravel and Adobe	......	60	44	82	48	......		17.7		
Las Cruces, N.M	3,850	32.17	Adobe.	25.02	59	46	77	38	2.95	42	7.2	18	4947
an, Ariz.	2,300	32.14	Sand and Gravel	27.50	69	50	88	42	3.20	44	12.0	57	3765
Phœnix, Ariz.	1,100	32.28	Adobe.	28.68	70	52	90	45	3.08	42	9.0	52	3380
Yuma, Ariz.	130	32.44	Sand.	29.90	72	56	96	46	3.22	43	3.1	18	4322

5

is little or no dust; the writer having recently entered a cottage which had been closed for nearly a year was very much surprised to find practically no dust; the cottage is situated in a broad hacienda where the alfalfa grows luxuriantly.

Applied Climatology.—The tubercular patient, properly selected, who is placed in the indicated environment under competent supervision, soon exhibits the following phenomena: 1. Cough is checked; expectoration increased (at first), and made easy.   2. The respirations are deeper and slower.   3. Febrile symptoms disappear.   4. A noticeable increase in chest development.   5. A diminished anemia.   6. Increased appetite with consequent gain in weight and feeling of well-being.

Flick has stated, " Climate itself is of little value in the treatment of consumption; it is the *outside* air which counts, and it makes very little difference where the outside air is got from, so it is got *every day,* and *all the day and night.*" (The italics are the writer's.)

The open air plan of treatment, boldly pursued in the arid region, *alone* makes possible this dictum. Osler has stated: " The cure of tuberculosis is a question of nutrition. Digestion and assimilation control the situation; make the patient grow fat and the local disease may be left to care for itself." Nowhere can the truth of this axiom be better exemplified than in the arid belt, where the possibilities of outdoor life are unlimited, where digestion waits on appetite and fresh air is a forerunner of both.

" If it be a good thing for a sick man to change his residence, it must be a proper thing for him to know what it is that he is avoiding, and what it is that he is to *acquire in exchange for it* in another place." If this trite remark of Scoresby-Jackson is in some small way realized through the medium of this article then, indeed, will the writer feel content.

BIBLIOGRAPHY.

1. Abercromby, Ralph—Weather.
2. Annual Reports U S. Weather Bureau, 1890-1903, incl.
3. Author's "On Tubercular Patients, whom to send and where to send them," *Journal A. M. C.*, March, 1900.
4. Ibid. "Climate Therapy." *Canadian Practitioner*, 1897.
5. Reference Handbook of the Medical Sciences.
6. W. F. R. Phillips, M.D., U. S. Weather Bureau, Washington.
7. Edward Osgood Otis, M.D., Boston.
8. Sally S. Edwin, M.D., Medical Climatology.

THE VIVISECTION PROBLEM: TWO VIEWS.

I.—VIVISECTION AND A HUMANE SPIRIT.

BY WILLIAM LAWRENCE,
Bishop of Massachusetts.

MANY people are puzzled to-day about the question of vivisection. Is it humane? Is it not cruel? Has any man the right deliberately to experiment on a hundred guinea-pigs in the hope of making some discovery? Granted that a discovery is made, is it worth the sacrifice of the lives of many dumb, helpless animals?

Perhaps it is a presumption on the part of any one who has not a scientific training to write upon the subject. I have thought, however, that some people might like an expression of opinion from a layman in science who has given some consideration to the question.

Some twenty-five years ago I was called to a family in my parish in which a terrible scourge held sway. Diphtheria had struck the home; one child lay dead, another with heartrending gasps was struggling for breath, another was in the early stages of the sickness; their lives were doomed. As one watched the mother's agony and the children's cruel sufferings, his thought was, "O for some relief from this dreadful scourge!" If, by the taste of a tender pigeon or chicken, life could be sustained, how quickly would we serve it! If twenty miles away there were a physician who could stay the disease, the father would ride his horse even unto death to fetch him. Other children near by were dying of the same scourge. What were the lives of a hundred pigeons or a hundred horses, if only the scores of children who were doomed to die of diphtheria in that city during that winter could be saved?

Twenty-five years have passed, and to-day, when diphtheria enters a home, lives are comparatively safe. Thousands, literally thousands, of children are playing in our homes, thousands of men and women are doing their part towards building up our nation, who, except for the beneficent discovery of antitoxin, would, so far as any one of us can see, be dead to-day. Many animals have been sacrificed in the progress of the discovery, to be sure. Horses are to-day put to discomfort and some slight pain in the manufacture of the material. But the free distribution of antitoxin among the poor of our great cities and its use in the hospitals are saving thousands of human lives. Mothers receive back their children to life again. I start with this discovery, for in it are suggested a few points that we need to keep in mind.

In the first place, I assume that we all agree that man depends for his life upon the use and sacrifice of animals. Every chicken and turkey on our dinner-tables tells us that. The milk that we drink is gained at the cost of the anguish of the cow which is bereft of her calf. The slaughter that goes on in our abattoirs is horrible to contemplate, if we put our mind upon it and dwell on the details; yet every one of us lives daily upon the results of the slaughter.

On the other hand, this is true: this generation is probably more sensitive to the thought of pain and suffering in animals than any other in history. The blessing of anesthetics has so released humanity from the awful terrors of suffering that we cannot endure even the thought of what our fathers passed through. Surgery has become so skilful and painless as to have lost much of its terror. Operations certainly fatal one year are comparatively safe the next year, and are almost without danger the year after; so marvellous has been the increase in the knowledge of the human body, and of the action of its organs and the intricacy of its parts. There never were so many people under the knife as there are to-day; there never have been so many lives saved by surgery and medicine as now; and there never has been so little suffering among the sick and injured. At the same time that these conditions prevail it is also the fact that vivisection was probably never before so much practiced.

The people demand, therefore, and rightly demand, that there shall be no unnecessary suffering laid upon even the lower animals. They will not allow cruelty or wilful injury in any form. The Societies for the Prevention of Cruelty to Animals and the stringent legislation against cruelty in this last generation are the efficient expressions of the feelings of modern society. No class of men, not even the leaders in science, are or should be exempt from these humane laws. Where there is cruelty, wilful injury, or unnecessary loss of life, there the State enters, arrests, and imprisons or fines the guilty.

Here, then, we have the situation. For the life and welfare of men, animals must be sacrificed; we all accept this fact when we sit down to our Sunday roast beef. The cruel or unnecessary sacrifice of animals is universally condemned.

The question in connection with vivisection is, How far have we a right to sacrifice animal life and to inflict pain upon animals for the welfare and life of man?

No one of us would undertake to say how many guinea-pigs could be set against the life of one little child. One? Ten? A thousand? How many against the lives of a thousand children? Clearly, child life and man's life are of high value. The practical question for all of us who desire the welfare of man and the saving of children's lives is, Which shall be sacrificed—men and children, or animals? For experimentation must go on, if lives are to be saved. Shall the experiments be on children or on mice and rabbits?

Shall we allow our children, thousands on thousands of them, to decline in health and become subject to all sorts of diseases through breathing the vitiated air of school-rooms, or shall we follow with interest the careful experiments with animals breathing vitiated air, thus discovering methods of purifying the air, and by the sacrifice, it may be of many, many mice and rabbits, protect and sustain the health of the children of our cities? Shall we allow our surgeons to experiment on the patients in our hospitals, killing man after man in the fruitless attempt to remove one kidney; or shall we encourage them to experiment again and again, and a thousand times again, if necessary, on all sorts of animals, that they may safely undertake the operation when the next sufferer at the hospital is brought to them?

All these things mean vivisection. So did the discovery of the circulation of the blood, on which all surgery and medicine rest; so also artificial respiration, skin-grafting, the alleviation of angina pectoris, and the cure of hydrophobia. To vivisection and experimentation on animals are due, at least in great part, our increasing knowledge of that terrible scourge, tuberculosis, and the means of preventing it. In the amputation of a limb, in these days almost bloodless and painless, nearly every step in the operation has been dependent upon the experience gained in experiments upon animals. The discovery and application of antiseptics have enormously reduced the death-rate in hospitals and sick-rooms, sufferings untold are avoided, and tens of thousands of valuable lives are saved. In his researches towards this discovery Sir Joseph Lister was dependent upon vivisection. In fact, one can hardly name a disease or form of suffering the partial relief of which has not had some relation to vivisection.

Could not these discoveries have been made without vivisection? Some would say " No," and they would have good reason for their answer. I would rather say, " I don't know," but I do know that they were not made without vivisection, and I am sure that without vivisection they would not be known *to-day*. And are not the hastening of the discoveries and thereby the saving of thousands of precious lives worth all that they have cost?

That some vivisection is probably necessary is, I think, the verdict of almost every one who thinks of the subject at all. Still, there are many questions and doubts lingering in the minds of the people. Perhaps I may put some of them in such form as they have come to me, with a few suggestions for consideration.

(1) " Is not vivisection attended with unnecessary cruelty?" it is asked. " We read of surgeons and students in Europe who do horrible things; we see illustrations that shock us." What may be done in Europe I do not know, though I have the impression that doctors and scientists there are, as a rule, humane men.

What is done in our own communities interests us more closely. Now, if there is any case where an animal is cruelly operated on, if it is put to unnecessary pain, it is time for those who have the evidence to call in the police. Our people will not tolerate cruelty.

It is well for us to remember that, with very rare exceptions, the subject of vivisection is completely under the influence of anesthetics. If the animal moves, however, by reflex muscular action, it is very difficult for some persons not to imagine that it is in pain. We are often told by those who deplore the practice that the subject writhes and struggles.

A bit of personal experience has helped me on this point. Called to undergo as a young man a slight surgical operation, I was etherized. They were not so skilful in giving ether in those days as now. In the midst of the operation I struggled and fought as in the utmost agony. I awoke to find myself on the floor with a rug on top of me, on which the doctor sat to hold me down. The operation was successfully over. My parents were in the utmost distress at the pain I must have suffered—a distress quickly relieved when I told them that my only sensation was a funny dream of a fight, in which I came off second best—not a suggestion of pain.

We need to keep in mind that a hundred dogs may be studied under vivisection and then killed, and beyond the discomfort attending etherization feel no sensation equal to the prick of a pin. And if a student or investigator allow one dog to suffer unnecessarily, he is liable to arrest for cruelty.

There are, as I have just suggested, very exceptional instances where anesthetics may interfere with the object of the experiment; even in those cases the slightest carelessness as to suffering or unnecessary continuance of pain is, under the law, criminal. Granted even that some pain and suffering are necessary, we must remember that these experiments are carried on with the sole purpose of so advancing science as to relieve men and women from far more suffering and agony than animals endure.

(2) Again, we are asked, "Why should medical students be allowed each one to experiment on animals? Why shouldn't they be shown in the hospitals how the work is done, and then sent forth to do it?"

Why should the motorman be compelled not only to understand the mechanism and see others handle the car, but also to handle it himself under direction before he is trusted with the lives of passengers? Because there is something in personal experience, in the touch, the sense of friction on grades and curves, which no lessons can give.

Medical science is concerned with life, and life must be studied at first hand. The body and its organs are marvellously intricate. Will a mother allow a young doctor to cut open her child's body, if he tells her that this is the first time he ever had a knife in his hand for action? She would let him know in no measured words that he could try his experiments on some one else first; and that is just what the medical student, under the careful direction of his teacher, does; he experiments, so far as is necessary and only so far, on animals, in order that he may not be compelled to experiment on children.

(3) A third question arises, "Why may not the State have an oversight of all these things, and employ agents to inspect and see that everything is done in a humane way?"

One is struck at first thought by the apparent good sense of the proposition. On second thought, one is prompted to ask why the State should take this responsibility and go to this large expense. And if it should, would the results justify the action?

The Harvard Medical School and, I take it, every medical institution are glad to welcome any disinterested and intelligent persons and show them all their methods. Is it worth while to hire agents to force doors that are already open? Are there authenticated cases of cruelty so bad or numerous as to demand inspection?

Again, agents would be required so skilled and advanced in scientific knowledge as to understand the purpose of the operation, its intricacies, and its relation to other operations. Can the State pay for such men? Agents ignorant of the subject would be worse than useless.

In England vivisection has been sharply restricted; the inspection system prevails. The work of science has been so hampered that, to the minds of some, the leadership in surgery at least is passing over to America and other countries Even Sir Joseph Lister, one of the great benefactors of his race, is said to have been compelled to leave England after the passage of the restrictive act of 1876, that he might carry on his investigations in behalf of the saving of human life.

The great safeguard against cruelty in vivisection is not legislation or inspection, but the high professional spirit of doctors and investigators. Taking them as a body, is there any set of men to whom we will more confidently trust our health and lives and those of our children? We find them tender and humane in our homes and in the hospitals. We cannot believe that they become brutes in the laboratory, or that they will countenance brutality. We must believe that their ruling motive in life is humane, the good of humanity; and for the good of humanity the sacrifice of animal life is necessary We men and woman, citizens, who are not doctors, have a vital interest in the subject. Public opinion is powerful.

We want to make the investigator realize that not a sparrow falls without the Father's care, and that he has no right to sacrifice even one humble animal more than is necessary for the good of man by the advancement of science. We want also to hold him so rigidly to his great and beneficent work that he will not hesitate to sacrifice one animal or a hundred if thereby science is so advanced that even one little child may not perish.

Whether men approve or disapprove of vivisection, all are, I believe, led to their opinions by a spirit of humanity On that common ground we all stand.

II.—FOR RESTRICTION AND LIMITATION.

BY ALBERT LEFFINGWELL, M.D.,

Author of "The Vivisection Question," Director of the American Humane Association, and of the Vivisection Reform Society.

It was about thirty-five years ago, in the city of New York, that I first saw a painful vivisection, performed by a distinguished physiologist for the purpose of impressing upon the memory of students certain physiological facts. Not long after, fortified by observation and personal experimentation, while engaged in teaching some of the elements of physiology to a class of young men, it occurred to me to avail myself of this method of instruction; and accordingly an invitation was extended to the class, or to any one who cared to be present, to come to my improvised "laboratory" at the close of the school session. To my gratification, every member of my class was present; and though a third of a century has passed, I still remember vividly the enthusiasm which my few experiments seemed to excite. Of course, to use present-day phraseology, " no more pain was inflicted than was necessary for the success of the experiment." I could honestly affirm, too, that " anesthetics were always used "; but nevertheless the accident of " incomplete anesthesia " occasionally happened during my demonstrations—just as I had seen it occur during the experiments of most accomplished vivisectors. Certainly I felt no compunctions; was I not helping forward, in some slight degree, the cause of Science?

It was a period of intellectual ferment, especially for young men. Brown-Séquard, one of the most cruel vivisectors that ever breathed, visited this country, gave a science talk in the lecture-room of Plymouth Church—where we were all proud to shake his hand—and vivisected a lamb, without anesthetics, before the students of a certain medical school, to illustrate his theories. The great names of Tyndall, Darwin, and Huxley were ever on our lips. The medical student of that day was accustomed to smile with significant contempt at any criticism of vivisection; painful or not, it concerned only the scientist. Possibly my vivisections continued for a year or two, during the winter terms.

But, one afternoon, the President of the Polytechnic Institute chanced to visit my laboratory after I had gone home. There he found some pigeons upon which I had performed, before my class, the celebrated experiment of Flourens on the brain. The next day there was remonstrance, with a request that vivisection immediately cease, and that use of the blackboard take its place. The protests of President Cochran deeply impressed me. Going abroad after graduation in medicine, I saw in Paris and elsewhere experiments so atrociously cruel, carried out with such complete indifference to the causation of agony for mere purposes of demonstrating what everybody knew, that the question of their utility and justification was constantly in mind. Admitting that the experiments helped a student to remember his lesson, was that sufficient to justify the agony they cost? I could not assert it. But everything was not painful. Would it not be possible, without impediment to scientific discovery, without injury to scientific teaching, to draw a line which should distinguish between what is permissible and what should be condemned? The extreme pro-vivisection advocates in this country demand that everything shall be permitted to an advanced student of physiology or a teacher of the science The anti-vivisectionists, on the other hand, as a rule, insist that all use of the lower animals for scientific purposes be legally forbidden. Each view has the merit of simplicity. Yet there are objections to each. And so, twenty-five years ago, I took the position, ever since maintained, that in this matter of vivisection there should be, not abolition of experimentation, but legal regulation.

Within the limits of a brief paper it is manifestly impossible to mention all the objections that exist regarding more radical views, or the arguments supporting a middle course. Some of these, however, may be briefly stated.

Let it be conceded, in the first place, that a law abolishing every form of experimentation upon animals, with heavy penalties for its infraction, would do very much to lessen the evils of vivisection, and particularly of painful vivisection. Of course it would not prevent the investigations of science, if any were deemed sufficiently important to warrant defiance of the law; it would simply place vivisection on a par with gambling which, although a crime, is nevertheless practiced to a greater or less extent in every large city. That that abolition would occasion any infinitely great injury to human interests, as is sometimes claimed, is most improbable. All the claims of utility are exaggerated when controversially necessary; I do not believe that the average length of human life would be diminished by an hour if never another painful experiment were made, or if all the drugs of Christendom—barring perhaps half a dozen— were dumped into the sea. The latter event is certainly remote, with human credulity as it is at present; so, too, is the abolition of all animal experimentation. Carried into legal effect, such abolition would prevent all painless demonstrations of scientific facts against which the charge of cruelty could not be urged; it would prevent researches which might be exceedingly useful at times in the detection of crime or the causes of disease. Some day, in the distant future, I believe that the human race will take into consideration its whole duty toward our lower kindred. But to-day, in a world of butchery of animals for food, for sport, for clothing, for outer adornment, and for convenience, to expect that society will prohibit even the *painless* forms of scientific research and let all the rest exist, is to expect the impossible. Nevertheless, an agitation which keeps alive a great ethical question cannot be in vain. The service which the abolitionist rendered to the cause of human freedom is the service which the anti-vivisectionist has rendered the cause of humaneness to the lower forms of life.

The position of the free-vivisection party is also simple. For the vivisector it claims absolute freedom from every form of legal regulation or supervision. If he wishes to perform a painless experiment, well and good; if he desires to perform the most excruciating of agonizing operations, merely to demonstrate some well-known fact—well and good also. "Hands off!" is the cry of the vivisector in America, as well as elsewhere. But there is a difficulty, When a leading professor in a great medical school tells the world that "a brief death by burning would be considered a happy release by a human being undergoing the experi-

ence of some of the animals who slowly die in a laboratory," and
that " the time will come when the world will look back to modern vivisection in the name of science as it does now to burning
at the stake in the name of religion," does one fancy that absolute
freedom to perform such experiments will be conceded without
inquiry or protest?

Assuming, then, the desirability of some reform, how may it
be effected without resort to absolute prohibition, and without
impediment to scientific progress? This is the problem of the
hour. Sometimes we are told that vivisection is already most
carefully restricted by the vivisectors themselves. Well, here is
a fair test. Suppose a European physiologist of eminence, whose
cruelty is world-renowned, to come to this country, and to be
invited by the director in charge of some American laboratory to
repeat an experiment involving the utmost degree of torture—
what would prevent? Any conceivable experiment may now be
performed, provided only that permission be accorded by the
director in charge of the laboratory. We cannot depend to-day
upon our superior humanity. Some of the worst vivisections
recorded in history have been made in an American laboratory
within the past ten years. " The law should interfere," said Professor Henry G. Bigelow, M.D., of Harvard Medical School, a
few years ago. " There can be no doubt that in this relation there
exists a case of cruelty to animals far transcending in its refinement and in its horror anything that has been known in the history of nations." I do not take Dr. Bigelow to mean that every
vivisector is cruel, or every laboratory a den of cruelty. He means
only this: that where there is no legal restriction *everything is
possible, because, somewhere, everything has been done.*

But how far can we go with State control of vivisection without detriment to scientific advancement? Limitations of space
prevent anything but the briefest outline of what may be done in
the direction of reform.

First. Every laboratory where vivisection may be legally
carried on should be licensed and placed under the charge of some
responsible director. This certainly can harm no one.

Second. The privilege of vivisection should be accorded only
to persons holding a State license, granted only upon some specified examination of qualifications, intellectual and moral.

Third. The director in charge of each place licensed for vivisection should cause to be kept a register, wherein should be recorded (1) the number and species of animals received for experimentation; (2) the number of experiments made, and the
species of animals upon which they were performed; (3) the
object of each experiment, whether for research or for instruction of students; (4) whether the experiment was painless, and

whether the animal was permitted to recover from the anesthetic. An annual report, giving facts and figures desired, should be required from each laboratory, and published for information of the public.

This is by far the most important condition of any reform. It does nothing but this: it removes the veil of secrecy behind which vivisection is now conducted. What objection to such publicity can possibly be urged by men who have nothing to conceal?

Fourth. No painful vivisection should be permitted simply as a demonstration of well-known facts; and, if at all, only for purposes of great utility and with every precaution against abuse.

Inasmuch as we are told that painful experiments are seldom, if ever, performed nowadays, why should there be any objection to this provision?

Finally comes the important question of laboratory inspection by a salaried officer of the State. To this the most strenuous objections have been urged. Some of these seem to me not unreasonable. If admission to all laboratories were freely accorded to certain classes, such as clergymen, physicians and members of the State Legislature, I am inclined to think that paid inspection could be given up. Others, however, regard something of the sort as of supreme importance. The late Dr. Bigelow, of Harvard Medical School, declared that " every laboratory ought to be open to some supervising legal authority competent to determine that it is conducted from roof to cellar on the humanest principles," in default of which it should be suppressed. Here, then, is opportunity for compromise. If we can once agree that it is desirable to prevent certain abuses of vivisection, there will be no long dispute as to the method.

Thus, briefly, I have attempted to outline the views of those who, despite considerable misunderstanding of their aims, are working simply for the legal regulation of vivisection in the United States.—*Outlook,* New York.

A NOTE ON THE TREATMENT OF SCIATICA.

BY ARTHUR H. BOSTOCK, L.R.C.P. (LOND.), M.R.C.S. (ENG.).

WHILE house physician at St. Bartholomew's Hospital, I was much struck with the number of cases of sciatica which were not amenable to ordinary methods of treatment, and the object of this note is to recommend the use of a remedy to which I have now given a thorough trial. It has been of most use in the cases of true neuralgia.

The drug is phenalgin (ammonio-phenylacetamido) dose 5 to

20 grs., and I find that this substance so given has no depressing action on the heart, neither does it expose the patient to the risks incurred in the use of such analgesics as opium and morphia. When a case is in the acute stage the patient should be placed in the recumbent position, and poultices should be applied locally. A commencement should be made with phenalgin in a dose of ten grains, repeated every three hours. After the first twenty-four hours, if the drug is acting, I reduce it to ten grains (four tablets) three times a day, and next day to three tablets (seven and a half grains) three times a day. I then leave a few tablets with the patient to take a dose of ten grains, should the pain show a tendency to recur. In my experience doses consisting of less than three tablets (seven and a half grains) are of no use at all.— *London Lancet,* April 15th, 1904.

JAMAICA, A LAND NEVER TOUCHED BY FROST.

THE BLOOM IS PERPETUAL AND THE NORTHERNER FINDS THE COUNTRY ONE WHERE CARE NEVER LINGERS.

SIMEON L. HARRELL, who has been to Jamaica on several occasions, has written an entertaining story on that land of perpetual bloom which has attracted a great deal of attention. Mr. Harrell believes that when Americans become more acquainted with the eastern paradise they will flock to the island and drink in its vast delights. Mr. Harrell's story of Jamaica follows:

Nature and history have combined to bring the islands of the Caribbean Archipelago into prominence in the eyes of the world at the present time. Travelers visiting these southern waters have always borne testimony to the tropical beauty of these islands and the lingering mediæval civilization of their towns and cities, but it is only recently that the tide of travel has turned in any volume to these attractive shores.

The war with Spain and subsequent relations with Cuba, Porto Rico and the United States, 'the recent terrible volcanic devastations in Martinique and neighboring islands of the Lesser Antilles, have awakened much interest in regard to these regions. Northern people have just begun to learn that almost at their doors, at the end of a short and delightful sea voyage, is a veritable "Garden of Eden," where there are no chilling winds or frosts, no blazing, heated days, or dull, hot, enervating nights, either in mid-winter or mid-summer; an almost changeless, ideal climate, with rich tropical fruit, foliage and vegetation, constantly in bloom. Such a spot is Jamaica, the largest and most important of the British West Indian possessions. It is situated

1,588 miles south of Boston, 92 miles south of Cuba, and 100 miles west of Hayti. The island is 144 miles long, varying from 21 to 49 miles in width, containing nearly 6,000 square miles. It lies in the path of the Gulf Stream, which it divides, causing a constant flow of mild, crystal blue waters all around it. It is also directly in the track of that mysterious air current—the Trade Winds—which blow steadily half the year from the north-east, and the other half from the south-west. There also extends nearly the entire length of the island a magnificent range of lofty mountains whose verdure-clad peaks tower from 1,500 to 1,800 feet above the sea, sloping frequently toward the sea on either side into lovely valleys, broad plateaus, covered with fertile, smiling plantations and villages. These geographical conditions all combine to cause this really tropical location to possess almost the entire year the delightful atmosphere known in New England as a " perfect day in perfect June," the thermometer ranging from 70 to 88 degrees.

Jamaica was discovered by Columbus in 1494, during the second voyage to the new world. In 1500 the first Spanish colony was founded. It remained 160 years in possession of Spain—until 1654—when it was captured by an English expedition sent out by Oliver Cromwell, and has since remained under British control.

• There were but few of the original Caribs found on the island when Columbus landed, but during the Spanish and a portion of the English occupation many thousands of negroes were brought here by the brutal slave traders, and were held in bondage until between 1834 and 1838, when Great Britain gradually abolished slavery in its colonial possessions. As freemen the negroes proved lazy and unreliable workers on the plantations, consequently the plan was adopted of bringing in thousands of coolies from India on five-year labor contracts, and they have proved valuable workers for the planters. The soil is so rich, producing so many kinds of nourishing foods, that the island sustains a population of over 700,000, about 10 to 15 per cent. of whom are white.

During the Spanish reign, Jamaica was the headquarters of all the pirates, buccaneers, free-booters, cut-throats and slave traders, who roamed the seas and pillaged the Spanish main. They made Dry Harbor and Port Royal their chief rendezvous. On the 17th of June, 1692, the town was shaken by a tremendous earthquake, whole streets, with their inhabitants and dwellings, also a fine cathedral, being swallowed up by the sea. Many of the ruins are now visible when the waters are quiet, and relics and valuables are frequently brought up by divers.

Kingston, the chief town and seat of government, contains a population of about fifty thousand, with several fine government buildings, a cathedral, fine stores, well kept hotels and boarding houses, chief of which are the Myrtle Bank and the Constant Spring House, the latter being about four miles out in the suburbs, at the end of an electric road. A steam railway extends from the western part of the island to Montego Bay, and another through a wild and interesting gorge to Port Antonio, which is the largest town located on the north-eastern end of the island, the headquarters and great shipping port of the United Fruit Company, formerly (the Boston Fruit Company) of Boston. This company has done a great deal to develop industry and increase the prosperity of Jamaica. They run, twice each week, their four elegant "Admiral" steamers from Philadelphia and Boston to Port Antonio, besides many freight steamers laden with bananas, oranges and other tropical fruits, the yearly traffic amounting to many million dollars. The company have also built an elegant American style hotel, called the Tichfield House. Owing to the increase of travel to Jamaica, and the deserved popularity of the Tichfield, the United Fruit Company have decided to very largely increase the capacity of the hotel and cottages so as to fully meet all demands for hotel accommodations next season. The views from the broad piazzas of this hotel toward the sea, as well as from the mouth of the harbor, taking in the town of Port Antonio and the lofty Blue mountain, clothed to the top with masses of tropical vegetation, is pronounced by many world-wide travelers as the most beautiful views of earth. A famous poet writes of this scene as follows:

> "Could you but view the scenery fair
> That now beneath my window lies,
> You'd think that Nature lavished there
> Her purest waves, her softest skies
> To make a heaven for us to sigh in,
> For bards to live and saints to die in."

There is a sea coast of nearly 500 miles frequently indented with safe harbors and lined with beautiful hard, white, sandy beaches, inviting you to bathe in the waters of the Caribbean, almost as warm as the air, amid shouts of laughter and play of children, and older ones as well, who bid farewell to cares in this ideal land of rest.

The government has built and maintains about 4,000 miles of smooth, hard, macadamized roads, 900 miles of wide paths, besides about 180 miles of railways. There are walks and drives through the banana plantations, along the rocky coasts, ever resounding to the music of the sea waves, up secluded valleys to places with such romantic names as "Golden Vale," "Hope Gardens" and "Paradise," names not inappropriate. If you have the courage to rise before the sun you can obtain a saddled horse for 50 cents an hour and climb into the mountains, with views hardly surpassed anywhere for beauty and grandeur. Up through banana groves and forests of cocoa palms you come to fields where sheep and cattle are grazing, down into a valley, then up higher hills you find yourself skirting the edges of steep cliffs half hidden by a profusion of tangled vines. The red hibiscus is intertwined with morning glories and roses and flowers of every hue. Here and there you pass cleared fields where peasants are planting yams or sweet potatoes.

To a northern person the most peculiar feature of the Jamaica climate is the absence of seasons. There seems to be no summer or winter, but one continuous blooming springtime. If any time is more delightful to visit the island than another it is from May to October, and we predict that it will not be long before the fashionable crowd will flock to this lovely isle instead of to Florida in winter, and the mountains and lakes of the north in summer, for here there is always a balmy air of rest for tired nerves and weak invalids. Another strange and almost anomalous feature of Jamaica is the absence of flies, mosquitoes, fogs, malaria and venomous insects and reptiles. In this respect it seems unlike any other tropical spot on earth, and a great improvement over many much vaunted northern summer resorts. For the student of botany, geology, or astronomy, this is indeed an ideal place for study and research. The moon and stars seem nearer and clearer than ever before, while that wonderful constellation, "The Southern Cross," shines in all its glory.

The voyage by sea from Boston of five days each way on the elegant "Admiral" steamers of "The United Fruit Company," is well worth the cost of $60 for the round trip. If you are longing for rest, or an entirely new and delightful experience, the writer would advise a summer trip to Jamaica—"The Gem of the Caribbean Sea."

The Canadian
Journal of Medicine and Surgery

J. J. CASSIDY, M.D.,
EDITOR,
43 BLOOR STREET EAST, TORONTO.

W. A. YOUNG, M.D., L.R.C.P.LOND.,
MANAGING EDITOR,
145 COLLEGE STREET, TORONTO.

Surgery—BRUCE L. RIORDAN, M D ,C M., McGill University; M D University of Toronto; Surgeon Toronto General Hospital; Surgeon Grand Trunk R R ; Consulting Surgeon Toronto Home for Incurables ; Pension Examiner United States Government ; and F N. G. STARR, M B , Toronto, Associate Professor of Clinical Surgery, Toronto University ; Surgeon to the Out-Door Department Toronto General Hospital and Hospital for Sick Children.
Clinical Surgery—ALEX PRIMROSE, M B., C.M Edinburgh University ; Professor of Anatomy and Director of the Anatomical Department, Toronto University ; Associate Professor of Clinical Surgery, Toronto University; Secretary Medical Faculty, Toronto University
Orthopedic Surgery—B. E McKENZIE, B A., M D , Toronto, Surgeon to the Toronto Orthopedic Hospital ; Surgeon to the Out-Patient Department, Toronto General Hospital ; Assistant Professor of Clinical Surgery, Ontario Medical College for Women ; Member of the American Orthopedic Association ; and H. P. H. GALLOWAY, M D , Toronto, Surgeon to the Toronto Orthopedic Hospital , Orthopedic Surgeon, Toronto Western Hospital; Member of the American Orthopedic Association.
Oral Surgery—E H. ADAMS, M.D , D.D.S , Toronto.
Surgical Pathology—T. H MANLEY, M D , New York, Visiting Surgeon to Harlem Hospital, Professor of Surgery, New York School of Clinical Medicine, New York, etc , etc.
Gynecology and Obstetrics—GEO. T. McKEOUGH, M D , M R C S Eng , Chatham, Ont ; and J. H. LOWE, M.D , Newmarket, Ont
Medical Jurisprudence and Toxicology—ARTHUR JUKES JOHNSON, M B., M R.C S Eng ; Coroner for the City of Toronto ; Surgeon Toronto Railway Co., Toronto ; W. A YOUNG, M D , L R C P Lond.; Associate Coroner, City of Toronto.
Pharmacology and Therapeutics—A. J. HARRINGTON M D., M R C S Eng , Toronto

Medicine—J. J CASSIDY, M D , Toronto, Member Ontario Provincial Board of Health ; Consulting Surgeon, Toronto General Hospital ; and W J WILSON, M D. Toronto, Physician Toronto Western Hospital
Clinical Medicine—ALEXANDER McPHEDRAN, M D., Professor of Medicine and Clinical Medicine Toronto University ; Physician Toronto General Hospital, St Michael's Hospital, and Victoria Hospital for Sick Children.
Mental and Nervous Diseases—N. H BEEMER, M. D., Mimico Insane Asylum; CAMPBELL MEYERS, M.D., M R C S. L R C P (L ndon, Eng), Private Hosp tal), Dee Park, Toronto , and EZRA H. STAFFORD, M.D.
Public Health and Hygiene—J J CASSIDY, M.D , Toronto, Member Ontario Provincial Board of Health ; Consulting Surgeon Toronto General Hospital , and E. H. ADAMS, M D , Toronto
Physiology—A. B EADIE, M.D., Toronto, Professor of Physiology Woman s Medical College, Toronto
Pediatrics—AUGUSTA STOWE GULLEN, M D., Toronto, Professor of Diseases of Children Woman's Medical College, Toronto ; A. R GORDON, M D., Toronto.
Pathology—W H PEPLER, M D., C.M., Trinity University ; Pathologist Hospital for Sick Children, Toronto ; Associate Demonstrator of Pathology T ronto University; Physician to Outdoor Department Toronto General Hospital ; Surgeon Canadian Pacific R R , Toronto , and J J MACKENZIE, B A , M B , Professor of Pathology and Bacteriology Toronto University Medical Faculty.
Ophthalmology and Otology—J M. MACCALLUM, M.D., Toronto, Professor of Materia Medica Toronto University ; Assistant Physician Toronto General Hospital ; Oculist and Aurist Victoria Hospital for Sick Children, Toronto
Laryngology and Rhinology—J. D THORBURN, M D., Toronto, Laryngologist and Rhinologist, Toronto General Hospital.

Address all Communications, Correspondence, Books, Matter Regarding Advertising, and make all Cheques, Drafts and Post-office Orders payable to "The Canadian Journal of Medicine and Surgery," 145 College St., Toronto, Canada.

Doctors will confer a favor by sending news. reports and papers of interest from any section of the country. Individual experience and theories are also solicited Contributors must kindly remember that all papers, reports, correspondence, etc., *must be* in our hands by the fifteenth of the month previous to publication.
Advertisements, to insure insertion in the issue of any month should be sent not later than the tenth of the preceding month. London, Eng Representative, W. Hamilton Miln, 8 Bouverie Street, E. C. Agents for Germany Saarbach's News Exchange, Mainz, Germany.

VOL. XVI.   TORONTO, NOVEMBER, 1904.   NO. 5.

Editorials.

THE PASSENGER CAR VENTILATION SYSTEM OF THE PENNSYLVANIA RAILROAD.

WE have received a pamphlet, written by Charles B. Dudley, Ph.D., chemist, and issued by the Pennsylvania Railroad Company, in which a description is given of a system of ventilating passenger coaches. This pamphlet, which also contains five ex-

6

planatory figures, can be understood by the ordinary reader, as it is free from technical terms.

No claim for originality in the general plan of ventilation is made. The fresh air is taken from the outside of a coach through two hoods, situated just above the lower deck roof, at diagonally opposite corners of the car; thence through the downtakes underneath the hoods to the spaces on each side underneath the car floor, bounded by the floor, the false bottom, the outside sill and nearest intermediate sill. These spaces which are in sections about 14 x 7½ inches, extend the whole length of the car. From these spaces the air passes up through the floor by means of proper apertures over the heating system and thence out into the aisles of the coach through 14 floor openings, 12 x 2 inches, and finally escapes from the coach through Globe ventilators, situated on the centre line of the upper deck roof. The means for introducing fresh air into the coach is identical with the one used in the ventilation of ships, in which by windsails and cowls turning towards the wind air is driven between the decks and into the hold. In using the wind in this way the difficulty is to distribute the air so that it shall not cause draughts. This is best done by bending the tubes at right angles, two or three times, so as to lessen the velocity, by enlarging the channel toward the opening in the interior of the vessel, by placing valves to partially close the tubes if necessary, and by screens of wire gauze. In the ventilation system we are considering valves are used in the down-takes and the cowls are screened, while there are three angles between the point where the fresh air enters the hood and the points where it issues into the coach. The heating system consists of pipe radiators. The pipes extend nearly the whole length of the car and are enclosed in a continuous boxing, 5½ x 8½ inches, inside dimensions. The heating substance is steam.

This ventilating plan provides for the hourly admission and escape of 60,000 cubic feet of air, while the coach is in motion; when at rest, as at a station, about one-third of that amount would be passed through the coach. The difference between the amount of fresh air supplied, when the coach is at rest and when it is in motion, measures the effect of the movement of the railroad train on the ventilating system in the coach.

From what has been said it appears that this ventilating system depends on the perflating power of the wind, as well as its aspirating power; it is a combination of the plenum and vacuum methods of ventilation. The hood, when the coach is in motion, acts as an injector and forces air into the coach; the Globe ventilators, of which there are seven to each coach, exercise an aspirating action and exhaust the air above the upper deck level of the coach.

Owing to the small cubic space available in a coach holding 60 passengers, about 66.66 cubic feet, per head, the supplying of 1,000 cubic feet of air per head, without inconveniencing the occupants of the car, is a notable achievement. It is true that 1,000 cubic feet of fresh air per hour is a small allowance for an adult male; but sometimes a coach is not half full, while frequently many of the passengers are women and children, who do not excrete carbonic acid in as large quantities as men, and who, therefore, do not require as large an amount of fresh air per head as men do. Thus, according to Parke, adult males, say 160-pound weight, excrete .7 of a cubic foot of carbonic acid per hour; females, say 120 pounds, .6 of a cubic foot, and children, say 80 pounds, .4 of a cubic foot. According to this calculation adult males should have 3,500 cubic feet of fresh air per hour; females, 3,000 cubic feet; children, 2,000 cubic feet; for a mixed community, 3,000 cubic feet. As already stated this system of ventilation supplies to a car holding 60 passengers 1,000 cubic feet per head per hour, but if there should be 25 passengers the amount of fresh air per head would be 2,400 cubic feet, while if there should be but 20 passengers in the ventilated coach, the ideal 3,000 cubic feet would be forthcoming.

All the air which escapes at the roof must pass through the Globe ventilators, as the ordinary movable deck sash is not used in the ventilated car, the deck sash being purposely made tight and immovable. This feature is said to improve the behavior of the lamps, which used to cause much difficulty, on account of cross draughts between the open deck sash. A further advantage of the fixed deck sash is the absence of cold air currents falling on the heads of passengers.

The heating of the ventilated car, even in cold weather, is satisfactory. Careful observations of temperature were made by a competent person during a trip from Philadelphia to Altoona, a distance of about 237 miles, with the thermometer outside at 2° to 5° Fahr. below zero, most of the distance. It was easy to keep the thermometer on the bell-cord hanger at 70° and above. It seems evident that more steam will be required for a ventilated coach than for an unventilated one; but the report shows that thus far no serious difficulty has been experienced in heating coaches. A few through trains, having from three to five ventilated cars in them, have been operated with perfect success for over a year.

Large cinders are excluded by the gauze netting over the hoods; small cinders, which pass the gauze netting, are deposited in the conduit between the sills. The location of the hoods at the top of the lower deck is thought to greatly diminish the possibility of dust from the track being a serious source of annoyance. The smoke from the locomotive is usually higher than the hoods, or it is diverted to one side of the train or the other by the wind. The report says: " This leaves only the conditions concomitant to long smoky tunnels to be provided for. The closure of the valves in the down-takes and the rapid change of air in the car by this system, only about four minutes being required to completely replace the air in a car, after it has passed the tunnel, so greatly mitigate this difficulty, that no serious trouble has thus far been experienced from the introduction of objectionable matter from without by the ventilating system."

It is also stated that " Practical experience with this ventilating system on the road has been very gratifying. Passengers, officers and trainmen seem to find the new system such an amelioration of conditions that it is not rare for them to pronounce it a marked success. The tendency to open the windows is very greatly diminished, and the possibility of running with closed doors in the heat of summer is clearly noticeable."

At the present time this system of ventilation is in use on 800 cars of the Pennsylvania lines east of Pittsburg and Erie. It is being applied to all new cars as they are built, and to the older cars in the equipment, as fast as conditions will warrant. It has not yet been applied to a sleeping car.

We feel pleasure in giving editorial prominence to the system of car ventilation which is here briefly described, and we think that the laboratory force of the Pennsylvania Railroad and their associates of the mechanical department deserve credit for their very scientific and practical method of improving the ventilation of passenger coaches. J. J. C.

WHAT SHOULD BE THE CONDUCT OF SANITARIANS TOWARDS PATIENTS WITH VENEREAL DISEASES?

WRITING on the prevention of venereal diseases, a physician of Western Ontario expresses the following views: " Medical practitioners are liable to fine and punishment if they neglect to promptly report mumps, measles and whooping cough or other simple diseases, affecting defenceless, innocent babes and children, while medical practitioners not only need not, but even dare not, report the moral imbecile, covered with syphilitic sores or saturated with gonorrheal discharges, whose foul presence obtrudes itself everywhere—the hotels, the Pullman, the theatre, church, ball, or even private homes."   This syphilitic or gonorrheal imbecile knows his security, and the medical practitioner, instead of properly and safely isolating the poisonous wretch, is compelled to appear disinterested and meet him anywhere and everywhere just as if the social leper were not the greatest menace to public health.'

The respected writer of this letter does not indicate the *modus operandi* of the quarantine which he suggests. No person will deny that the isolation of gonorrheal patients is a desirable thing, but the method of doing it adequately is as yet unknown. Probably the principal reasons for the actual condition of public opinion on this question are that the disease is common and thought to be of little moment; while, at the same time, people of both sexes, who have this disease, are most anxious to keep their unhappy possession a profound secret. If a physician were legally bound to report his cases of gonorrhea to the M. H. O., and were to comply with the law, his practice among the " moral lepers " would soon reach the vanishing point.

But, for argument's sake, let us suppose that every physician and druggist in Ontario were to unite in obeying a law which would call for the reporting of gonorrhea. Unless it were made an absolute condition that every gonorrheal patient would be compelled to retire to an hospital and remain interned until cured, the reporting of some cases would not extinguish gonorrhea.

It would be certainly in the interest of the public health if gonorrheal cases were segregated in an hospital. It would also be in the interest of the patients themselves. Treated by modern methods uncomplicated cases would be cured in, let us say, eight weeks and the complications which sometimes arise from imperfeet or unsafe methods of treatment would not occur at all. The required treatment would be more thoroughly carried out than it can be in a private house, or even at a physician's office; the patient's diet could be supervised, and, in all probability, the disease could be arrested in a period of time less than what has been observed in cases of this disease occurring in private practice.

Instruction could also be given the patient, verbally, or by leaflet, as to the dangers of gonorrhea to other persons, and an educational campaign could be tried, in order to prevent its spread to innocent persons. It is quite probable, likewise, that the dread of quarantine would powerfully assist in controlling the behests of lust, so much, indeed, as to induce even lechers " to assume a virtue if they have it not."

The quarantine of syphilis would be much more difficult. Instead of a quarantine of eight weeks the syphilitic patient would have to be interned for one or several years. Should a syphilitic patient be quarantined during the primary, as well as the secondary stage of the disease? Prior to answering this question we revert to the already quoted letter of the Ontario physician. He writes: " A patient comes to my office at 6 p.m., from a local bank. He is in a most foul condition from syphilitic disease. At 11 o'clock the same evening I arrive at a society ball, and imagine my surprise to find my recent patient, the Johnny two-step from the bank, quite the lion among pure and innocent young girls and apparently sane matrons."

To this we say: The bank clerk could communicate primary syphilis by the sexual act, but that method of contagion would be unlikely in the case of decent women. If his disease were in the secondary stage he would be more dangerous to the opposite sex, and he should be debarred from flirting with pure and innocent girls until his disease is cured. We have treated two cases in which chancre of the lip was communicated to innocent girls by men who had mucous patches of the mouth, and the literature of syphilis contains many similar cases. Men or women exhibiting signs of secondary syphilis, viz., mucous patches or condylomata of the mouth or anus, and syphilitic eruptions of the

skin, should be quarantined. Neither should children exhibiting the well-known signs of hereditary syphilis be allowed to associate with healthy children until their disease has been cured.

Theoretically these counsels as to gonorrhea and syphilis would
be the part of wisdom; practically we do not think they could be
carried out. Vanity, conceit and self-interest would conspire to
defeat them. The course advised at the Congress of Venereal
Diseases, held at Frankfort, Germany, during the present year
seems preferable. At that congress it was determined to send
to every physician a leaflet or slip, in which reference is made to
the precautions to be taken by venereal patients in order to prevent
the extension of their disease to other persons.

During the present year, also, a committee of three has been
appointed by the President of the Conference of State and Provincial Boards of Health " To prepare a leaflet that would be
acceptable to physicians to give to their patients, setting forth
the precautions to be taken by one suffering from a venereal disease, to prevent its communication to others, and to make such
other suggestions as it may deem proper," etc.

A quiet, persistent campaign of an educational character, conducted by a physician with an auditory of one, will accomplish a
good deal in keeping down venereal diseases, though it would be
less sensational than notification and quarantine. We quite agree,
however, with the contention of our confrere in the far west of
Ontario, that it is galling to a physician's sense of justice to see
a man with gonorrhea or syphilis enjoying his untrammelled
liberty, while a patient with measles must be quarantined.

J. J. C.

CAWTHRA MULOCK'S GIFT.

THE trustees of the Toronto General Hospital have accepted the
generous offer of Mr. Cawthra Mulock to erect an out-patient
building at a cost of $100,000. Mr. Mulock's letter to Mr. J. W.
Flavelle, Chairman of the Board of Trustees, read as follows:

" With reference to the various conversations regarding the
present position of the Toronto General Hospital, it has been made
evident that, while the present buildings have in the past
served the purpose for which they were intended, they have now
become entirely inadequate to perform the duties required of a
great hospital in a growing city like Toronto.

" To me it appears that the most urgent need at the moment, however, is an out-patient building, in which those who are too poor to pay for hospital service can be properly treated, and in which the clinical teaching so necessary for the School of Medicine in connection with the university can be carried on to the satisfaction of the faculty of medicine.

" In the hope that a general plan for the gradual rebuilding of the whole hospital establishment will be the eventual outcome, I am prepared to build, equip and furnish at an expense of $100,-000 a separate building or wing for such an out-patient department. I do not desire to make any conditions which would embarrass the Board of Trustees of the Toronto General Hospital, but I shall hope that the effect of my gift will be to produce the two results already suggested, namely, the free services to the poor of an out-patient department, and the provision of satisfactory clinical teaching for the University School of Medicine."

Upon the question as to the best site for the proposed new building medical opinion is divided. A number of the profession feel that, as in the big cities of England and the United States, such buildings are usually situated as close as possible to the centre of population, a central site somewhere near old St. John's Ward should be chosen, and they point out that in addition to meeting the wants of the poor it would better serve the purpose of clinical teaching for the University School of Medicine.

Others think that the new building should adjoin the present Toronto General Hospital if it is to be utilized for clinical teaching. They contend that all students are more or less identified with hospital work, and to have the new building close at hand would be a great convenience.

As far as we are concerned, we feel that the trustees should consent to " go easy " in the matter, and rather delay a little now than choose the site too hastily, only to regret the same after the foundation is laid. If we are not mistaken, some important news as to increased hospital accommodation in Toronto is forthcoming very soon, and we would not be at all surprised if before the next twelve months elapse, a still further building appears in the Queen's Park in the shape of a hospital in direct connection with, and controlled entirely by, the Medical Faculty of Toronto University.   w. a. y.

A NEW PRISON INSPECTOR.

THE resignation of Dr. T. F. Chamberlain, Inspector of Prisons and Public Charities, was recently accepted by the Provincial Secretary's Department, to take effect October 1st. Dr. Chamberlain's health during the past six months has been such as to necessitate his taking this step. He has been succeeded by Dr. R. W. Bruce-Smith, up till recently assistant physician at the Asylum for the Insane at Brockville.

Dr. Smith formerly practised in Seaforth, and a few years ago accepted the position of President of the Ontario Medical Association. Prior to going to Brockville, he was assistant physician at the Hamilton Asylum. Dr. Smith is highly thought of by the profession, and we heartily congratulate him upon this deserved recognition of his executive ability, and feel certain that he will perform his duties to the eminent satisfaction of not only the Ontario Government, but those with whom he will be brought into contact.

Dr. J. C. Mitchell, of the Toronto Asylum staff, has been appointed assistant physician at Brockville, to succeed Dr. Smith, and will occupy that post till the new buildings at Woodstock are ready next year; and Dr. Harris, at present relieving officer for the public institutions, has been appointed to the position vacated by Dr. Mitchell.

Dr. Chamberlain graduated M.D. at Queen's University in 1862, and practised his profession at Morrisburg. He held a variety of municipal and other offices, including the Reeveship of Morrisburg and the Wardenship of Stormont, Dundas and Glengarry. He was also Superintendent of Public Schools. He sat in the Ontario Legislature in the Liberal interest for Dundas from 1886 to 1888, since which time the constituency has been represented by Mr. J. P. Whitney. He was appointed Inspector of Prisons and Public Charities in September, 1889. During the past summer Dr. Chamberlain was critically ill, and, although he has considerably improved, he is still far from well, and contemplates spending the winter in the South.　　　　W. A. Y.

EDITORIAL NOTES.

WE regret exceedingly not, in this instance, being able to keep faith with our readers and give them the benefit this month of Mr. Mayo Robson's address at the Vancouver meeting of the Canadian Medical Association, the manuscript arriving too late.

The Explanation of Some Marvelous Cures, which are Advertised in the Papers.—In an editorial note which appeared in the *New York Medical Journal* and *Philadelphia Medical Journal,* August 27th, 1904, we observe an Associated Press communication, showing one of the methods by which the patent medicine manufacturers obtain their glowing testimonials:

Remarkable testimony has been obtained by the post office department as to the ways in which testimonals are obtained by some of the big concerns engaged in this business. One large firm admitted, that it had agents out seeking persons who had formerly occupied prominent positions in the community, but had suffered financial reverses and were harassed by debts they were unable to settle. The agents would obtain possession of the unpaid accounts, and would then apply pressure to the unfortunate victims, demanding immediate payment in full. Finally, after long persecution, the desperate victim would be invited or commanded to call at the office of an attorney, where he would be given to understand, that, if he would sign and swear to a testimonial, a receipt in full for the claims against him would be given. This seems incredible, but the facts are now on file in the records of the post office.

The cruelest part of the joke is that the article in the Associated Press communication is headed " Methods of Medical Men."

Auto-Intoxication in Nervous Diseases.—Roger alludes, in his book, " The Introduction to the Study of Medicine," to experiments which show the effects of auto-intoxication in cases of mental diseases. Generally in these cases the toxicity of the urine is increased, and sometimes it shows particular characters, relating to the state of the patients. Brugia holds that the urine of patients suffering from mental excitement produces convulsions, while the urine of others, who suffer from mental depression, produces lowness of spirits and a considerable reduction in temperature. In studying a paroxysmal disease, epilepsy, Dr. Féré shows that the urine of an epileptic before the seizure is very toxic, and causes convulsions if injected into rabbits, but that after the attack, the urine is not toxic, and shows little tendency to cause convulsions. Mairet and Ardin Delteil show that the toxicity of the perspiration collected during and immediately after an epileptic seizure is most marked. Sajous says, Vol. L, p. 777: " Some cases of acute mania, for instance, may require stimulation of the adrenal system, simply because the engorgement of the neurons may find its cause, not in an exogenous poison, but in accumulation of physiological toxics, which, as in the case of epilepsy, tetanus, etc., give rise to sudden exacerbations of adrenal activity, *i.e.,* to explosions of functional activity calculated to rid the organism of the morbific agencies by a process of active combustion." As Féré's experiments seem to show that idiopathic epilepsy is caused by auto-intoxication, there is a certain resemblance between epilepsy and uremia. In the former, however, the toxic agent is produced at variable intervals, and the quantity or continuance of its production are not sufficient to destroy life, offering, in this respect, a strong contrast to uremia. If this pathological view be correct, knowledge of the nature and source of the toxic agent which produces the convulsive seizure in epilepsy may be acquired, and its elimination from the organism might, as we may hope, render this disease controllable.

Clinical Examination of the Sputa in Children.—The difficulty of obtaining sputa from young children is in one sense a blessing, as they do not contribute to the spitting nuisance. Neither do they spread pneumonia or pulmonary consumption by expectoration. As in suspected cases of tuberculosis, the bacteriologic test is of paramount importance, and as a physician, when treating a child for broncho-pneumonia, may wish to strengthen his diagnosis by a bacteriological test of the sputum, a simple and efficient means of obtaining the sputum is of the first practical importance. A practice which obtains in the French hospitals consists in covering the finger with gauze and passing it into the aperture of the child's glottis. The irritation thus excited causes the little patient to cough, and the mucus expectorated is caught on the gauze and subsequently examined.

Barbers' Shops and Contagious Skin Diseases.—An English surgeon writing to the *British Medical Journal,* August 27th, 1904, claims that he contracted impetigo contagiosa after a shave at one of the leading shops in a suburb of London. He says, that for ten years he had scarcely entered a hairdresser's shop, preferring to shave himself and submit his hair to the amateur ministrations of his wife. But as he was dining out, and was pressed for time, in a luckless hour he went to a barber's shop, and was shaved. Five days afterwards a pimple developed, and impetigo subsequently developed. He was obliged to have a locum tenens, nearly poisoned himself with drastic mercurial ointments, and generally felt a wreck. That shave, he says, will cost him $250. In his opinion, compulsory antiseptic precautions ought to be enforced in barbers' shops. When one considers the various diseased and unclean conditions existing on the faces of the patrons of a shaving parlor, one is struck with wonder that more of them are not inoculated with virulent germs, more particularly if the barber uses a dull razor, shaves off a bit of epidermis, or decapitates a pimple. The sterilization of the barber's razor with boiling water for thirty seconds after shaving a customer, and the washing of his own hands, before passing to another customer, should be obligatory. His shaving brush should be placed every night in a closed box, in which it is exposed to the vapor of formalin. If gentlemen of cleanly habits believe that such precautions are necessary, they should not hesitate to ask for them. However, a surgeon, of all men, should be able to shave himself. If he will not do it, the teachings of his profession require, that the razor, shaving brush and soap, used on him by the barber, should be free from infection.

Red Light in the Treatment of Smallpox.—The treatment of smallpox by red light has been described in glowing terms in Scandinavian medical journals, and optimistic views have been expressed in Europe and America as to the curative influence of this agent. In London, as we learn through the *Medical Press*, August 17th, 1904, this method of treating smallpox has been tested and found wanting. Dr. Ricketts, the Medical Superintendent of Joyce Green Smallpox Hospital, made the test and published his experience in the Annual Report of the Metropolitan Asylums Board. A small ward was set apart for the purpose, the windows being covered with ruby fabric, and the ward doors hung with thick curtains of Turkey twill. Illumination was supplied by a red lamp. In this room one or two patients were placed at a time, all of whom were subject to careful selection. Those chosen were in the early papular stage of attacks which seemed likely to run an ordinary suppurative course. In all some twelve cases were treated, in none of which was the development of the stages of the papules in any way different from what might have been naturally expected. Three patients died and several were badly pitted. In Dr. Ricketts' opinion the red light treatment for smallpox is a dead failure. Smallpox has been successfully treated with red light by Drs. Krohn, Mygind, Peronnet, Abel, Backmann, and others. Dr. Ricketts may, inadvertently, have neglected to observe some important minutiæ of Finsen's treatment, total exclusion of the chemical rays of light being the main feature.

Mercurial Injections in Syphilis.—A series of articles on the treatment of syphilis appeared in the July number of the *London Practitioner.* In what may be regarded as the most important paper in the series, Louis Wickham says that the hypodermic method has the great advantage of sparing the stomach. It favors the more direct penetration of the mercury into the blood, a more complete utilization of the dose administered, and permits of exact dosage. If the state of the kidneys is carefully watched and the cleanliness of the mouth maintained, large doses of mercury can be given without causing inconvenience. The initial dose should be small, and then raised gradually, but persistently, as long as no reaction ensues. It is best to raise the dosage to a considerable amount rather than to use a moderate average dose, which may prove quite insufficient in particular cases. It must be remembered that an attack of syphilis which at first appears benign may develop into a grave case. In cases of gravity it is natural to employ large doses, but every case must be looked on as potentially grave, and treated as such. Collateral remedial measures, such as tonics and local dressings, must be carried out; in some cases such measures assume a dominant position. In cases where the weakness of the patient is marked, injections of physiologic serum, apart from the daily injections of mercury, are excellent. The best site for the injection is the buttock, at the point of intersection of two lines, one horizontal line passing through the junction of the upper quarter with the lower three-quarters of the buttock, the other a vertical line through the junction of the inner third with the outer two-thirds of the region. The injections can be made in an area having a radius of 2 c.m., the point of intersection of the two lines being its centre. Because of the irritation produced by salts of mercury, the injections are almost always intramuscular. In those subjects in whom gluteal, intramuscular injections are not well borne, and in whom it may be necessary to attack the disease vigorously, the intravenous route may be chosen. The injections may be made at the bend of the elbow into the cephalic or basilic nerve on either side. The usual antiseptic precautions must be observed. The salt used is a cyanide of mercury, the largest dose hitherto employed being 0.01 gram daily. J. J. C.

PERSONAL.

Dr. A. A. Macdonald has purchased No. 341 Bloor St. west, and will remove there immediately.

We congratulate Drs. G. B. Smith and W. F. Bryans of Toronto, on the result of the suit entered against them by one Mrs. Stickle.

Dr. N. H. Beemer, of Mimico Asylum, is to be congratulated upon the marriage of his daughter, three weeks ago, to a New York gentleman.

Dr. Geo. Elliott, General Secretary of the Canadian Medical Association, removed two weeks or more ago from the corner of John and Nelson Streets to his new home, 203 Beverley Street (corner of Cecil Street).

OPENING LECTURE OF THE MEDICAL FACULTY OF TORONTO UNIVERSITY.

PROFESSOR J. ALGERNON TEMPLE gave the opening lecture before the Faculty and students in medicine of the University of Toronto, on the evening of October 5th, in the gymnasium building. He made an appeal for private beneficence and a more generous public support of medical and scientific education.

In opening he said that the experience of the past year had demonstrated beyond peradventure the wisdom of federation. The Faculty of Trinity became convinced that it was no longer possible to support by private enterprise a medical school that could do the work demanded for the present time. They saw that medical science must rely on the hope of both Government and private assistance.

Dr. Temple continued: If this country is to retain its prowess the Government must recognize more fully the commercial value of scientific education and scientific work; and the makers of wealth must value more highly those institutions of learning to which is due in a large measure their success in the amassing of money. It now remains for the Government to establish chairs in bacteriology, hygiene and pathology. Public opinion in Canada is scarcely what it should be in regard to education, and it is, therefore, hard to arouse the interest of public men on this question. The emphasis of public opinion in Canada cannot be said to be placed on things of the intellect. The man who is the best shot or the champion sculler receives marked attention. Among the people of the United States there is an intense belief in education. There is an amazing liberality on the part of their public men. Canadians should have more enthusiasm for culture and education, for the reason that the emphasis given to them is a fair criterion of a country's civilization. When the mass of the people are more anxious for quacks and patent medicines than for scientific treatment the condition is not satisfactory. The public press teems with disgusting advertisements that are a disgrace to the public prints. I can't understand why they are admitted.

No other profession is so deeply concerned with the life of the people as the medical profession. It is, therefore, important that the standard be kept high. I hope that the recent generous gift of Mr. Cawthra Mulock will stimulate other citizens to emulate his example. I trust, concluded Dr. Temple, he will live long enough to see the splendid results of his gift.

Dean Reeve presided, President Loudon, who was to have been in the chair, having been seized with a sudden indisposition shortly after his arrival. He was compelled to go home. At a late hour he was reported as better.

Dr. McPhedran announced that as a mark of approval of the single-mindedness of Dean Reeve the Faculty had decided to continue the Dean Reeve scholarship for research, and through the generosity of Mr. P. C. Larkin they were enabled to do so. The announcement was received with loud applause. The Dean replied briefly and with feeling.

Dr. Primrose announced that provision had been made for instruction in experimental physics for first year men, and for laboratory work in the fifth year.

The Dean made the interesting announcement that 134 had registered in the first year, and that the whole registration exceeded the record of any previous year.

THE MISSISSIPPI VALLEY MEDICAL ASSOCIATION.

THE Thirtieth Annual Meeting of the above Association was held in Cincinnati, O., on the 11th to the 13th _ult., when the following papers were read:

Address of the President, Hugh T. Patrick.

Address in Medicine. By C. Travis Drennen, Hot Springs, Ark.

Address in Surgery. By W. J. Mayo, Rochester, Minn.

Spleenless Men: Report of Two Successful Cases of Splenectomy. By J. H. Carstens, Detroit.

Reflection Upon the Origin of Hallucinations of Sight and Hearing. By Charles J. Aldrich, Cleveland, O.

Prevention of Conception and the Evils Thereof. By William F. Barclay, Pittsburg, Pa.

Relative Dangers of Craniotomy and Cesarian Section. By James M. Barnhill, Columbus, O.

Treatment of Diabetes Mellitus. By R. Alexander Bate, Louisville, Ky.

Prognosis. By John M. Batten, Downington, Pa.

Foreign Bodies in the Esophagus. By Carl E. Black, Jacksonville, Ill.

Acute Anterior Poliomyelitis. By Sanger Brown, Chicago.

A Case of Bilateral Tic Douloureux Treated by Intra- and Extra-Cranial Neurectomy. By W. O. Bullock, Lexington, Ky.

Pathologic Changes Resulting from Prostatic Enlargement. By Charles E. Burnett, Fort Wayne, Ind.

Treatment of Tubercular Pleuritis. By James G. Burroughs, Asheville, N.C.

Pseudo-Membranous Croup. By Robert E. Carlton, Latonia, Ky.

Cranial Injuries. By Shelby C. Carson, Greensboro', Ala.

Echinacea. By C. S. Chamberlin, Cincinnati, Ohio.

The Value of the X-Ray to the General Practitioner. By James E. Coleman, Canton, Ill.

Report of Some Unusual Surgical Cases. By A. H. Cordier, Kansas City, Mo.

Loss of Consciousness and Automatism in Inebriety. By Thomas D. Crothers, Hartford, Conn.

The Relation of Trauma to Hernia. By Daniel N. Eisendrath, Chicago, Ill.

The Typic (Anatomic) Operation for the Radical Cure of Oblique Inguinal Hernia. By Alex. Hugh Ferguson, Chicago, Ill.

Two Factors in the Pelvic Diseases of Women: Their Prevalence, Result and Prevention. By J. H. Firestone, Freeport, Ill.

A Plea for Better Feeding of the Patients in our State Hospitals for the Insane. By W. B. Fletcher, Indianapolis, Ind.

Perilous Calms of Appendicitis. By Robert Wallace Hardon, Chicago, Ill.

Prophylaxis of Appendicitis. By William M. Harsha, Chicago, Ill.

Factitious Eruptions. By M. L. Heidingsfeld, Cincinnati, Ohio.

Infectious Diseases: Their Communicability, Quarantine and Prevention. By Henry D. Holton, Battleboro, Vt.

Formalin in the Treatment of Amebic Dysentery and Kindred Affections. By John L. Jelks, Memphis, Tenn.

Report of a Case of Brain Abscess of Otitic Origin, with Some Observations. By George F. Keiper, LaFayette, Ind.

Report of Two Cases of Amputation of Both Legs; Recovery. By F. D. Kendall, Columbia, S. C.

Report of Two Cases of Pancreatic Cyst. By VanBuren Knott, Sioux City, Iowa.

Extra-Uterine Pregnancy. By Florus F. Lawrence, Columbus, O.

Report on Operative Work through the Cystoscope. By Bransford Lewis, St. Louis, Mo.

Insanity in Relation to Obstetrics and Gynecology. By Henry F. Lewis, Chicago, Ill.

A Contribution to the Plastic Surgery of the Urethra. By G. Frank Lydston, Chicago, Ill.

Ectopic Gestation. By H. B. R. McCall, Kansas City, Mo.

The Mamma: Its Physiological Purposes and Finer Anatomy. By Thomas H. Manley, New York, N.Y.

Radium: Its Therapeutic Value. By M. Metzenbaum, Cleveland, O.

Protection of the Axillary Nerves and Vessels after Dissection of the Axillary Space. By J. B. Murphy, Chicago, Ill.

The Obstetric Significance of the Transverse Diameter of the Pelvis. By Joseph B. DeLee, Chicago, Ill.

Hereditary Predisposition to Tuberculosis. By Charles Louis Mix, Chicago, Ill.

A Clinical Study of the Mental Disorders of Adolescence. By Frank C. Norbury, Jacksonville, Ill.

Hospital Construction in American Cities. By A. J. Ochsner, Chicago, Ill.

The Treatment of the Morphine Habit. By Curran Pope, Louisville, Ky.

What Shall be Done with the Criminal Insane? By John Punton, Kansas City, Mo.

Strictures of the Urethra. By A. Ravogli, Cincinnati, O.

Foreign Bodies in the Cornea. By Dudley S. Reynolds, Louisville, Ky.

The Transverse Fascial Incision for Operations in the Pelvis, with Report of Cases. By Emil Reis, Chicago, Ill.

Why So Many Errors in the Diagnosis of Graves Disease? By J. H. Stealy, Freeport, Ill.

Association and Antagonism of Diseases. By Albert E. Sterne, Indianapolis, Ind.

Suppuration of Nasal Accessory Sinuses; Symptoms and Treatment. By J. A. Stucky, Lexington, Ky.

The Recognition of Important Eye Lesions by the Practitioner. By George F. Suker, Akron, O.

Valvotomy *versus* the Clip for Cure of Obstipation. By Sterling B. Taylor, Columbus, O.

Internal Hemorrhoids and Their Treatment. By Wells Teachnor, Columbus, O.

A Clinical Experience. By W. W. Vinnedge, La Fayette, Ind.

Needles, Ligatures and Sutures; Their Uses and Abuses. By H. O. Walker, Detroit, Mich.

The Combined Method in the Arrest and Cure of Tuberculosis. By H. B. Weaver, Asheville, N.C.

Tenotomy of the Tendo Achillis in Partial Amputations of the Foot in Compound, Comminuted Fractures of the Tibia and Fibula. By J. R. Webster, Chicago, Ill.

Subjective *versus* Objective Requirements in Surgery. By Otho B. Will, Peoria, Ill.

Radical Cure of Hernia. By Hal C. Wyman, Detroit, Mich.

Acute Intestinal Surgery, with Remarks on Technic. By John Young Brown, St. Louis.

ITEMS OF INTEREST.

The American Medical Association.—The date set for the next session of the American Medical Association is July 11-14, 1905.

University Convocation Hall.—It is reported that the tenders for the erection of the University Convocation Hall call for an expenditure of $174,000. The amount provided was $100,000. It is not yet decided whether the plans will be changed or an effort made to collect more funds.

Three Hundred Physicians will be needed in Panama to preserve the health of the workmen on the isthmus. This is the preliminary estimate made by Colonel W. C. Gorgas, the chief sanitary officer, who sailed from New York on Tuesday to assume charge of the sanitary works there. These physicians, it is expected, will be drawn from civilian ranks, though quite a number of government surgeons will have the higher posts.— *Med. Age.*

An Unfortunate Error.—On page lxxx of our October issue we published the clinical aspects of a case of amenorrhea, that had recently come under the notice of Dr. M. T. Runyon, of Oberlin, Ohio, which he treated with mechanical vibratory stimulation. Through an error on the part of our printers, but part of the abstract appeared. The instrument used was the " Chattanooga " Vibrator, as made by the Vibrator Instrument Co., of Chattanooga, Tenn. If our readers will kindly refer to the report they will see the method of treatment adopted by Dr. Runyon, and the results, viz., that menstruation became again established normally, thus proving the value of mechanical vibratory stimulation. We tender to Dr. Runyon our regrets for the unintentional mistake and seeming carelessness.

Toronto Medical Society.—An "open" meeting of this society was held in the new medical buildings on October 6th at 8.30 p.m., and was attended by a large number of the profession. The president's (Dr. J. Hunter) address was entitled "The Medical Society." Dr. W. J. Wilson's paper on "The Treatment of Typhoid," which will appear in our next issue, was discussed by Drs. Thistle, Fotheringham, W. P. Caven and others. Dr. A. A. Macdonald gave a talk on his visit to the Canadian Medical Association's meeting in Vancouver, B.C. A most enjoyable evening was spent, and we trust that, under Dr. Hunter's guidance, the Toronto Medical Society will enter upon a new era of success.

Toronto University Senate Elections.—The entire ticket which we supported for appointment to the Senate of Toronto University at the elections held last month received the support of the electors throughout. The graduates in medicine elected the following, who received from a total poll of 1,189 votes the number indicated: Dr. Bingham, Toronto, 812; Professor I. H. Cameron, 799; Dr. Adam Wright, 789; Prof. J. Algernon Temple, 774. Of these, Dr. Bingham and Dr. Temple are new members. Dr. W. H. B. Aikins, 712, and Dr. James M. MacCallum, 356, are defeated candidates. The two latter had previously served on the Senate. Though Dr. MacCallum had announced his intention of not running at all, his announcement was received, however, by the Registrar too late, and therefore largely accounts for the small vote polled in his behalf.

Radio-active Wool.—A new method of employing radium in medicine has been described by E. S. London, a Russian physician, which consists of using cotton-wool which has been submitted to the reaction of radium emanation. The result of a series of experiments seems to justify the conclusion that the effects of the radium emanation and of the direct action of the radium are the same, consisting in an inflammation of the skin and a destruction of protoplasm. Wool so treated, which is convenient for easy distribution over the body, when packed in hermetically sealed jars or other containing vessels, loses its radioactivity very slowly, and can be sent to any distance desired. From a few miligrams of radium a large quantity of wool may be prepared, and thus widely extend the use of a small amount of radium, whose cost is so great as to interfere with its widespread use. Radio-active wool, therefore, may become a stock pharmaceutical preparation, but it still remains for the medical profession to determine its therapeutic value.

Extensive Counterfeiting in Proprietary Medicines in New York.—After immense outlay financially and a tremendous amount of work by the most astute detectives in the country, who were employed by them, The Farbenfabriken Co., of Elberfeld (New York City), have succeeded in running down the worst gang of criminals in the United States, who have for a long period been manufacturing (?) the pharmaceutical products of this well-known house and putting them upon the market through some fourth-rate druggists, under the names of phenacetin, sulphonal, trional, etc. The manufacturers have been on the track of the gang for a long period, but never succeeded in running them to earth till the middle of last month. They sold those medicines under false labels at ruinous prices and have done immense injury to the originators, who are well known as manufacturers of preparations of merit. We are pleased to know that the counterfeiters have been caught red-handed, and trust that long terms of imprisonment will be promptly meted out to them.

Rockefeller Institute Plans.—Plans have been filed for the new laboratory building to be erected on Exterior Street, east of Avenue A, for the Rockefeller Institute of Medical Research, of which Dr. William H. Welch, of Johns Hopkins University, is President, and Dr. S. Flexner, Resident Director. It is to be a five-storey edifice, 136 x 60, with a facade of lime-stone and brick. It will be decorated with pilasters of brick, and have a porch entrance flanked with decorative columns for the support of electric lights. The first floor will be an assembly hall, with a library and study and directors' room. The upper floors will contain large general and special laboratories and research rooms. The fifth will have a dining hall and living quarters, and the roof a special operating room and quarters for the animals under examination. Adjoining the main building will be a two-storey building for the animals used by the doctors, and power-house. The cost of the buildings is estimated at $325,000.—*Med. News.*

New Surgical Building Dedicated.—The new surgical building at the Johns Hopkins Hospital will be dedicated October 5th. The programme will consist of addresses by several prominent American and foreign physicians, and a large number of eminent medical men, including those gathered at St. Louis this month, will be invited to attend. After dedication it will be inspected and a luncheon will be served. In the afternoon a bronze tablet erected to the memory of Dr. Jesse W. Lazear, who lost his life from yellow fever in Cuba while investigating that disease there in 1900, will be dedicated in one of the amphitheatres. The building cost $150,000, is of brick and four stories high. Sanitation and ventilation are important features. All the floors are of tiles, every room and hallway used by patients being also wainscotted with glazed white tiles. The stairways are of marble and iron, and there are toilet rooms and baths on each floor. A surgical amphitheatre, forty feet high, also has extensive tiling, marble work and a wide hall with lights composed entirely of wired glass. There are a number of consultation rooms. On the first floor will be emergency rooms for accident cases, minor operation rooms and the orthopedic department. Two large vaults of brick and cement are provided for surgical records.— *Jour. A. M. A.*

Dr. Charles R. Dickson was at St. Louis, September 10th to 20th, returning by Chicago. While in St. Louis he took part in the International Electrical Congress, held in the Coliseum, in connection with the Louisiana Purchase Exposition, being a delegate from the American Electro-Therapeutic Association, and attended the annual meeting of the latter body also, at the Inside Inn. Before a joint session of the Congress and Association he read by invitation a paper on " Some Observations upon the Treatment of Lupus Vulgaris by Phototherapy, Radiotherapy and Otherwise," and at the Association he presented a paper, entitled " Some Aspects of Phototherapy," and was elected a member of the Executive Council for the fifth time. Both meetings were most successful, and very enjoyable. Among the Congress festivities held on the World's Fair Grounds were a reception by the St. Louis Committee at the New York State Building, a reception by the Associazione Electrotecnica Italiana at the Italian National Pavilion, a luncheon tendered by the Engineers' Club at the Palace of Electricity, followed by participation in the Electricity Day Parade of the grounds in autos, a reception by electrical exhibitors in the Palace of Electricity with special electrical effects in the decorations of the building, grand basin and electric launches for the occasion, a reception by the Commissioner-General of Great Britain and Mrs. Watson at the British National Pavilion, a banquet in honor of foreign members of the Congress at the German National Pavilion, and many lesser, though not less enjoyable functions. Delegates were tendered free use of telegraph and telephones, including long distance services, and all visitors were made to feel that for the time they practically owned the electrical department of the Fair. In addition, a reception was tendered the members of the Association at the Missouri State Building. It was a never-to-be-forgotten week of constant activity and enjoyment. The attendance of so many distinguished foreign delegates lent an added charm.

The American Medical Society for the Study of Alcohol and Other Narcotics was organized June 8, 1904, by the union of the American Association for the Study of Inebriety and the Medical Temperance Association. Both of these societies are composed of physicians interested in the study and treatment of inebriety and the physiological nature and action of alcohol or narcotics in health and disease. The first society was organized in 1870, and has published five volumes of transactions and twenty-seven yearly volumes of the *Quarterly Journal of Inebriety,* the organ of the association. The second society began in 1891, and has issued three volumes of transactions and for seven years published a *Quarterly Bulletin,* containing the papers read at its meetings. The special object of the union of the two societies is to create greater interest among physicians to study one of the greatest evils of modern times. Its plan of work is to encourage and promote more exact scientific studies of the nature and effects of alcohol in health and disease, particularly of its etiological, physiological and therapeutic relations. Second, to secure a more accurate investigation of the diseases associated or following from the use of alcohol and narcotics. Third, to correct the present empirical treatment of these diseases by secret drugs and so-called specifics, and to secure legislation, prohibiting the sale of nostrums claiming to be absolute cures, containing dangerous poisons. Fourth, to encourage special legislation for the care, control and medical treatment of spirit and drug takers. The alcoholic problem and the diseases which centre and spring from it, are becoming more prominent, and its medical and hygienic importance have assumed such proportions that physicians are called on for advice and counsel. Public sentiment is turning to medical men for authoritative facts and conclusions to enable them to realize the causes, means of prevention and cure of this evil. This new society comes to meet this want by enlisting medical men as members, and stimulating new studies and researches from a broader and more scientific point of view. As a medical and hygienic topic the alcoholic problem has an intense personal interest, not only to every physician, but to the public generally, in every town and city in the country. This interest demands concentrated efforts through the medium of a society to clear away the present confusion, educate public sentiment, and make medical men the final authority in the consideration of the remedial measures for cure and prevention. For this purpose a most urgent appeal is made to all physicians to assist in making this society the medium and authority for the scientific study of the subject. The secretary, Dr. T. D. Crothers, of Hartford, Conn., will be pleased to give any further information.

Obituary

DEATH OF DR. ERNEST WILLS, OF CALGARY, N.W.T.

We feel that the profession, as a body, sincerely regrets the death at Calgary, N.W.T., of Dr. Ernest Wills, on Sept. 22nd, especially those who had the pleasure of his immediate friendship. Dr. Wills established not long ago Calgary Sanatorium, and had succeeded in securing quite a nice patronage from the profession, especially throughout the West. Mrs. Wills writes us to say that the sanatorium will be continued as before under the superintendency of a competent physician, who is well acquainted with all of Dr. Wills' methods and will follow them throughout.

DR. A. E. MALLORY'S DEATH.

Dr. Albert E. Mallory, registrar of East Northumberland, died October 5th at his home in Colborne. Dr. Mallory was of U. E. L. descent, and was born at Cobourg, February 1st, 1849. He was educated at Albert College, Belleville, graduated in medicine at McGill University, and started practice at Warkworth, Ont. He was licensed by the Royal College of Surgeons, Edinburgh, and obtained a certificate of British registration in 1878.

Dr. Mallory was for many years one of the most effective speakers the Liberals, then in Opposition, had, and he was a prominent figure in political life in Ontario. He was elected for East Northumberland at the general election in 1887, but unseated, and afterwards defeated at the bye-election. In the one session he sat in the House of Commons he gave great promise as a member. In 1889 he was appointed registrar by the Ontario Government. Dr. Mallory was a member of the Methodist Church. He married a daughter of the late Sheriff Waddell, of Chatham. Mr. C. A. Mallory, the Patron leader, is a brother.

The Physician's Library.

BOOK REVIEWS.

A Text-Book of the Diseases of Women. By CHARLES B. PEN-
ROSE, M.D., Ph.D., formerly Professor of Gynecology in the
University of Pennsylvania. Fifth edition, thoroughly
revised, octavo volume of 539 pages, with 221 fine original
illustrations. Philadelphia, New York, London: W. B.
Saunders & Co. 1904. Canadian agents: J. A. Carveth &
Co., Limited, 434 Yonge Street, Toronto. Cloth, $3.75 net.

We have frequently referred to a copy of the fourth edition
of Dr. Penrose's text-book of Diseases of Women, and always with
satisfaction. The author writes happily and presents the newest
ideas and best methods of gynecology. The fifth edition, which
appears three years after the fourth, speaks eloquently for the
author's popularity with medical students and practitioners. In
its revised form the work continues to be an admirable exposition
of gynecology. J. J. C.

A Hand-Book of Pathological Anatomy and Histology, with an
introductory section on post-mortem examinations and the
methods of preserving and examining diseased tissues, by
FRANCIS DELAFIELD, M.D., LL.D., Emeritus Professor of
the Practice of Medicine, College of Physicians and Surgeons,
Columbia University, New York; and T. MITCHELL PRUD-
DEN, M.D., LL.D., Professor of Pathology and Director of the
Department of Pathology, College of Physicians and Surgeons, Columbia University, New York. Seventh edition,
with 13 full-page plates and 545 illustrations in the text in
black and colors. New York: Wm. Wood & Co. 1904.

Part First of Delafield and Prudden's Hand-book is devoted
to the study of autopsies, the lesions caused by certain forms of
death, *e.g.,* asphyxia, strangulation, hanging, etc., and the general
methods of preserving pathological specimens and preparing them
for study. Though this covers but 60 pages of the book, we think
that Section 1 is alone worth the price charged for the volume.
There are too few of our younger practitioners who know how to
correctly perform an autopsy and turn in to a coroner a proper
report of the same, and if such will but study the first part of this

volume, they will naturally benefit and find the work thereafter not only much simpler, but vastly more interesting to themselves. Part Second is devoted to general pathology, inflammation, animal and plant parasites, infectious diseases and tumors. Part Three consists of over 500 pages and covers special pathology. We find that Dr. Prudden has wisely extended his footnotes very much throughout the book, rendering the study much more interesting by " pointing the student to other publications in which a fuller bibliography may be found." Quite a number of new illustrations have also been added.   w. A. Y.

The Doctor's Series. By CHAS. WELLS MOULTON, General Editor. Vol. IV., " The Doctor's Red Lamp," a book of short stories, concerning the doctor's daily life. Selected by Chas. Wells Moulton. 1904. Akron, O., Chicago and New York: The Saalfield Publishing Co. Canadian agents, Chandler & Massey, Limited, Toronto, Montreal and Winnipeg.

Vol. IV. is composed of 22 chapters, each made up of short stories of events occurring in the daily walk and conversation of a busy physician's life. The volume we hardly think just as interesting as its predecessors, but makes withal most enjoyable light reading. The frontispiece, " The Village Doctor," from the painting of H. Kretzschmer, is splendidly executed, and the illustration, " A Spoonful Every Hour," on page 88, is clever in the extreme. To pass away an hour after a hard day's work, we especially recommend as a prescription Chapter VIII., entitled " The Various Tempers of Grandmother Gregg." It is true to life, amusing and clever.

Radiotherapy and Phototherapy, including Radium and High Frequency Currents; their Medical and Surgical applications in Diagnosis and Treatment for Students and Practitioners. By CHARLES WARRENUE ALLEN, M.D., Professor of Dermatology in the New York Post-Graduate Medical School, etc. With the co-operation of Milton Franklin, M.D., Lecturer on Electro-Radiotherapy, New York Polyclinic Medical School, and Samuel Stern, M.D., Radiotherapist to Dr. Lustgarten's Clinic at the Mount Sinai Hospital. Illustrated with 131 engravings and 27 plates in colors and monochrome. New York and Philadelphia: Lea Brothers & Co. 1904.

This is an attempt, and a very successful one, to collect the mass of knowledge regarding the therapeutic value of radiant energy, and to present it in a usable form. The practical and technical side of radiography is treated briefly, nearly all the space being devoted to a discussion of therapeutic indications and methods of treatment. The history and character of the X-ray is considered in Part I., and medical and surgical diagnosis by means of the rays in Part II. In Part III. radiotherapy is fully discussed under such headings as the treatment of cancer, skin, and other diseases. The remaining four chapters are given up to light, actinotherapy, radiotherapy and high frequency currents. The therapeutic value of the X-ray in cancer and other diseased conditions of the skin is emphasized by many good cuts, showing the condition and appearance before and after treatment. The various kinds of instruments and apparatus used in treatment are illustrated, and fully described, and the author is careful to point out the fact that harm as well as good may be done by their application, and precautionary directions are given. The book is full of interest from first to last · and we are sure that everyone who reads it will be delighted with it, and will be well repaid for his labor.   A. E.

The Utero-Ovarian Artery; or, The Genital, Vascular Circle. Anatomy and Physiology, with Their Application in Diagnosis and Surgical Intervention. By BYRON ROBINSON, B.S., M.D., Chicago, Ill., author of "Practical Intestinal Surgery," "Landmarks in Gynecology," etc. Chicago, Ill.: E. H. Colegrove. 1903. Price, $1.00.

This monograph of 182 pages contains over 100 illustrations, many of them in color, showing the origin and course of the utero-ovarian artery in the formation of the so-called genital, vascular circle. The author says that much time has been spent in securing accurate and reliable illustrations from nature, and that the labor in producing the illustrations has many times exceeded that of the text, which is largely explanatory. The illustrations show the course and relations of the utero-ovarian artery as it is in the adult, as it exists before puberty, and after the menopause. They also include the genital, vascular circle in the guinea-pig, dog, cat, rabbit, leopard, cow, sheep, pig, horse, monkey and baboon.

The whole monograph is designed to be a useful help in diagnosis and a topographical aid in surgical work; but, besides this, it helps to solve many of the problems relating to the vascular supply of the uterus and ovaries which affects so largely the functional activity of these organs.   A. E.

The Principles and Practice of Gynecology for Students and Practitioners. By E. C. DUDLEY, A.M., M.D., President of The American Gynecological Society; Professor of Gynecology, Northwestern University Medical School; Gynecologist to St. Luke's and Wesley Hospitals, Chicago; Corresponding Member of the Société Obstetricale et Gynecologique de Paris, etc., etc. Fourth edition, revised. With 419 illustrations in colors and monochrome, of which 18 are full-page plates. Philadelphia and New York: Lea Brothers & Co. 1904.

Dr. Dudley's volume is divided into six parts, the first being devoted to general principles; the second to infections, inflammations and allied disorders; part three to tumors, tubal pregnancy and malformations; four to traumatisms; five to displacements of the uterus and other pelvic diseases, and six to disorders of menstruation and sterility. It will thus be seen that the author has followed out a very wise plan in arranging the subjects " in pathological and etiological sequence." In this manner, the reader will realize at once how much more valuable this method is to that so frequently carried out, viz., grouping in each part all the diseases of any particular organ. This we consider a most valuable point in Dr. Dudley's work, and the plan might well be followed by other authors with considerable advantage.

The book has been very largely revised and re-written, some chapters condensed, while others have been enlarged; all the most recent advances in gynecology having been introduced, bringing the volume up-to-date and modernised in the fullest sense of the word. We cannot refrain from referring to the color plates as being the best we have seen in any volume for quite a time. If publishers were, as a rule, to pay more attention to this department, their books would be much more valuable, scientifically and commercially. W. A. Y.

A Text-book of Pathology for Practitioners and Students. By JOSEPH MCFARLAND, M.D., Professor of Pathology and Bacteriology in the Medico-Chirurgical College, Philadelphia; Pathologist to the Philadelphia Hospital and to the Medico-Chirurgical Hospital, Philadelphia. With 350 illustrations, a number in colors. Philadelphia, New York, London: W. B. Saunders & Co. 1904. Canadian agents: J. A. Carveth & Co., Toronto.

We anticipated much pleasure and interest as we commenced reading Dr. McFarland's work on pathology, and our greatest expectations have been fully realized, for the book is excellent, indeed.

The author's long experience as a teacher of this subject, besides his extensive personal researches in the laboratory, have well qualified him to write a text-book on pathology. Unlike most works, this subject is treated not from the professors' but the students' point of view in a succinct and intelligent form.

Well-known facts are presented as such, while others not thoroughly understood are dismissed after a brief mention.

Two types of print are used to prevent a common evil, viz., over-voluminousness.

The book is worthy as regards both text and illustrations. Of the latter there are a number of beautiful ones in colors printed directly in the text. Quite a few works on pathology have come to our desk within the past few years, but none have reached a higher standard of excellence. w. h. p.

A Reference Hand-book of the Medical Sciences, embracing the entire range of scientific and practical medicine and allied science. By various writers. Edited by Albert H. Buck, M.D., New York City. Volume VIII. Illustrated by chromo lithographs and 435 half-tone and wood engravings. New York: Wm. Wood & Co. 1904. Canadian agents: The Chandler & Massey Limited, Toronto, Montreal and Winnipeg.

This is the last volume of the new edition of the " Reference Hand-book," and comprises almost everything included in the letters Amb. to Zym. The undertaking on the part of Dr. A. H. Buck and his collaborators has been a very considerable task, and they certainly deserve congratulation upon the successful conclusion of their work. In order to see the enormity of their self-imposed labor, all one has to do is to refer to the list of authors and their contributions, as given at the end of Volume VIII. To each and all the greatest credit is due, the new edition of the " Reference Hand-book " being one of the most voluminous and complete works on the medical sciences issued for many years. The author very nobly attributes the kindly reception accorded to his work by the profession generally to the earnest and sincere efforts of his staff of collaborators, one and all having contributed their honest share of toil towards the end in view. We take this means of conveying to Dr. Buck our congratulations, and bespeak for his " Hand-book " the reception it richly deserves.

The Surgical Treatment of Bright's Disease. By George M. Edebohls, A.M., M.D., LL.D., Professor of the Diseases of Women in the New York Post-Graduate Medical School and Hospital; Consulting Surgeon to St. Francis' Hospital, New York; Consulting Gynecologist to St. John's Riverside Hospital, Yonkers, N.Y., and to the Nyack Hospital, Nyack, N.Y; Fellow of the New York Academy of Medicine and of the American Gynecological Society; Honorary Fellow of the Surgical Society of Bucharest; Permanent Member of the

Medical Society of the State of New York, etc. New York: Frank F. Lisiecki, Publisher, 9 to 15 Murray Street. 1904.

Dr. Edebohls has been a regular contributor to current medical literature in America and Europe for twenty years, the list of his papers filling three pages of the present work. His most important paper, entitled "The Cure of Chronic Bright's Disease by Operation," was published in the *Medical Record,* May 4th, 1901, page 601. Since then Dr. Edebohls has published ten articles on the subject of renal decapsulation and the surgical treatment of nephritis. In the present work clinical records are given of the 72 cases of this disease which have been treated by the author. His final conclusion is that "The evidence submitted," in the author's opinion, "not only justifies the surgical treatment of chronic Bright's disease, but establishes surgery as at present the main, if not the only, hope of sufferers from a hitherto incurable malady." The clinical histories of the cases reveal the causative influences of gout, scarlatina, typhoid fever, malaria, measles, influenza, and exposure to cold or wet in the order given. In the majority of the cases a cause is not assigned. Alcoholism appears once, peritonitis once, pneumonia once, fever once and rheumatism once. The bibliography enables the reader to trace the expression of opinion on renal decapsulation in the medical journals of Europe and America. Thus the editorial we published in THE CANADIAN JOURNAL OF MEDICINE AND SURGERY, 1902, XI., 313-317, and the original article by Dr. Primrose, THE CANADIAN JOURNAL OF MEDICINE AND SURGERY, 1902, XI., 143-152, are mentioned. The work is creditable to Dr. Edebohls' literary talent, showing that he is as familiar with the pen as the scalpel. We bespeak for it a large sale among the profession.

J. J. C.

Text-Book of Nervous Diseases and Psychiatry, for the use of students and practitioners of medicine. By CHAS. L. DANA, A.M., M.D., Professor of Nervous Diseases and (*ad interim*) of Mental Diseases in Cornell University Medical College; Visiting Physician to Bellevue Hospital; Neurologist to the Montefiore Hospital, etc. Sixth revised and enlarged edition, illustrated by 244 engravings and 3 plates in black and colors. New York: Wm. Wood & Co. 1904.

The name of Charles L. Dana is well known throughout the continent, and any work on neurology, bearing his name as author, must, almost of necessity, carry with it considerable weight and literary ability. The author has revised most of his books, which to-day comprises nearly 700 pages, and it may safely be said that though the study of insanity and similar conditions as a rule makes somewhat dry reading, Dr. Dana's book presents the subject in as succinct a style as could be wished for, many parts being quite interesting.   He has followed, in his description of the types of insanity, the scheme of classification used by Kraepelin. The views held by Dr. Dana are the result of his own experience and study in asylum practice, and he is a strong believer in making as few people as possible insane.   A special chapter has been added on psychological terms, which is quite valuable to the reader.

Practical Materia Medica for Nurses.   With an appendix containing Poisons and Their Antidotes, with Poison Emergencies: Mineral Waters; Weights and Measures; Dose List, and a Glossary of the terms used in Materia Medica and Therapeutics.   By EMILY A. M. STONEY, Graduate of the Training School for Nurses, Lawrence, Mass.   Second edition, thoroughly revised.   Philadelphia, New York and London: W. B. Saunders & Co.   1904.

This little volume of three hundred pages is well adapted to the needs of nurses in training.   It contains much practical and useful matter relating to the source, action, uses and dosage of the various drugs usually described in works on materia medica. Its usefulness is increased by a carefully prepared chapter on poison emergencies, in which are given the symptoms and the appropriate treatment for ordinary cases of poisoning.

A System of Practical Surgery.   By PROF. E. VON BERGMANN, M.D., of Berlin; PROF. P. VON BRUNS, M.D., of Tubingen, and PROF. J. VON MIKULICS, M.D., of Breslau.   Volume IV., Surgery of the Alimentary Tract.   Translated and edited by William T. Bull, M.D., Professor of Surgery, College of Physicians and Surgeons, Columbia University, New York; Edward Milton Foote, M.D., Instructor in Surgery, College of Physicians and Surgeons, Columbia University, New York; Carlton P. Flint, M.D., Instructor in Minor Surgery, College of Physicians and Surgeons, Columbia University, New·York; and Walton Martin, M.D., Instructor in Surgery, College of Physicians and Surgeons, Columbia University, New York.   New York and Philadelphia: Lea Brothers & Co.   1904.

The fourth volume of this admirable system of surgery is fully abreast of its excellent predecessors.   The subjects dealt with are discussed under the following headings: malformations, injuries and diseases of the esophagus; injuries and diseases of the abdominal wall; injuries and diseases of the peritoneum: laparotomy; malformations, injuries and diseases of stomach and

intestine; hernia; injuries and diseases of the liver and biliary
passages; injuries and diseases of the spleen; injuries and diseases
of the pancreas.

Two or three decades ago an exhaustive digest of all the really
valuable knowledge pertaining to the surgery of the alimentary
canal could have been presented in much less space than the seven
hundred and fifty pages contained in this volume. But this field
has become so vast within recent years that its literature would
fill a good-sized library. Bearing this in mind, instead of being
disappointed with the comparative brevity of the discussion of
certain topics, the fair-minded critic should rather feel gratified
that so much really excellent and up-to-date material is presented
in such concise and readable form. It is safe to say that the
reader who desires to acquaint himself with the present status of
surgical opinion in regard to the subjects which come within the
range of this book, is likely to feel well repaid for the time expended in reading its various sections.

Many excellent illustrations are introduced, and the reader
will often experience a peculiar satisfaction in having before his
eyes, just where they are most needed, reproductions of familiar
anatomical cuts with which to refresh his memory regarding the
normal anatomy of parts under consideration from the surgical
standpoint.   H. P. H. G.

A Text-book of Human Physiology. By ALBERT P. BRUBAKER,
    A.M., M.D., Professor of Physiology and Hygiene in the
    Jefferson Medical College; Professor of Physiology in the
    Pennsylvania College of Dental Surgery; Lecturer on Physi-
    ology and Hygiene in the Drexel Institute of Art, Science
    and Industry. With colored plates and 354 illustrations.
    Philadelphia: P. Blakiston's Son & Co., 1012 Walnut Street.
    1904. Canadian agents: Chandler & Massey Limited,
    Toronto, Montreal and Winnipeg.

" The object in view in the preparation of this volume was the
selection and presentation of the more important facts of physiology in a form which it is believed will be helpful to students and
to practitioners of medicine. Such facts have been selected as
will not only elucidate the normal functions of the tissues and
organs of the body, but which will be of assistance in understanding their abnormal manifestations as they present themselves in
hospital and private practice."

This is a new work, and it contains the latest reliable teaching
on the subject. It contains a large number of good illustrations,
but the author was wise in excluding those illustrations which

refer to purely technical subjects, such as physiologic apparatus and the like.

We believe it will be a very popular text-book with medical students, and can recommend it as a useful and handy book of reference for those in practice. w. a. y.

The Urine and Clinical Chemistry of the Gastric Contents, the Common Poisons and Milk. By J. W. HOLLAND, M.D., Prof. of Medical Chemistry and Toxicology, Jefferson Medical College, Philadelphia. Forty-one illustrations. Seventh edition, revised and enlarged. Philadelphia: P. Blakiston's Son & Co., 1012 Walnut Street. 1904. Price, $1.00.

This is a very useful work for the student or general practitioner for laboratory or office use. It contains all the best tests used in the examination of urine, gastric contents, common poisons and milk in a very convenient form. It is a compilation, and, consequently, is brief. There are several cuts of apparatus used, and microscopic findings of casts, crystals, etc. The book opens from the end like a notebook and has every other page blank for memoranda. We have much pleasure in recommending this work, which is now in its seventh edition, to our friends. w. j. w.

A Practical Treatise on Diseases of the Skin, for the use of students and practitioners. By JAS. NEVINS HYDE, A.M., M.D. Professor of Skin, Genito-urinary and Venereal Diseases, Rush Medical College, Chicago; Dermatologist to the Presbyterian, Augustana and Michael Reese Hospitals, of Chicago; and FRANK HUGH MONTGOMERY, M.D., Associate Professor of Skin, Genito-urinary and Venereal Diseases, Rush Medical College, Chicago; Professor of Skin and Venereal Diseases, Chicago Clinical School. Seventh and revised edition, illustrated with 107 engravings and 34 plates in colors and monochrome. Philadelphia and New York: Lea Bros. & Co. 1904.

The revised edition of Hyde and Montgomery consists of a volume covering over 900 pages. It is prefaced with a colored plate, beautifully executed, of Xeroderma pigmentosum (from a painting in oil), and which in itself is a work of art. The authors present now a volume that may be said to have been thoroughly revised, covering fully the subject of Dermatology. They have also eliminated a good deal of material that has become what might be termed out-of-date, and have added quite a number of most creditably colored plates and engravings. "Hyde and Montgomery" may be looked upon as a work on skin diseases of no small merit, full yet concise, thoroughly up-to-date, and altogether a most reliable exponent of the subject which it covers.

8

A Treatise on Obstetrics for Students and Practitioners. By EDWARD P. DAVIS, A.M., M.D., Professor of Obstetrics in the Jefferson Medical College, Professor of Obstetrics in the Philadelphia Policlinic, etc., etc. Second edition, illustrated with 274 engravings and 39 plates in colors and monochrome. Philadelphia and New York: Lea Bros. & Co. 1904.

The revision of Dr. Davis' work on Obstetrics has resulted in its very considerable enlargement, making it now a volume of about 800 pages. The second edition is a great improvement on the first, and it takes but a short time to recognize the fact that the author has put in a great deal of time in his revision. He now presents to the profession a book that will compare favorably with any in print, there being no branch in medicine in which greater advances have been made than obstetrics. Dr. Davis' volume is the more valuable because it is practical and largely the results of his own experience.

The Principles of Hygiene. A Practical Manual for Students, Physicians and Health Officers. By D. H. BERGEY, A.M., M.D., Assistant Professor of Bacteriology, University of Pennsylvania. Second edition, thoroughly revised. Handsome octavo volume of 536 pages, fully illustrated. Philadelphia, New York, London: W. B. Saunders & Company. 1904. Cloth, $3.00 net. Canadian agents: J. A. Carveth & Co., Limited, 434 Yonge Street, Toronto.

Great advances in preventive medicine have resulted in modified views in certain particulars. In Chapter xvii. (Vital Causes of Disease), the author describes the vegetable and animal organisms, which may exist on the human host, and by their presence or through the production of toxins cause disease. A list is given of the bacteria, which are pathogenetic to man and the specific organisms of diseases belonging to the vegetable kingdom, with the date of discovery and the name of the discoverer, *e.g.*, 1863, bacillus of anthrax, Davaine; 1879, micrococcus of gonorrhea, Neisser, etc., etc. The important question of immunity and susceptibility is discussed at considerable length, descriptions being introduced of the different theories advanced by Pasteur, Chauveau, Metschnikoff, Buchner, Pfeiffer, Bordet and Ehrlich to explain these phenomena. The antitoxic sera, bactericidal immune sera, the prevention of infection by inducing immunity, showing the influence of vaccination in restricting smallpox and Haffkine's sera in the prevention and treatment of typhoid fever, cholera and bubonic plague are likewise explained. The prevention of malaria and yellow fever is also explained. The pathogenic influence of rats, bedbugs, flies, mosquitoes, fleas, and roaches is also discussed under different heads, and means for removing or destroying these pests given. Trypanosomiasis, helminthiasis and uncinariasis are briefly described, and finally, this chapter winds up with the vegetable parasites, viz., the Tricophyton fungus, the microsporon furfur, actinomycis bovis, Oidiomycosis, etc. The quarantine laws of the United States are given in full. The metric system is used throughout the book. The reader will also find all the subjects usually found in such books—air, water, food, disinfection, etc.—well described. Quite an up-to-date book and the author has handled the multifarious material at his disposal with great skill. J. J. C.

Lectures to General Practitioners on the Diseases of the Stomach and Intestines, with an account of their relations to other diseases, and of the most recent methods applicable to the diagnosis and treatment of them in general; also " The Gastrointestinal Clinic," in which all such diseases are separately considered. By BOARDMAN REED, M.D., Professor of Diseases of the Gastro-intestinal Tract, Hygiene and Climatology in the Department of Medicine of Temple College, Philadelphia; Attending Physician to the Samaritan Hospital, etc., etc. Illustrated. New York: E. B. Treat & Co., 241 and 243 West 23rd Street. 1904.

We think that we are correct when we state that there is no work, except the one under review, in the English language which in one volume treats of diseases of both the stomach and intestines. This will, therefore, recommend Dr. Boardman Reed's text-book to many. It cannot be said that there is a great multiplicity of books dealing with this subject, so that the publication of Dr. Reed's lectures does·not come amiss, especially as his book contains brief concise descriptions of the tests most easily applied by practitioners in studying the derangements, displacements and diseases of the digestive organs, or abdominal viscera. We like the book for the reasons stated, and feel that it will be received well by the profession, especially by those who prefer not too bulky a volume, but one that is " boiled down," and, therefore, to the point.

The Practice of Medicine. A Text-Book for Practitioners and Students, with Special Reference to Diagnosis and Treatment. By JAMES TYSON, M.D., Professor of Medicine in the University of Pennsylvania and Physician to the Hospital of the University; Physician to the Pennsylvania Hospital; Fellow of the College of Physicians of Philadelphia; Member of the Association of American Physicians, etc. Third edition, thoroughly revised and in parts re-written. With 134 illustrations, including colored plates. Philadelphia: P. Blakiston's Son & Co., 1012 Walnut St. 1903. Canadian agents: Chandler & Massey Limited, Toronto, Montreal and Winnipeg.

It is but seven years since Dr. Tyson published the first edition of his " Practice of Medicine,' since which time he has re-written it twice. His third edition may be said to represent in the highest degree the present state of modern medicine. The subject of medicine is a most extensive one, and exceedingly difficult to attempt to cover in one volume of 1,200 pages, so that it cannot be expected that any author will not in some ways fall short of the mark. Dr. Tyson, however, has succeeded admirably, and in his third edition has presented the profession with a volume second to none in print. As would be expected, the part in which the most extensive changes will be found is that devoted to infectious diseases, our knowledge of them becoming more comprehensive every day. The volume is divided into fourteen sections, viz., infectious diseases; diseases of the digestive system; respiratory system; diseases of the heart and blood vessels; diseases of the blood and blood-making organs; of the thyroid gland; urinary organs; constitutional diseases; nervous system; muscular system; the intoxications; effects of exposure to high, though bearable, temperature; animal parasites and the conditions caused by them; and Section XIV. devoted to a summary of symptoms following overdoses of poisons. We congratulate the author upon the result of his labors.   W. A. Y.

A Manual of the Practice of Medicine. By FREDERICK TAYLOR, M.D., F.R.C.P., Senior Physician to, and Lecturer on Medicine at, Guy's Hospital; Consulting Physician to the Evelina Hospital for Sick Children; President of the Clinical Society; Examiner in Medicine at the University of London; late Examiner in Medicine at the University of Durham and the Royal College of Physicians, and in Materia Medica and Pharmaceutical Chemistry at the University of London. Fourth edition. London: J. & A. Churchill, 7 Great Marlborough Street. 1904. Canadian Agents: J. A. Carveth & Co., Toronto.

As one would naturally suppose, this is an up-to-date manual of the Practice of Medicine. It is the fourth edition of a work, the first edition of which was issued in January, 1890, or a new edition every two years. It is a manual and is a handy volume which one can comfortably hold in one's hands without the aid of a table.

The author devotes " most attention to the description of the symptoms, to diagnosis, to prognosis and to treatment, feeling that they are the divisions of the subject which most answer to the idea of practice.

" Dr. Taylor has not devoted much space to the discussion of theories, finding that the facts of medicine are amply sufficient to fill, and more than fill, a volume such as this, and being convinced that these facts require to be seized and held fast by the beginners in medicine, not only for the sake of diagnosis and treatment, but also for the right estimation of the various theories which are advanced."

The subjects now introduced for the first time into the book are sleeping sickness and trypanosomiasis; family periodic paralysis; diseases of the conus medullaris and cauda equina; diseases of the thymus gland; arsenical poisoning; infective arthritis; myelopathic albumosuria, and some of the rarer diseases of the skin.

It may also be stated that at the end of the work there is a treatise on diseases of the skin. There are a good many illustrations scattered through the book. We have read several articles in this work and have been much pleased with the lucidity of the author's statements. The article on neuritis is particularly good, and the presentation of the motor symptoms of hysterical paralysis very instructive. The book is printed in large, readable type, and is neatly bound. J. J. C.

Appleton's Medical Dictionary. An illustrated dictionary of medicine and allied subjects, in which are given the derivation, accentuation and definition of terms used throughout the entire field of medical science. Edited by FRANK P. FOSTER, M.D., Editor of *The New York Medical Journal* and *Philadelphia Medical Journal,* consolidated, of a reference book of practical therapeutics, and of Foster's Illustrated Encyclopedic Medical Dictionary. New York and London: D. Appleton & Co. 1904. Canadian agents: The Morang Co., Limited, Toronto.

If we wished to sum up in a word or two a suitable and true description of " Appleton's Medical Dictionary," we could not do better than use the Latin expression, " *Multum in parvo.*" As the author himself says, it " is in no sense a compilation, but the outcome of an extensive course of independent reading." It takes but a few minutes to realize the enormous amount of work such a volume has entailed. In many respects Appleton's Dictionary eclipses some others in print, though, on the other hand, in other ways Gould and Dunglison are superior. It is a pity that the publishers did not give us the benefit of a thumb index, which is exceedingly handy in volumes of this size, naturally alphabetical in arrangement. Again, we think that a considerably greater number of illustrations would have rendered the book more valuable; but altogether, Dr. Foster has given the profession and student population a magnificent volume and one that should have a ready sale.

A Text-Book of Materia Medica, including Laboratory Exercises in the Historic and Chemic Examinations of Drugs. For Pharmaceutic and Medical Schools, and for Home Study. By ROBERT A. HATCHER, Ph.G., M.D., Instructor in Pharmacology in Cornell University Medical School of New York City; and TORALD SOLLMANN, M.D., Assistant Professor in Pharmacology and Materia Medica in the Medical Department of the Western Reserve University of Cleveland. 12mo volume of about 400 pages, illustrated. Philadelphia, New York, London: W. B. Saunders & Co. Canadian agents: J. A. Carveth & Co., Limited, Toronto. 1904 Flexible leather, $2.00 net.

We strongly recommend the students, now entering their winter's studies at Toronto University, to purchase Dr. Hatcher's Materia Medica, as we feel that it will very materially assist them in their laboratory work. The text-book goes fully into laboratory exercises, a method of teaching that is far ahead of the older didactic system, especially applied to materia medica.

Medical Jurisprudence, Insanity and Toxicology. By HENRY C. CHAPMAN, M.D., Professor of Institutes of Medicine and Medical Jurisprudence in the Jefferson Medical College, Philadelphia. Third edition, thoroughly revised, greatly enlarged and entirely reset. Handsome 12mo volume of 329 pages, fully illustrated, including four colored plates. Philadelphia, New York, London: W. B. Saunders & Co. 1903. Canadian agents: J. A. Carveth & Co., Limited. Cloth, $1.75 net.

This work is based on the author's practical exprience as Coroner's Physician of the City of Philadelphia for a period of six years. Dr. Chapman's book, therefore, is of unusual value to the medical and legal professions, presenting, as it does, the information gained from active participation in medico-legal cases. This third edition, enlarged by the addition of new matter to the extent of seventy-five pages, has been entirely reset, and it is evident that in its preparation every page has undergone a careful scrutiny, so as to include the very latest advances in this very important branch of medical science. Much of the matter has been rearranged, the text has been more fully illuminated by additional references to cases, and a number of new figures and tables have been added.

In reviewing this excellent work, we have found that it covers the field completely and thoroughly, nothing of practical importance to the physician or lawyer having been omitted. In our opinion, there is no doubt that the work will meet with as great favor as the previous edition—a popularity which it certainly deserves.

Medical Monograph Series. No. IX., Adenoids. By WYATT WINGRAVE, Physician and Pathologist, Central London Throat and Ear Hospital. Pp. 128, crown 8vo. Price 2s. 6d., net. London: Bailliere, Tindall & Cox.

At the Central London Throat Hospital one may, any afternoon, rain or shine, see an interesting gymnastic performance in the removal of tonsils and adenoids under nitrous oxide anesthesia. True, it needs a dextrous surgeon, a somewhat husky nurse to hold the struggling patient—but they do it just the same. The private opinion publicly expressed by the older patients as to the surgeon's character are somewhat interesting, too; but then, what will you?

Of Dr. Wingrave's experience there can be no question, and he has treated the whole question of adenoids in a very readable and thorough manner. He devotes a chapter to the question of recurrence, so that evidently it is not unknown to him, for nitrous oxide anesthesia conduces to aerobatic surgery rather than thoroughness. M.

Kirke's Hand-Book of Physiology. Hand-book of Physiology, revised by FREDERICK C. BUSCH, B.S., M.D., Professor of Physiology, Medical Department, University of Buffalo. Fifth American revision, with 535 illustrations, including many in colors. New York: Wm. Wood & Co. 1904.

Kirke's Physiology has for many years been looked upon as a standby for both student and practitioner, and, judging from Dr. Busch's revised edition just to hand, it will be many years before it will be replaced as a college text-book. The book has been carefully gone over and revised, some parts having been condensed and others extended, so that the profession have now a thoroughly modern work on physiology, written in an interesting and concise manner.

Charts Received.

(1) The Relations of the Segments of the Spinal Cord and Their Nerve Roots to the Vertebræ. Mechanical Vibration Chart. (2) The Sympathetic Nerve. Vibration Chart. Copyrighted by M. II. L. Arnold Snow, M.D. 1904.

Books Received.

Thirtieth Annual Report of the Secretary of the State Board of Health of the State of Michigan, for the fiscal year ending June 30th, 1902. By authority. Lansing, Michigan: Robert Smith Printing Co., State Printers and Binders. 1903.

Twenty-second Annual Report of the Provincial Board of Health of the Province of Ontario (Canada), for the year 1903. Printed by order of the Legislative Assembly of Ontario, Toronto. Printed and published by L. K. Cameron, Printer to the King's Most Excellent Majesty. 1904.

The Canadian
Journal of Medicine and Surgery

A JOURNAL PUBLISHED MONTHLY IN THE INTEREST OF
MEDICINE AND SURGERY

VOL. XVI.   TORONTO, DECEMBER, 1904.   NO. 6.

Original Contributions.

COMPLICATIONS OF FRACTURES AND AMPUTATIONS.

BY THOMAS H. MANLEY, Ph.D., M.D.,
Visiting Surgeon to Harlem and Metropolitan Hospitals, New York.

IT has been my custom in hospital and private practice to endeavor to demonstrate that conservatism is not only the most humane, but the safest course to pursue, when a limb has been so shattered that the question of amputation may arise; and adopt those means by which, when properly utilized, primary amputation may be abandoned altogether in civil life. The mangled limb has been cleansed, hemorrhage subdued, and comfortable dressings applied, and our patient placed in bed. We wait and observe the limb, for, in many cases, time alone will determine its fate. Now, in order to afford our patient the best prospects, not only is it necessary to clearly understand what the phenomena of mortification and gangrene are, but to anticipate their onset; and should they appear be prepared to intelligently interpret the signs which precede them.

It is likewise highly important that the various phases of asphyxiation or decomposition about to set in are early recognized and actively treated, on such lines as the changes in the anatomical elements indicate. Without being thus prepared for the rational and skilful management of such cases, probably our patient's prospects would have been equally as good, or better, had the damaged limb been immediately sacrificed after injury. It may be observed that immediately after a grave injury to a limb, there are no symptoms or signs by which it is possible to estimate with precision the degree of vitality remaining.

4

The limb in common with the whole body is cold; after reaction sets in, heat may return completely or partly. It may remain icy cold. When this frigid state of the limb persists more than forty-eight hours, it is a certain precursor of mortification.

Dupuytren was the first who called attention to the importance of this symptom in prognosis here. He found by the use of the thermometer that the temperature in a limb about to mortify is lower than that in the dead body, and that of the surrounding atmosphere. When along with this abstraction of heat, sensation is lost, a greenish-gray color covers the skin, and a gaseous crepitation is felt under it, the parts are hopelessly mortified, and decomposition is advancing.

Happily in a considerable number this advent of mortification is not so sudden, the temperature gradually lowers; here and there are other significant symptoms that will warn us of its approach. A gradual diminution in sensation, with changes of color in the skin, especially near the toes, with total loss of power in the damaged limb, is often a forerunner of mortification when the lower extremity is damaged. But it is important to know that the behavior of a gravely traumatized limb, in the beginning, varies; a badly injured limb is much like a grave injury of the body, of which it is but an appendage.

For example, in some instances, one is killed outright; in others, after a varying period, deep shock passes off and the patient recovers; in others, again, full reaction never sets in, but collapse gradually deepens and the patient sinks.

So in some crushes of a limb; it may be killed outright, as it were, animation never returning. In others, the member is but temporarily devitalized; there is a species of " suspended animation," the circulation returning after varying intervals. In another class there is but an imperfect return of the vital processes, and death of the limb sets in. This last type, in my experience, is alarmingly mortal to the tissues and calls for prompt amputation.

Traumatic Gangrene.—This type of diseased action is frequently encountered after nearly every description of serious injury of an extremity or any of its appendages. As it is dependent on a variety of causes, so it presents a considerable diversity of phases. Its fundamental etiological factors are chiefly two: (1) Violence to the tissues, mechanical disorganization; (2) chemicoseptic changes consecutive to injury. As an illustration, great violence being applied to a limb, its main arterial trunk is damaged and the vitality of the parts is imperilled by anemia and impending asphyxia, until the collateral circulation is established, which is not enough, perchance, to preserve and nourish all the distant parts. The too tight application of a splint, in a fracture, may shut off the lumina of the larger vessels, when the parts supplied by them maintain thereafter a feeble existence or perish. In certain fractures, a spicula of bone crushes through the trunk of a large artery, and thereby so impedes the circulation to parts beyond that the surface tissues may part with their vitality.

In another class, violence favors the development of gangrene by impairing the vitality of the parts on which it falls; vessels are torn open, nerves lacerated and muscles severely contused. Therefore, an injury, *per se,* is an active cause of gangrene, varying in its effects, according to circumstances.

But in a large member, force is only the proximate cause. The deep parts are opened; a stagnant congested state of the circulation exists over the seat of injury, inflammatory changes have begun. The tissues are but feebly resistant to eccentric influences, and changes of decomposition commence; toxic elements have penetrated from without. There is undoubtedly toxic infection; bio-chemical or microchemical changes are in operation. Whether, indeed, the entrance of some specific germ is the first step in gangrenous changes, or it is brought about through chemical influences stimulated into activity through the action of the atmosphere on feebly vitalized tissues is immaterial.

Modern bacteriological studies would seem to prove that infection of pathogenic germs is alone responsible for the primary pathological changes; but it is well known that the atmosphere plays an important role, as does also the general condition of the patient; above all, in diabetes and in tubercular subjects.

The symptoms which indicate the approach of traumatic gangrene in a limb in serious injuries are general and local. With the onset of those inflammatory changes which precede the sloughing or devitalization of the tissues, a well-marked chill, is experienced, the temperature rises and the pulse quickness; the appetite is lost and thirst is urgent. General debility is marked and the patient sleeps little. These are the usual concomitant disturbances noted, though there are occasional instances in which gangrene sets in, in the most subtle, insidious manner. The day before, the limb may have presented all the signs of a healthy vitality, but, after an interval of twenty-four, or forty-eight hours, on removing the dressings, we are appalled to find an extensive area cold, insensitive and dead. Such cases, however, are very rare indeed; and if we investigate them we discover, as a rule, that some oversight has been committed, that nature's danger signal, great pain, was blunted or destroyed by over-dosing with morphine; that the case was injudiciously treated, or neglected, until too late.

Of the local subjective symptoms, there is one whose significance is of more importance than all the others combined. That symptom is *pain,* not of a moderate, intermittent description, but a grinding, excruciating, incessant agony. It racks and agitates the whole frame. The pain of incipient acute gangrene is always of a most intense and excruciating character. We read it in the deathly pallor of the patient. Indifference to, or a disregard of this symptom on the part of the medical attendant has resulted in the needless sacrifice of many a limb which should have been spared. In every variety of fracture or traumatic disorganization of the soft parts overlying the osseous structure, when severe persistent pain sets in, of such severity as to make comfortable rest impossible, and to provoke markèd constitutional disturbances, we should act promptly in exposing the parts and endeavor to ascertain its cause. Besides this symptom there are other signs, which, when correctly interpreted, will generally point with precision to the' true character of the lesions. Along with the *coolness* of the toes, when the leg or foot is traumatized, we will notice a blueness of the nails, an edema of the tissues and a limited anesthesia. Pulsation of the arteries has ceased, and we will observe that when we press the blood out of the subcutaneous capillaries, they fail to refill. But it is necessary to observe caution in all cases at the onset, at least, that we do not prematurely condemn and amputate what might be saved; for we will sometimes see the tissues covered with blebs, congested, purple and boggy, which, after the active institution of local remedies, suddenly undergo the most remarkable, salutary changes.

Under certain circumstances, surface appearances will deceive us. For example, the foot or hand has been crushed; swelling with active inflammation ensues, in vain we apply local remedies to reduce them, and wait; assuming that inasmuch as the integument is sound the deep parts are intact; but in time, deep suppuration becomes evident; we open the tissues, and, behold! loose dead bone, with large sloughs, broken down tissues in every direction. How it comes that a car-wheel may pass over a foot or leg, or it may be violently struck a concussive blow, yet have its bones extensively shattered thereby, and other deepeer tissues disorganized, while the cutaneous investment escapes extensive laceration, is not easily explained; but more than once have I seen the bone-shaft crushed into fragments, while the overlying skin was unbroken.

Gangrene, as we have seen, is a disease, which is characterized by its tendency to advance into healthy tissues, and destroy, as it extends; the necrotic rotten residue which it leaves we designate " sphacelus."

In mortification, after reaction has become established, changes of decomposition involve the dead tissues, when they are clearly separated from the living by a distinct, demarkating line, as a general rule. This is most commonly witnessed in traumatic gangrene.

Gangrenous processes may spread far up, through, and under the muscles, while the *integument remains whole and free.* It may, on the other hand, even involve but *one set of muscles,* and spare the others. The following short note on a case will illustrate this: A boy of ten years came under my care, who had sustained a fracture between the condyles of the right knee and a compound fracture of the upper third of the fibula. His limb had been caught between the spokes of a moving cart-wheel, and had suffered great violence. It was evident that the posterior tibial artery had been seriously crushed, for the parts supplied by it soon showed signs of incipient gangrene. For several days the limb presented a threatening aspect; but, in time, communicating branches became competent to carry on the circulation, and limited function returned. The fragments united, but through an opening just posterior to the middle of the shaft of the fibula, the macerated, gangrenous, fleshy parts of the peroneus-longus and flexor-longus digiterum were discharged, completely disconnected, with their osseous origin and tendinous termini. The little fellow finally escaped with a fairly useful limb, though there was a marked linear depression over the area occupied by expelled muscles. This was the first instance of muscular gangrene I had ever seen.

Everyone knows that gangrenous processes may attack and destroy one tissue alone, after any injury, while all the others escape. This is called *necrosis,* and probably is the most common type of the process we encounter. Every surgeon whose practice brings him in contact with serious traumatisms is familiar with the fact that vast areas of the integuments become the seat of gangrene, and fall off in stiff, charred casts, leaving all the tissues underneath with their vitality unimpaired; when the limb may possibly be amputated for no other purpose than to secure a skin flap, above, to cover in the denuded surfaces.

Treatment of Mortification and Gangrene.—Strictly speaking, in their etymological sense, the two terms, mortification and gangrene, are integral parts of the same process; the one kills and the other deals only with disintegration, and disposing of the dead tissues. But clinically and pathologically the distinction is wide, and a knowledge of this fact has an important bearing on a rational therapy. In the one case, we see a finger, hand or arm, a part of which has been quite totally destroyed; but it preserves its connection with the body. Cold, bloodless and senseless, we are quite certain it has perished; its vascular supply has been destroyed, and decomposition is quite certain to speedily follow. *Mortification* sets in now. For the purpose of separating the dead from the living, a vitalized wall is thrown around the limb, **at** which point all the vessels are stenosed or obturated, and spontaneous severance begins. The process is a *limited* one. We can see that therapeutic effort is futile in the way of restoring vitality. Therefore, we have done our full duty when we have staunched all hemorrhage, placed the damaged limb in a comfortable position, sterilizing or cleansing the injured parts with thoroughness, and applying antiseptic dressings. This line of practice is generally observed by myself in all serious crushes of a limb, instead of having recourse to immediate amputation. It is true that we make no impression on vital changes; but we give our patient time to recover from the grave general shock which almost invariably attends these traumatisms, while the damaged part is slowly preparing to elide itself from the body corporate which it so long aided to maintain. Besides, as time pencils off the dividing line above, the sphacelated tissues, we know precisely the point at which we will make resection, or employ the amputating knife.

Mortified tissues are *bloodless.* As strangulation of the circulation and consecutive asphyxia invariably lead to it, it is, therefore, clear that inflammatory action is absent in the invaded tissue, and we have no occasion to make provision against hemorrhage.

Our treatment of mortification in its early stages, at least, must bear the stamp of extreme conservatism. If we would carry our case to a successful issue, we should direct a large share of attention to our patient's general condition. Let us look closely to environment, diet, and psychic influences. Opium, that peerless mental exhilarant and unrivalled antidote to pain, is more valuable than all other medicinal agents, given in any description of serious traumatism. Let no one heedlessly discard this by the seductive claims of other medicaments, for *none* can equal it.

But let it be *opium,* and not morphine, codeine, or other of the alkaloids, for they are all more dangerous, and none can be substituted for it in this class.

Certainly it will not be administered at all, if the indications for a narcotic or a sedative are not urgent, and under all circumstances must its employment be governed by strict attention to its effects.

Mechanical or artificial interference comes in as a *finale* to mortification, simply for the purpose of hastening a process that it had initiated, and amputation is called for.

Gangrene.—Gangrene being a much more complex process than mortification, and its course being influenced by a diversity of causes when produced by trauma, no fast or fixed lines can be drawn in its treatment. The clinical history of *traumatic gan-*

grene presents many distinguishing and definite characteristics, which lead me to believe they should be considered apart from those which go with mortification. The causes of traumatic gangrene are determining or constitutional, and direct or local. With one suffering from atheromatous arteries, or whose tissues present a feeble vitality, a slight abrasion or a moderate contusion may fail of repair, or may be followed by gangrene.

Subjects of diabetes mellitus are specially prone to gangrenous change following trauma. It is no doubt through this cause that sometimes, after simple incisions into healthy tissues, they suddenly become putrescent, foul, and rapidly decompose.

Dr. Robert Taylor, of New York, has reported a case, in which, after a simple urethrotomy, performed with every precaution, gangrene spread into the perineum, advanced into and attacked the pelvic viscera, rapidly proving fatal.

Last autumn a large heavy man, 55 years old, very fat, was operated on by me for an incarcerated inguinal hernia. The operation was not difficult, every precaution was taken against contamination of the wound. The fourth day after the operation everything in the vicinity of the wound was one mass of putrescence, and the patient succumbed.

An old man, of a fine physique, who some years before had injured his right popliteal artery, now while removing an ingrowing toe-nail accidentally nicked the skin with the blade. A gangrenous sore followed, which soon threatened the outer half of the foot. A prominent surgeon called in declined amputation, because the patient's urine was highly saccharine. In a state of great distress he sent for me, when I amputated the infected member. But within forty-eight hours, gangrene returned, and in the course of one night after the onset, it overspread the whole foot and threatened the ankle. Another amputation was promptly performed, this time close to the knee joint. Fortunately primary union and recovery followed. I am not sure, however, whether glycosuria in these cases is a cause of gangrene *de novo* or a coincidence. In my hernia case there was no trace of sugar in his urine; and many times have I operated in well-marked glycuronic cases, when the wounds have done well. But there are constitutional disturbances and conditions which exert a positive influence, both in the origin and spread of gangrene. These predisposing and determining factors should be allowed their full weight when deciding our course, when the disease presents itself. Some of them may be eliminated and others are quite beyond our reach.

The local phenomena which gangrene presents, are not uniform, but vary according to circumstances. In severe contusions of the toes we may find the circulation exceedingly languid or temporarily suppressed; the nails are blue, and the integuments cool, but in healthy young subjects, by the aid of artificial heat and rest, in a while warmth returns, and vitality is restored. In other similar cases, severe pain sets in with active inflammatory changes; lividity is not so marked, but the toes are puffed and exquisitely sensitive. At a varying rate this condition extends back into the body of the foot, the pain in the meanwhile continuing very severe, with marked constitutional disturbances. Gangrene may advance along on one side of the foot, or the other, or it may creep up across the entire width at once. Gangrenous processes may suddenly cease in their incipient stages, and resolution so completely follow that no trace of them remains. Inflammation ceases, the extravasated blood and inflammatory deposits are resorbed, the staining of the integument is bleached out, sensation returns and full function is restored.

For the above type of traumatic gangrene, resulting from contusion, various lines of treatment must be adopted, but they in the main equally apply to gangrene, from puncture or septic intoxication.

One has sustained a deep puncture through the pulp of a finger or toe, little is thought of it, and the parts are well in a few days; but in another, the finger festers, swells, and becomes intensely painful. Inflammation spreads and the other fingers become involved, as the condition spreads, and crosses the webbing line below.

Gangrene may follow from the bite of an animal or venomous reptile; some sort of a deadly ferment is deposited in the tissue, which not only destroys the vitality of the part into which it is injected, but it spreads upward towards the body and destroys with appalling rapidity, if the part which was primarily infected be not promptly amputated. Cadaverous poison acts in a similar manner.

A man came under my care, seven years ago, who was stung the evening before by a rattlesnake, which he was exhibiting. Immediately he lost sensation in the first joint of the index finger, which was stung; in less than an hour the whole finger was cold, numb and black; by midnight (he was stung at eight in the evening), all the fingers and the whole hand were cold, stiff and inanimate. When I saw him at eight o'clock the following morning the whole arm and shoulder were in a state of advanced gangrene. The pulse at the wrist was gone; the arm cold, black and bloated. The blade of a scalpel could be passed painlessly in anywhere from the wrist to the shoulder. A greenish-black, horrible smelling ichor exuded. The immediate application of a constrictor over the forearm, with prompt amputation, might have saved this man's arm and life. The incipient signs of gangrene must be met by radical measures, but not necessarily operative.

For the tumefied congested tissues, probably nothing will afford so much relief and put a stop to its course as numerous incisions, the free abstraction of blood with a thorough immersion of the parts in a solution of carbolic acid. This is to be preferred to any other antiseptic, because of its sedative effects on the exposed surface. Warm, moist, sterilized dressings are then applied. It is unnecessary to say that " prevention is always better than cure," and that in all complicated fractures we should never apply rigid bandages or dressings until inflammatory symptoms have subsided, and the danger of strangling the circulation is past.

The question when to amputate in traumatisms can be decided rather by experience than by any formulated set of rules. In mortification, when the line of demarkation is formed, it is answered. But we have no such guide in gangrene. Though more than one author lays it down as a rule, that we should not amputate in this condition until the line of demarkation is formed, and then we should carry the blade through the circle, by a strict observance of this rule, serious evil is certain to result.

In incipient gangrene of a toe or finger, for example, after being assured that gangrene has commenced in a contusion, or a punctured wound, which has become infected, if we hope to cut short its march, one or more of the phalangeal joints must be immediately amputated. Possibly so extreme a measure may be obviated by the substitution of some other less radical operation; but at all events what is done must be done early before other neighboring parts are contaminated, and long before any demarkating line is apparent. The older writers used to say that we should not amputate in " hot gangrene," but Larry, Guthrie, Hennan, McClintock and others of great experience contradict this view. The rule, however, will hold good in what is known as *senile gangrene* and mortification, succeeding a traumatism which destroys part of a limb. In peripheral gangrene commencing in a finger or toe, which endangers a limb through septic diffusion along the lymph channels, we entirely disregard this rule, and make a severance through such a line as we believe preserves its vitality. The dread of not going high enough up, beyond the infected tissues, and the chances of a fresh infection seizing on the divided tissues was what inspired this precept. My experience has not confirmed this view; on the contrary, in my earlier hospital service, by a sort of a religious observance of it, I have seen this death-dealing malady slowly creep close to the trunk, while we waited for the *line of demarkation,* and then only interfered when the whole limb was imperilled. A timely amputation, a thorough disinfection of the flaps and stump, with free drainage, will call a halt on the course of gangrene, with as much certainty as extraction will annul a toothache.   But the work of eradicating all infected tissues must be thorough, and the surroundings must be favorable to recovery.   It is almost unnecessary to say that much of one's success in these cases will depend on the general condition of our patient.   Under any circumstances as far as local treatment of the case goes, if we have one with a broken-down constitution, in insanitary surroundings, inadequate diet and nursing, our case is quite certain to do badly, whatever the course we adopt.   A nourishing diet, with plenty of stimulants, if there be great bodily weakness, pure air, and cheerful surroundings, are most effective, constitutional antidotes to consecutive gangrene.   For medicine, quinine, the bitter barks; acids and iron, with small doses of mercury, if there be a specific taint, are called for.

If we would have the wound do well, we must look diligently after our patient's general condition, attend carefully to his digestion and his emunctories.

THE MEDICAL SOCIETY: ITS PLACE AND EQUIPMENT.*

BY JOHN HUNTER, M.D.,

Physician, Toronto Western Hospital.

A WRITER says, " There is, for every one of us, a place and also an equipment that, taken together, ensure success. It is our duty to find our place, and to use our equipment." ، The wisdom of this statement may be taken as indisputable. I shall, therefore, with some license use it as a text on which to base a few remarks that you will please accept as an instalment on the debt which, as president, I owe to the members of this society for the honor conferred upon me. It has the merit, too, of being a fairly orthodox text, for it can be said that it naturally divides itself into two heads: The Place and The Equipment.

THE PLACE.

The medical society was begotten, and has ever been perpetuated, by one of the most meritorious inspirations that govern the physician's life, namely, the desire for more knowledge, wider experience and greater skill. A glance over the names enrolled in the membership of a medical society shows the place it holds in the estimation of medical men. There you find the names of men distinguished alike for the highest professional attainments in technical knowledge and skill, and also for the noblest attributes of character. The fact that the medical society can gather into it such a class of men is very positive evidence that it has a place. Another equally strong proof of its right to claim a place is the fact that the progress in the science and art of medicine is very largely due to the work which has been done in the medical society. Where else can papers be presented and discussed to better advantage? The medical journal is a great medium for the distribution of knowledge. But what physician, who has listened to the words and studied the play of emotions, as expressed in feature and gesture of some of our great medical teachers, would exchange that experience for a perusal of the same article in the quiet of the library, however interesting and instructive a careful reading might prove to be? Would the apostles have accomplished as much for Christianity if they had read the words of its Founder instead of hearing them from His lips? Was it not the impress of a personality that made these men invincible? What surgeon could listen to Lister without receiving an inspiration to do all his work more aseptically for all the days to come? Those of us who had the pleasure of hearing Osler's address at the meeting of the Canadian Medical Association, in Montreal, treasure that occasion as one of the most inspiring of the reminiscences of life. To these two names each one of us could add many others, of men to whom we have listened with the greatest pleasure and profit. But some may say, that often they have neither been pleased nor edified by the manner in which papers and addresses have been given in the medical society. This suggests another feature that may be very briefly referred to, viz., that the medical society is a place for moral and social development.

High attainments in technical knowledge and skill may be grievously impaired if associated with irascible tempers and boorish manners, which ruthlessly lacerate those tender feelings that constitute the "woof and warp" of our sentiments. A medical society is a school in which anything incongruous in language or manner is likely to be rebuked and corrected. In what other place do sharp tricks, dishonorable intrigues, or petty jealousies seem so small and contemptible to us as when we are convened in a medical society? Here we meet in a quieter and serener atmosphere, where the heat and discomfitures that arise from the friction and collisions of the every-day struggle for existence or pre-eminence are not felt, and where we can estimate more justly the work and worth of our fellows.

Time will not permit me to dwell any longer on this phase of my subject; but I wish, *en passant,* to refer briefly to those who are not members of any medical society. These men belong chiefly to one or another of three groups: The egotists, who are deluded by the belief that they are the incarnation of all knowledge, and, therefore, cannot be taught anything by their fellows; the indolent and indifferent—quite too numerous a class; and, perhaps, the most pitiable of all, those who cling to the delusion that they must cherish a real or imaginary grievance against some member or members of the society. These feel their loss keenly, but still hold that it is their duty to immolate themselves on the altar of revenge. Some may say, "Well, if these do not wish to attend, let them stay away; we can get along without them." Could we dispose of these classes in this cursory manner, it certainly would be an easy way to get rid of them. But can we do so? These men are members of our profession, and the old adage holds true in our case as in all others, that "a chain is no stronger than its weakest link, a fleet no swifter than its slowest vessel, nor a fortress any stronger than its weakest point." A majority of the cases of sickness fall into the hands of the nearest physicians; and, if any of these be less competent because they will not avail themselves of the help a medical society can render, their incompetency and ignorance imperil life and bring opprobrium on an honorable profession. Have those of us who can speak from experience of the value of the medical society no missionary work to do among these classes who do not attend its meetings? Should we leave egotism, ignorance, indifference and petty jealousies to exercise their baneful influence? Is there any better way to get rid of evils than to expose them? " Is not he who is afraid to see, and dare not mention the wrong-doing of himself and his colleagues, his profession's worst enemy?" Should we not govern our own lives, and, as far as lies in our power, help others to govern theirs, by the abstract truths that "right is right, wrong is wrong, and duty is duty?" Unless the wisest, most cultured and upright men have erred in judgment, or have been deceived by experience, their actions prove that the medical society is the right place for every medical man, inspired with any desire for more knowledge, wider experience and greater skill.

THE EQUIPMENT.

The question of equipment is always involved in the character of the work to be done. Upholstered furniture would not be an essential part in the equipment of a dissecting room. It might represent surplus wealth or a morbid type of refinement; but strong tables and adjustable stools would answer much better. So in a medical society, learned papers and discussions on mere abstract theories might exhibit mental acumen, but the record of everyday experience would be of much greater utility.

The equipment of a medical society, in so far as the place of meeting is concerned, and the frequency with which the meetings are held, must be governed by special conditions. The rooms should be centrally situated, suitably furnished, well ventilated and lighted. Experience fully proves that meetings held weekly or bi-weekly are much better attended than those held at longer intervals. The meetings should open at the appointed hour. They should not, as a rule, extend over two hours, as long hours exhaust vitality and impair the interest in the proceedings. I suppose it is a matter of individual opinion as to whether or not we should retire immediately after the session is over, or spend a few minutes socially over some light refreshments. Personally, I prefer the latter, as it affords an opportunity for the members to become better known to each other, and, as a result, to become better friends.

We come now to consider the most essential part of the equipment of the medical society—the papers, discussions, and the presentation of cases, pathological specimens, photos, instruments and surgical appliances.

Before entering upon the discussion of these, permit me to make a short digression, for I wish to state as emphatically as I can, that there is an imperative obligation resting upon every member of a medical society, not only to attend its meetings as regularly as possible, but also to take an active part in the work. The function of a medical society is not to nurture drones and parasites, but to be a school in which all are experts and zealous students, imparting and acquiring knowledge.

PAPERS.

In preparing a paper, at least three features should be most religiously kept in view. It should be practical, tersely and concisely written in technical language, and brief. In a society like this one, which includes the whole field of medicine and surgery, the writer of a paper has a great variety of subjects to choose from. When a choice has been made, the writer should strive to imitate the true artist—stamp his individuality on his work. He should never leave it possible for anyone to say that his paper was simply a mere repetition of what has been written in books or journals. Before writing his article, he should read every book and journal that can aid him; but his paper should be as characteristically his own as are his features or tone of voice. What one reads and hears should be to the mind what wholesome food is to the body. The cantatrice transforms her food into musical symphonies that are enchanting, and the statesman his dinner into words that are lustily cheered by his followers. If this be true of physical nutriment (and it is a scientific fact that without the proper assimilation of food we could have neither song nor speech), why not make as great a transformation in our mental pabulum? The auditory and ocular centres were never intended to be mere wayside storehouses out of which the same thoughts should pass again, but rather to be switchboards, flashing the impressions on to the psychic laboratories, whose functions are to discover and interpret these impressions as they come, and then stamp them with personality and send them forth again to delight others and to increase the common fund of knowledge. It does not necessarily follow that the work of each one of us will equal in importance that of a Harvey, a Hunter, a Jenner, or a Lister, but it should represent the best that the opportunities of our age, our experience and our mental endowments can produce.

So much for the intrinsic worth and character of a paper, and now a few words about the form and manner of its presentation. An instrument may have considerable value in its design, but be of such poor workmanship that its worth is seriously impaired. In like manner, a paper may show much originality of thought, and yet be so carelessly arranged and so poorly read that its real merit is lost to the audience. The writer of a paper should take under his " most careful consideration " the fact that an audience has only a limited amount of time and energy to spend on any one paper, and so should be extremely conservative of both. The scope of his subject should be clearly outlined in title and headings, and the language concise and technical. He should exercise all his elocutionary powers, the tone of voice being made pleasant and the pitch such as to be easily heard by all present. It is the speaker's duty to make himself heard, not the duty of the audience to have to strain their attention to hear him. How can one expect an audience to be interested in his subject when he buries his face in his paper and mutters away to himself? Papers should be of no greater length than is necessary to present the subject intelligently. It is as bad to overfeed an audience as it is to overfeed a baby. Too long a paper causes a wave of anguish to sweep over the faces of those who have to listen, and also a constant shifting of positions in order that they may be able to endure the affliction and mitigate their suffering as much as possible.

THE DISCUSSIONS.

These, like the papers, should bear the impress of the speaker. It is well to be able to quote authorities, but better still if able to qualify them from personal experience. This by no means excludes the younger members from taking part in the discussions; for how often it happens in earlier years, that cases are met which furnish an experience rarely, if ever, duplicated. The youngest member may thus be able to contribute something of as great value to the society as the old veteran can, and, if you will allow a slight digression here, I would say that this is pre-eminently the young man's age, and I wish to extend to all such a most cordial invitation to take a large share in our work. In doing so I am sure I express the feelings of all, not only of those in the strenuous period of mid-life, but also of those of us labelled with the serener graces of maturer years.

CLINICAL MATERIAL.

In this contingent of our equipment are included clinical cases, pathological specimens, photos, instruments and appliances. However valuable good papers and discussions may be, yet these do not seem to meet all the requirements. We rather long for something that we can see, feel and handle. The appearance presented by the morbid condition, the sounds elicited by percussion or heard through the stethoscope, the sensation produced by touch, can scarcely be overestimated as aids in furnishing information. In the absence of patient or morbid specimen, good photos are of great service, and no description of instruments or appliances can equal the act of examining and handling them.

I must not violate some of the precepts I have laid down, so will briefly summarize this phase of my subject as follows: The equipments of a medical society are, a home in a central locality with suitably furnished, well-lighted, properly ventilated rooms; weekly or bi-weekly meetings, beginning sharp on time, and of about two hours' duration; short, practical papers and discussions, bearing the impress of originality and personality; presentation of clinical cases, pathological specimens, instruments and appliances; a large membership, with punctual and regular attendance.

In conclusion, am I not justified in saying that any physician who makes it his business to join the Toronto Medical Society, or one of its sister societies, will find a place and an equipment that, taken together, will insure his success; not always, it may be, if judged from the pecuniary standpoint alone, but assuredly success in that far worthier achievement, the ability to do good work?

BY F. V. TREBILCOCK, M.D., ENNISKILLEN.

"AN extraordinary anemia" is an exclamation which comes to
the lips of every one of us who keeps his eyes open for any short
space of time, for housed away in every hamlet in our land is some
poor body of whom folks say, "She looks like a ghost." I say
"she" advisedly, for in the villages in which it is my duty and
pleasure to visit, such cases are usually of woman-kind. Generally speaking, these patients present problems which are only
soluble in part, and the most any man can hope to win is a very
moderate amount of relief from distressing symptoms for his
patients and a long season of unrewarded worry for himself.

I have wished to bring before you in the few minutes which
are mine, the clinical aspects of such a case, which has lately come
under my notice and care. I do this with the more diffidence because I am unable to give you the laboratory data which picture
the individual blood-cell; but as I desire my words to be re-
minders of old things rather than teachers of new ones, I trust
they may arouse some discussion in a field which may be of interest and profit to all of us.

I visited an unmarried woman, aged — years, for the first
time three months ago. Though she lived not a mile from me, I
had seen nothing of her for more than a year, and remembered
her only as being ghastly white, with a history of having been so
for a long time.

She sat in her chair showing the intensest air-hunger; tried
to say "Good-morning" to me, but found the sentence too long
to speak unbroken. At my bidding she remained perfectly quiet
where she was, and I began my examination.

Her hair was exceedingly sparse and much coarser than
natural; her face uniformly broadened, and, with the exception
of the under eyelids, which were noticeably bagged and soft,
was very firm under pressure. All expression was lost in the
diffuse swelling. The countenance was a pale yellow white, without the faintest trace of pink, even on the severest friction and
pinching; the ears translucent, so that heavy newspaper print was
distinguishable through the lobes. The alæ of the nose were
vibrating rapidly with the forced respiration. The whites of the
eyes were slightly muddy, and they themselves expressionless.

The neck was uniformly enlarged, with no special swelling to
be made out; the thyroid body not palpable, and no marked pulsation visible anywhere. The trunk was uniformly enlarged.
Her sister assured me that the back was broader than usual, and

---

* Read at meeting of the Ontario Medical Association, Toronto, June, 1904.

the abdomen more prominent. Careful examination showed no displacement of any organ, nor any enlargement. The cardiac impulse was just as turbulent as might be looked for.

The arms were swollen and hard to the touch, though not to the same extent as the legs, which were swollen until every curve was lost; no pitting could be seen, even after the severest pressure.

The skin was exceedingly dry and inelastic, and had been so for months; in fact, she remarked that she had not perspired since last summer, no matter how hot the room might be. There was no rash, only a diffuse scurfiness and a history of occasional spells of intense itching.

The oral mucous membrane was extremely pale; the tongue clean, and nothing extraordinary in the physiology of the alimentary tract except a marvellously large appetite, which had been noticed all winter. There was no distress after meals, nor any sign of undigested food in the stools. The latter were as frequent as could be expected from her habit of sitting so much. A mild laxative once a week kept her fairly regular, but lately she had noticed the stool becoming foul-smelling.

The circulatory system showed changes only in the pulse-rate and in the more tumultuous heart-beat. On my first visit the rate was 160, accompanied by no bruit or murmur, pulse faintly distinguishable in the tibial artery. No symptoms subjective or objective showed any interference with the normality of the genito-urinary system.

The muscles seemed to do their work as usual, except for the intense lassitude and fatigue.

On walking across the room nothing was to be seen abnormal in the gait, though the motion was very difficult on account of the intense dyspnea. The air-hunger was constantly marked, the upper chest heaving visibly so as to be easily seen through the clothes; the respirations were 70 per minute while sitting at rest. Physical examination of the chest showed nothing irregular in front, but low down behind were some fine mucous rales, probably edematous.

She complained of a sensation of dry burning, and I found a fever of 101 deg. F. She had been sleeping well, though ten hours' rest made not the slightest difference to the swelling anywhere, except in the eyelids, which were usually more puffed in the morning.

Having now gone over the symptoms as thoroughly as possible, I encouraged her to talk a very little. She had been ailing for ten years, having periods of intense anemia, when the legs would swell during the day but would return to their normal size in part, after a period of rest, and were never stony-hard as now. At times the dyspnea was intense, but never so severe as now. This present undoing began about a year ago, when she noticed herself getting exceedingly white and dyspneic; also noticed the eyes puffing some. The skin had never been dry like this before, nor had the hair gotten coarse until last winter. Every bad sign was so very bad that I sent her to bed at once and left her.

As I thought over the case, wondering how any woman could live in such a state as she said she had been in for ten years, I could not see that her anemia could be pernicious. So much of her symptom-story suggested myxedema, that I began to wonder if just at present that phase might not outweigh the pure anemia. At any rate the symmetrical bulkiness of the face associated with the general increase in size in back, arms, and legs, the element of edema being not compressible, and the rapid falling out of the hair, with growing coarseness in what was left, suggested a thyroid complication. Any lessening of mental power noticed was not severe enough to assist in the diagnoses, nor was there any red blotching over nose or cheek.

To what extent irregular thyroid physiology may interfere with blood formation or cause anemia, I could not then nor cannot now say, and it is largely to call out some ideas upon this point that I have spoken of this patient.

Another phase of the case which has interested me, takes us back ten years to the first beginning of this anemia, and may be etiological. This woman took care of her mother who died ten years ago as a result of a very severe ulcering facial epithelioma. For six months it was my patient's duty to dress the sloughing surface, and so marked was the stench that she made a bag to cover her own nose and mouth—a sort of respirator—in which she kept pieces of gum camphor. She assures me that she would be at least half an hour each day for half a year dressing the wound and breathing the camphor fumes, which would often cause her mouth and nose to be quite sore. Her anemia began before those six months had passed.

Very briefly—I sent her to bed under strict hygienic nursing, simple food, fresh juice pressed daily from beef, abundance of fresh air, and daily alcohol baths. Ordered her compound syrup of hypophosphites, with gradually increasing doses of arsenic. Also I began at once the exhibition of thyroid extract.

The improvement has been gradual but sure, and now, though still very weak and anemic, her face, trunk, and arms are perfectly normal and only slight hardness in the legs, the skin being soft and moist, except the leg below the knee.

The points I wish to raise for short discussion are:

1. What influence, if any, does the thyroid body exert in keeping up the normal blood-tone?

2. Was it probable that this grave condition followed the silly use of camphor?

3. Are we justified in thinking of any such case as pernicious?

URINARY ANTISEPSIS IN GONORRHEAL URETHRITIS.

BY E. REINHARDT, M.D., NEW YORK,

Admitting Physician, Lebanon Hospital.

To a great extent the internal treatment of gonorrhea, so popular in former years, has been supplanted by local measures, having for their object the destruction of the gonococcus.   There is no doubt that the expectant policy formerly pursued of waiting for the acute symptoms to subside before resorting to local treatment was responsible for many of these cases assuming a chronic character.   It has often been claimed that if a person suffering from his first attack of gonorrhea is put upon a bland liquid diet, as in other inflammatory conditions, the disease would often be cured without the necessity of resorting to other measures.   However that may be the plan is impracticable in the vast majority of cases.

It seems to me, however, that in the predilection for local remedies the value of conjoint internal treatment is too much underestimated.   Aside from rendering the urine less irritating by the use of alkalies very little attention is usually paid to the above point.   In my recent cases I have endeavored to ascertain what effect upon the gonorrheal process could be exerted by administering an internal urinary antiseptic.   The remedy selected by me for this purpose was the anhydromethylencitrate of hexamethylen-tetramin, known as helmitol.   This drug splits off formaldehyde in the urine, which thus becomes sterilized, and the urine charged with formaldehyde would seem to exert an antiseptic action in its passage over the infected urethral mucous membrane.

One of the great advantages of helmitol is that it can be administered in good-sized doses without fear of disturbing the stomach or of irritating the kidneys, and besides it is very palatable.

Having tested the drug in acute, subacute, and chronic cases of gonorrhea, I have thought it would be of interest to report typical cases of each variety, with a view of illustrating its manner of action and the results obtained.

CASE 1.—C. K., 24 years old, had gonorrhea since August, this being his first attack.   He stopped treatment as soon as the discharge ceased, and experienced no inconvenience until the latter part of November, when he felt a peculiar burning-like sensation in the urethra, and again presented himself.   On examination I found him suffering with a posterior urethritis with involvement of the bladder, as shown by the urine, both specimens being cloudy, but containing no albumin.   Helmitol, 15 grains, was prescribed, four times daily, and the urethra and bladder irrigated with a 1 per cent. solution of protargol. He reported two days later and examination of the urine showed it to be turbid and alkaline. He no longer complained of the burning sensation, and did not have to get up at night to void his urine more than once, while previously he had to do so twice at the least, and sometimes three or four times. The same treatment was continued, and in ten days the turbidity had cleared up entirely, although shreds were still present. Injections of protargol solution, 1 per cent., with Ultzmann syringe, were now made twice a week for four weeks, at the end of which time no gonococci could be found.

CASE 2.—E. P., aged 20 years, contracted gonorrhea about a month ago. He came to me after having tried the prescriptions of various druggists, complaining of a great desire to pass his water, which was very painful. He was compelled to get up at least ten times during the night. The urine was cloudy, containing shreds, and the scanty urethral discharge contained gonococci. Helmitol, 15 grains, was prescribed, four times daily, but on the following day he stated that he had been unable to sleep all night because of the frequent necessity of having to void his urine. After two days' treatment the urine was somewhat clearer, and the frequency of urination was much lessened, although he still had to get up three times at night. Injections of protargol, 1 per cent., were now added to the treatment, and after seven days the tenesmus had completely disappeared. The urine was now fairly clear, but gonococci were still present. The treatment was continued, and at the end of 29 days the discharge had entirely ceased; the urine was free from shreds and no gonococci were present.

CASE 3.—L. B., aged 30 years, had had four previous attacks of gonorrhea, which he claimed to have cured himself with injections of red wine. This remedy, however, proved ineffective in the present attack, and he appealed to me for assistance. He complained of a severe burning sensation when urinating, which he did very frequently. The urine was turbid, with a trace of blood in the second portion. He also had a discharge, which, however, was not marked. Helmitol, 15 grains, four times daily, produced some improvement after 48 hours, and at the end of another two days the urine was much clearer, with no sign of blood, and the ardor urinæ had completely subsided. I now commenced injections of protargol solution, 1:400, and reduced the dose of helmitol to 10 grains, t.i.d. Later the strength of the protargol solution was increased to 1:300 for three days and the helmitol continued. A relapse occurred with considerable ardor urinæ, and on inquiry I found that he had been drinking whiskey. The dose of helmitol was increased to 15 grains, and continued for 48 hours, when the burning had ceased and the urine had become clear, with the exception of some shreds. I now gave injections of protargol,

1:100, continuing the internal treatment, and two weeks later discharged the patient cured. A very satisfactory feature of this case was the rapidity with which the tenesmus yielded to the administration of helmitol, and the rapid disappearance of the gonococci, although it was a marked type of urethritis.

CASE 4.—J. S., aged 37 years, had been suffering for some time from chronic posterior urethritis, with enlarged prostate. The urine was turbid in both portions, but contained no albumin. The treatment consisted of helmitol, 15 grains, three times daily, with posterior injections of a 2 per cent. solution of protargol, later followed by massage of the prostate and the use of electricity. In this case the urine did not become clear until the end of ten days, and it required 40 days for the last remnant of shreds to disappear. The dose of helmitol was diminished to 10 grains at the end of ten days, and the drug continued for a week and a half longer.

CASE 5.—I. R., aged 27 years, presented himself with a severe form of gonorrheal urethritis, complicated with epididymitis and orchitis. Both portions of urine were turbid, and he complained of intense pain when urinating. Owing to the marked vesical symptoms I gave him helmitol, 30 grain doses, t.i.d., with but little improvement until the sixth day, but with entire absence of gastric irritation. At the end of that time the urine was much clearer, and the dose of helmitol was reduced to 15 grains, three times daily. Improvement continued, the burning ceased, and I now began injections of protargol, 2 per cent. solution. The urine, however, did not completely clear up for more than two weeks, at which time there was still present some discharge containing gonococci, which disappeared entirely after three weeks' treatment with protargol solutions.

This case showed that large doses of helmitol had no deleterious effect either on the stomach or on the kidneys.

CASE 6.—K. C. G., aged 42 years, strong, overfed man, widower, had contracted gonorrhea two weeks before. After applying to his druggists without relief, he came under my care, especially because of the severe pain on urinating. Examination of the urine showed it to be very turbid in both portions, containing albumin and a slight trace of blood, shreds, gonococci, and some pus cells, besides sugar. I put him on antidiabetic treatment, and for the relief of the tenesmus gave helmitol 20 grains, four times daily, but without much relief, the urine remaining turbid. Under strict diabetic regimen, however, in connection with the continued administration of helmitol, improvement was noticed at the end of three weeks, and the urine began to clear up. During the second week the dose of helmitol had been increased to 25 grains, t.i.d., and I continued this amount for a week when it was reduced to

20 grains. Four weeks from the beginning of treatment the urine was quite clear, containing only shreds. Helmitol was now discontinued, and injections of protargol, 1 per cent. made. The urine again became cloudy, and helmitol was resorted to, 15 grains, t.i.d., after which it became clear. The gonococci had entirely disappeared at the end of 54 days from the commencement of treatment.

CASE 7.—F. R., aged 37 years, had gonorrhea about eight months ago, for which he was treated, but discontinued his visits to the physician when the discharge stopped. About a month ago he noticed a slight stickiness at the meatus, which developed into a scanty discharge, so that he thought he had contracted another clap. On examination I found the discharge full of gonococci and the urine cloudy. The following prescription was administered: Methylen blue, 1½ grains; copaiba and oleoresen of cubebs, of each 10 grains; three times daily, about an hour before meals. Some improvement was obtained during the first three days after which he had a relapse, with severe scalding of the urine, which became markedly turbid. The capsules were, therefore, discontinued, and helmitol administered in 20 grain doses, four times daily. After three days the urine appeared much clearer, and the ardor urinæ had ceased. At the end of a week the urine was clear, and irrigations with warm permanganate of potash solutions were now begun. Under this treatment progress was slow, the shreds persisting in the urine, and for this reason protargel, 2 per cent. solution was resorted to, with the result that the shreds began to disappear more rapidly, although the case is not yet cured.

POINTS ON ENDOMETRITIS.

The *Clinical Review* of May, 1903, published an interesting article by F. H. Martin, M.D., on endometritis. In outlining the local treatment for uterine engorgement, endometritis and chronic urethritis, the writer believes it well nigh impossible to state definitely where one of these conditions ends and the other begins, so closely are they associated. In discussing treatment, we must consider the condition to be met; the endometrium presenting its varied stages of congestion, inflammation, degeneration of membrane with its putrefactive concomitants, according as types change from acute to chronic. In acute form, the discharge is catarrhal in character, and as the disease becomes chronic, we see the discharge turn to a greenish-brown color, and very offensive. In this stage, frequent hot vaginal douches of Glyco-Thymoline, in twenty-five per cent. strength, to encourage rapid depletion of the membrane, together with rest, will generally suffice. When the chronic stage is met, we must look more carefully into the cause; if displacement is present, it must be corrected, if old lacerations are shown, they must be aided in repair. Dilatation of the cervix will generally show us a turgid congested membrane, thickened from one-eighth to one-half inch by inflammatory process, in varying degrees of decomposition which demands radical treatment. There are those who hold against any local intra-uterine treatment, others disapprove of the curette, but the ideal treatment now recognized generally, is one which promptly rids the cavity of all agents that are producing toxins, the absorption of which might endanger sepsis. To thoroughly remove this broken-down membrane, the curette is used when irrigation will not suffice. The sharp variety is condemned as unnecessary and dangerous. An irrigating curette, with a dull spoon, is acknowledged to be the best. This instrument contains a small cannula which, when attached to a fountain syringe, permits the flow of an antiseptic solution such as Glyco-Thymoline, during the entire operation. The danger of the curette comes largely from the fact that unless used with precaution, it tends to destroy the lymph barrier, or reaction layer, which Nature has erected in her ideal method of combating this disease. Uterine phlebitis is aggravated by the rough use, and at times the walls have been punctured. When sepsis is present the curette is worse than useless.   Depleting antiseptic measures are our only hope.   Glyco-Thymoline used in fifty per cent. strength as an irrigation, rapidly reduces the inflammatory engorgement, checking further absorption of toxins, drawing outwardly through the capillaries the products of inflammation, and exerting a powerful influence in reducing temperature.

In the typical case of endometritis, after thorough curettage, the intra-uterine cavity should be flushed with a fifty per cent. solution of Glyco-Thymoline, and the vagina tamponed with a well-saturated Glyco-Thymoline gauze.   This should be removed in twelve hours, and vaginal douches of twenty-five per cent. Glyco-Thymoline hot ordered three times a day.

PROPRIETARIES.

DURING the meeting of the American Medical Association, held at Atlantic City last June, representatives of the State medical journals conceived and promulgated the idea that mutual interests would be better served, a bond of sympathy and good-will created between themselves, and the profession at large benefited by an association termed " The American Association of State Medical Journals."

One of their number whose bump of wisdom was more normally developed than that of some of those present, succeeded in having final action on the project deferred until the meeting of the A. M. A. at Portland, Ore., next year.

The points of special interest in their declaration of principles are: (1) No journal of this association shall accept an advertisement of a medicine which is not ethical, and " ethical " shall mean that the product advertised must have published with it not only the names of its constituent parts, but also the amount of such constituents, so that a definite dosage can be determined. Further, such product must not be advertised in the secular press, to the laity.   (2) If a product is marketed under a copyrighted name, the manufacturer shall furnish with it the proper chemical name, and if not patented, then also the process of its manufacture. (3) All advertisements not covered by the above paragraphs, or which contain extravagant or improbable claims, shall be submitted to the Executive Committee for approval before they can be accepted.

If the representatives present had any desire or wish for anything further they did not express it, and it is fair to presume that they do not want anything more.   Were an excessive or inordinate desire for gain present they might have demanded a share of stock in each company who patronized them, or levied on a portion of their patrons' receipts—pabulum for the "kitty," as it were—but as nothing of this sort was done, they cannot be accused of having had the slightest mercenary or other improper motives when their declaration of principles was formulated.

If they are ever put into actual operation, the "bond of sympathy" ought to be ordered exceptionally strong, as it is not difficult to foresee that the demands made upon it will be unusually heavy.

There is probably no question but that State medical journals, at least the more influential ones, can be conducted without a loss, without a page of advertising matter, as members of the State associations are in a measure morally bound to pay their subscriptions, if, in fact, the State association does not set aside a dollar or two from the annual dues of the members as a reserve for the expenses of their official organ, but the question of profit had better not be discussed.

It is also true that many independent medical journals could be issued regularly from month to month from the amounts received from subscribers, but it is safe to assume that medical editors and publishers "live not by glory alone," and do, undoubtedly, depend upon the commercial side for their maintenance and profit, to a considerable extent.

Notwithstanding the enormous circulation of some of the great daily papers of our large cities, but a small proportion of the excellent service we all enjoy is due to the amount received from subscriptions, and were it not for the general advertiser, the modern newspaper, with its foreign news department as completely served as its domestic, its elegant press work and fine illustrations, brilliant and lucid editorials, written by men whose salaries run into five figures, would dwindle to a mere job sheet, more despised than read.

As this project is scheduled to lie over until the next annual meeting of the A. M. A., there is ample time for a thorough consideration of the subject, and although no prophet, nor the son of a prophet, we venture the prophecy that its consummation will never be accomplished—unless suicide is contemplated, and that the Executive Committee who are delegated to pass upon the propriety of proposed advertisements, will not be compelled to shorten their office hours, nor curtail their outside work in order to perform their duties.

Medicinal preparations of a proprietary nature possess a distinctive character as marked as that of individuals, due to the process of manufacture and fixed composition. Many of the better known preparations would not suffer by the publication of their exact formulæ, as, for example, when certain complicated laboratory machinery is required for their perfect manufacture, but this is not true of many well-known preparations whose nature is that of a simple compound.

It is, however, also true that if the exact formulæ of certain proprietary remedies were known and taken to a number of skilled pharmacists for compounding, the results would differ in nearly every instance.

A common example is the preparation Essence of Pepsin. Every druggist can make it, and practically all do make it, all perhaps using the standard formula, yet, write ten prescriptions and compare the results! Compound Syrup of Hypophosphites is another example; this preparation can be found on the shelf of every drug store in the country, yet in appearance, taste and action all differ, and in many instances materially.

It is not to be supposed that a preparation can always be duplicated, providing the formula is known, but such a procedure would encourage substitution to an alarming extent, and in this fact lies the greatest danger. While substitution is probably not practiced as generally as some writers would lead one to believe, especially by the retail druggist on individual prescriptions, there is another form of substitution which, while in a sense not deceptive nor fraudulent, is nevertheless an imposition upon the original manufacturer and a source of positive financial loss to him.

This form of substitution is found in the drug stores presumed to be of the higher grade, the store located on the principal street and the most prominent corner. The proprietor has a certain percentage more brains than his up-town or down-town competitor; he has the ability to develop his one-time drug store into a department store with a drug department; he is patronised by the *elite,* and the high-priced doctors send their prescriptions to him for compounding.

Does this druggist substitute? Not much! He has sufficient intelligence to see beyond the extra dime or quarter profit he might make by using a cheap substitute for a high-priced proprietary; he argues that he charges good prices for his prescriptions and can afford to buy all the high-priced chemicals and compounds that the doctor may write for, but his keenly developed mental equipment soon reaches the conclusion that there is a shorter road to wealth than by the prescription, *via* proprietary remedy, route.

By the aid of his knowledge of chemistry and pharmacy, and a few timely hints by the editor of his drug journal, he soon perfects an elegant imitation of a certain proprietary, which, strange to relate, often possesses more virtue and curative power than the original. (?)

He now calls upon Dr. So and So and the others who have favored him with their business, thereby conceding evidence of their confidence in him and mutely acknowledging their belief in his superior ability, and in a few well-chosen words convinces the doctor that it is foolish to pay one dollar an ounce, or one dollar a pint, for a remedy that can be duplicated for less than half the amount, as he supposes. The doctor's attention is called to the fact that he, as an intelligent and educated physician, can, of course, readily see that nothing is gained by adhering to the old and genuine preparation, and the result is, he prescribes the druggist's imitation product more or less afterward. By continual efforts in this direction, worthy of a nobler purpose, doctors are constantly imposed upon through a want of a proper knowledge of the facts, but who believe the statements repeatedly made by the interested parties.

That harm frequently results from lack of precaution on the part of physicians, there can be no doubt, yet, the remedies prescribed are not always absolutely indicated, and in many cases the expected results are not obtained, even when genuine remedies are dispensed, but when this is the case under the best possible conditions, what can one expect from the use of imitations that are known and prescribed as such?

Apart from therapeutic views, it is unfair, venal, dishonest. Persons who further their own interests by appropriating the discoveries of others, and who confiscate the products of the brains of their superiors, are conducting their business along lines which the self-respecting and conscientious physician cannot follow with profit to himself, nor advantage to his patient.

Anything done that will make substitution easy, or which will enable the skilled but dishonest pharmacist to become a party to the deception of physicians, cannot but be looked upon as a step decidedly unwise, and in direct opposition to true progress and meritorious advancement.

The outcome of the plans proposed by the A. of S. M. J. will be watched with interest.—*Albright's Office Practitioner.*

MARTINDALE GOODS NOW PROCURABLE IN TORONTO.

Messrs. The W. Lloyd Wood Co., Toronto, Canadian agents for W. Martindale, of London, England, have received the following shipment of that firm's goods:

Lysoform.—A non-poisonous, non-corrosive antiseptic, which is a powerful deodorant and is stainless. They also have soluble pessaries medicated with Lysoform, solutions of Lysoform toothpaste, mouth-wash and toilet soap.

Unguentum Rusci Co.—A combination of birch tar with cala-
mine and resin ointment, specially indicated in eczema and
psoriasis.

Syrup Iodo-Tannicus, containing two grains of iodine to each
teaspoonful.

Lithion.—A granular salt, being a combination of lithium
citrate, magnesium sulphate and sodium sulphate.

A full assortment of the well-known Martindale sterules have
arrived. The assortment consists of atropine sulphate, one per
cent.; cocaine hydrochlor, two per cent.; dionin, one per cent.;
adrenalin, 1 in 1,000; pilo-carpine nitrate, two per cent.; protargol, ten per cent.

They are also supplied with a full assortment of oculist bottles,
sterile bandages, gauze and wool tissues, hygienic moss towels
and moss felt dressings.

Physicians can procure any of the above goods by telephoning
Main 1361,' or their prescriptions can be filled at cor. Gerrard and
Church Streets, Toronto.

WHY I GIVE PREFERENCE TO BUFFALO LITHIA OVER OTHER MINERAL WATERS.

BY VALDEMAR SILLO, M.D., PH.G.

WHILE I was a student in Bellevue Hospital Medical College
some fifteen years ago, such frequent reference was made to
Buffalo Lithia Water by the teachers and lecturers in the various
departments of that institution, that when I began the practice
of medicine later on, I regarded that water as one of our most
valuable therapeutic agents. And many years of active practice
have only served to confirm this high opinion of the many virtues
and make its place more permanent in my medical armamentarium.

In the earlier years of my practice many old " chronics " fell
to my lot, as in the experience of every beginner. Many of these
cases were the victims of chronic, articular, and muscular rheumatism and gout. Of course, they " had been the rounds of the
doctors," who had put them through the usual course of salicylates,
iodides, etc., with indifferent results.

From the very beginning I put these cases on Buffalo Lithia
Water, instructing them to drink it freely day and night, " as
much as they could hold." Some of them drank a full half-
gallon in every twenty-four hours. The only other treatment was
an occasional laxative, with specific directions as to diet and
exercise. As the specific action of this water is a little bit slow at

the beginning of its use, I had considerable difficulty in keeping some of my cases "up to their drink." The results in this class of ailments were all that could be desired, and I soon found my waiting-rooms filled with a most desirable class of patients.

The excellent effects of Buffalo Lithia Water in rheumatism and gouty conditions seem to be due to its diluent and eliminating properties. It seems not only to eliminate from the system all traces of uric and lactic acids, but it also prevents the formation of these substances by "beginning at the Beginning," and correcting all errors of digestion and assimilation. In fact, its action evidently extends throughout the alimentary tract as well as to the liver, kidneys and skin.

Its decided action on the stomach and its secretions, as is evidenced by its excellent effects in gastro-intestinal dyspepsia, should secure for this water a high place in the estimation of any intelligent practitioner of preventive medicine. It neutralizes excessive acid secretions before and during the taking of food, and in the various stages of digestion, thereby rendering the latter physiological process easy of accomplishment. It also undoubtedly stimulates the secretions in the alimentary tract immediately below the stomach, thereby stimulating intestinal digestion and assimilation.

By the employment of no other therapeutic agent have I been able to secure such permanent and lasting benefits in renal, hepatic and urinary calculi, as by the liberal use of Buffalo Lithia Water. These calculi seem to become porous, break down or disintegrate and pass out through their normal exits under the action and influence of this water.

Indeed, I have had many cases of urinary calculi, where it seemed nothing short of the knife promised relief, yield promptly to this water, and pass *via* the urethra in the form of a fine sand, which could be detected only by a most careful examination. In these cases the irritation and inflammation due to the presence of calculi in the bladder rapidly subside and leave the patient wholly comfortable and able to enjoy a much-needed and most refreshing sleep.

Equally satisfactory results are also secured by the free use of this water in the most violent attacks of kidney colic. I always urge my patient to drink freely of the water, as hot as he can take it, in the earliest stage of attack; the kidneys are quickly flushed, the parts are gently relaxed, and the calculus is soon forced from its lodgement in the ureter and carried into the bladder where it is rapidly disintegrated and soon voided.

In catarrhal conditions of the bladder, whether due to calculi, gonorrheal or catheter infection, or other causes, I have found Buffalo Lithia Water an indispensable remedy; in fact, I give it the preference over all other therapeutic agents, and it never fails me. It quickly relieves the distressing symptoms, such as irritability and tenesmus, and enables the organ to throw off and expel any pus, calculi or other detritus which may be present and responsible for the painful disturbance.

In Bright's disease it seems to give relief by its gentle but positive action on the kidneys, promoting a flow of urine and carrying off dropsical effusions. It diminishes the quantity of albumin and the number of granular and hyaline casts and gives tone and energy to the kidneys, thus affording positive relief to the patient. And while I am not prepared to state positively that it will cure this disease, I am satisfied that it would, in many cases, if administered in its early stages, arrest it entirely and prolong the life of the patient for many years.

In the albuminuria of pregnancy, I have used Buffalo Lithia Water with remarkably good effect. It is my habit to give the water freely during the last half of the gestation period and thus ward off albuminuria, but if I am asked to take charge of a case in, say the seventh or eighth month, and find albuminuria present, I proceed to administer the water in liberal quantities and keep it up until every trace of albumin has disappeared. In this way I always avoid puerperal eclampsia and bring my patient through a safe and easy delivery. Under no other conditions in the practice of medicine is it more important to resort to preventive measures and agencies than during the period of gestation and confinement, hence I would urge my professional brethren to see to it that Buffalo Lithia Water is kept in the home of every pregnant woman, and freely used by her during this important period. Not only will it insure her against puerperal eclampsia, but it will also prevent the nausea and vomiting of pregnancy and many of the smaller ills peculiar to that interesting period.

The extraordinary therapeutic and eliminative value of Buffalo Lithia Water in typhoid fever has long been appreciated by the medical profession in this country. I am not prepared to say whether the water exerts a germicidal influence in this disease, but we do know that it soothes the inflamed glands and holds the temperature in check while the process of repair is facilitated throughout the length of the small intestine. It also allays thirst and stimulates the kidneys, skin, and other excretories, thereby ridding the system of the many waste elements peculiar to this disease. I always allow my typhoid fever patients to drink this water ad libitum.

In the earlier years of my practice I learned the value of Buffalo Lithia Water in pneumonia, having been taught to administer it, with fresh milk, for the purpose of nourishing and sustaining the strength of my patients throughout the entire course of this distressing and trying malady. It seems to assuage the thirst and control the temperature, as in typhoid. I find that the good effects obtained by a liberal use of this water, in the various conditions which I have attempted to describe, are permanent and lasting.—*Mass. Medical Journal.*

THE IMPORTANCE OF CAREFUL GENERAL PREPARATION OF THE PATIENT FOR SURGICAL OPERATION.

DR. AUGUSTIN H. GOELET, of New York, in a paper read by invitation at the sixth annual session of the Tri-State Medical Association of the Carolinas and Virginia, at Danville, Va., Feb. 24th, 1904 (*International Journal of Surgery,* May, 1904), says that, unless immediate operation is imperative and will not permit delay, no surgical procedure of any importance should be undertaken without sufficient preparation to secure normal activity of the intestinal tract and to restore normal action of the liver, kidneys and skin; also, that it is the surgeon's duty to minimize the risk of his operations, as well as the anesthetic, and this cannot be done without the most careful preparation of the patient.

He lays stress particularly on the importance of re-establishing normal activity of the liver, which, if properly done, improves nutrition and does away with the intestinal distention so often a hindrance at the time of operations within the abdomen, and which is a source of so much discomfort during convalescence. This, he contends, cannot be accomplished with one or two doses of calomel or the cathartics usually employed.

The importance of testing for and recognizing the presence of bile in the urine as a guide to the proper functionating of the liver is particularly emphasized, and he does not consider the patient ready for operation as long as there is a trace of bile in the urine, since this shows that it is not being discharged normally into the intestinal tract, but is being absorbed into the circulation and is being eliminated by the kidneys.

For restoring functional activity of the liver he employs Sulpho-Lythin, a sulpho-phosphate of sodium and lithium, which, he says, is the most satisfactory and reliable hepatic stimulant he has found. It does not irritate the intestinal mucosa, and does not cause depletion, and may be given continuously without injury.

Careful regulation of the diet, baths and exercise, he regards as important essentials also in the preparation for operation.

The Canadian
Journal of Medicine and Surgery

J. J. CASSIDY, M.D.,
EDITOR.
43 BLOOR STREET EAST, TORONTO.

W. A. YOUNG, M.D., L.R.C.P.LOND.,
MANAGING EDITOR.
145 COLLEGE STREET, TORONTO.

Surgery—BRUCE L. RIORDAN, M.D.,C M., McGill University; M D University of Toronto; Surgeon Toronto General Hospital; Surgeon Grand Trunk R.R.; Consulting Surgeon Toronto Home for Incurables; Pension Examiner United States Government; and F N. G. STARR, M.B., Toronto, Associate Professor of Clinical Surgery, Toronto University; Surgeon to the Out-Door Department Toronto General Hospital and Hospital for Sick Children.

Clinical Surgery—ALEX PRIMROSE, M.B., C M. Edinburgh University, Professor of Anatomy and Director of the Anatomical Department, Toronto University; Associate Professor of Clinical Surgery, Toronto University; Secretary Medical Faculty, Toronto University.

Orthopedic Surgery—B. E. MCKENZIE, B A., M D., Toronto, Surgeon to the Toronto Orthopedic Hospital; Surgeon to the Out-Patient Department, Toronto General Hospital; Assistant Professor of Clinical Surgery, Ontario Medical College for Women; Member of the American Orthopedic Association; and H. P. H. GALLOWAY, M D., Toronto, Surgeon to the Toronto Orthopedic Hospital; Orthopedic Surgeon, Toronto Western Hospital; Member of the American Orthopedic Association.

Oral Surgery—E H. ADAMS, M.D, D.D.S, Toronto.

Surgical Pathology—T. H MANLEY, M D., New York, Visiting Surgeon to Harlem Hospital, Professor of Surgery, New York School of Clinical Medicine, New York, etc, etc

Gynecology and Obstetrics—GEO T MCKEOUGH, M D, M.R C S Eng., Chatham, Ont; and J. H LOWE, M.D., Newmarket, Ont

Medical Jurisprudence and Toxicology—ARTHUR JUKES JOHNSON, M.B., M R C S. Eng; Coroner for the City of Toronto; Surgeon Toronto Railway Co, Toronto; W. A. YOUNG, M D, L.R.C.P. Lond.; Associate Coroner, City of Toronto.

Pharmacology and Therapeutics—A. J. HARRINGTON M.D, M R C S.Eng, Toronto

Medicine—J J. CASSIDY, M D, Toronto, Member Ontario Provincial Board of Health; Consulting Surgeon, Toronto General Hospital; and W. J. WILSON, M D. Toronto, Physician Toronto Western Hospital.

Clinical Medicine—ALEXANDER MCPHEDRAN, M D., Professor of Medicine and Clinical Medicine Toronto University; Physician Toronto General Hospital, St Michael's Hospital, and Victoria Hospital for Sick Children.

Mental and Nervous Diseases—N. H. BEEMER, M. D., Mimico Insane Asylum, CAMPBELL MEYERS, M.D., M.R C S.. L R C P (London, Eng), Private Hospital, Deer Park, Toronto; and EZRA H. STAFFORD, M.D

Public Health and Hygiene—J. J CASSIDY, M D., Toronto, Member Ontario Provincial Board of Health; Consulting Surgeon Toronto General Hospital; and E. H. ADAMS, M D., Toronto.

Physiology—A B EADIE, M D., Toronto, Professor of Physiology Woman s Medical College, Toronto

Pediatrics—AUGUSTA STOWE GULLEN, M D., Toronto, Professor of Diseases of Children Woman's Medical College, Toronto; A. R GORDON, M D., Toronto.

Pathology—W H PEPLER, M D., C.M., Trinity University; Pathologist Hospital for Sick Children, Toronto; Associate Demonstrator of Pathology Toronto University; Physician to Outdoor Department Toronto General Hospital; Surgeon Canadian Pacific R R, Toronto; and J. J. MACKENZIE, B.A., M.B, Professor of Pathology and Bacteriology. Toronto University Medical Faculty.

Ophthalmology and Otology—J M. MACCALLUM, M.D., Toronto, Professor of Materia Medica Toronto University; Assistant Physician Toronto General Hospital; Oculist and Aurist Victoria Hospital for Sick Children, Toronto

Laryngology and Rhinology—J D THORBURN, M D., Toronto, Laryngologist and Rhinologist, Toronto General Hospital.

Address all Communications, Correspondence, Books, Matter Regarding Advertising, and make all Cheques, Drafts and Post-office Orders payable to "The Canadian Journal of Medicine and Surgery," 145 College St., Toronto, Canada.

Doctors will confer a favor by sending news, reports and papers of interest from any section of the country. Individual experience and theories are also solicited   Contributors must kindly remember that all papers, reports, correspondence, etc., *must be* in our hands by the fifteenth of the month previous to publication.

Advertisements, to insure insertion in the issue of any month. should be sent not later than the tenth of the preceding month. London, Eng. Representative, W. Hamilton Miln, 8 Bouverie Street, E. C. Agents for Germany Saarbach's News Exchange, Mainz, Germany.

VOL. XVI.   TORONTO, DECEMBER, 1904.   NO. 6.

Editorials.

THE SURGICAL TREATMENT OF GOUT.

PROFESSOR RIEDEL, of Jena, reports in *Deutsche Medicinsche Wochenschrift,* two cases of gout, which he treated by surgical operations.   The first occurred in 1882, the patient, a previously healthy man of forty-five, being attacked with acute inflammation of the metatarso-phalangeal joint of the right great toe.

6

The patient had passed the day previous to the attack, afoot, in hunting, and the seizure occurred during the succeeding night. As there was a slight hallux valgus of the joint and no history of disease in it before, Professor Riedel made a diagnosis of acute suppuration of the bursa over the joint of the great toe, with which it might have a communication. After removal to an hospital, the patient was operated on for removal of the diseased bursa. Incision of the skin failed to disclose the presumed serous bursa, and incision of the subjacent tissues opened up the articulation, which presented the typical appearance of a gouty joint: deposits of urates in the joint, with tophi encrusted on its capsule.

After recovering from his astonishment, Professor Riedel curetted away the urates, which were not deeply attached to the articular surfaces, and, in order to clean the joint, extirpated the articular capsule, removing, at the same time, some tophi, which surrounded the sesamoid bones at the base of the first phalanx of the great toe. The wound was not closed. On the same evening the patient was free from fever and pain. The surgical wound healed in a few weeks. This patient's after-history is interesting from a medical standpoint. He never had another attack of podagra; neither did he have pain in the joint which had been operated on. The joint also acquired a certain degree of mobility. In the year 1896, fourteen years after the operation, he contracted an arthritis of the vertebral column, and died in April, 1897.

The second case was a lady seventy years of age, who was attacked suddenly, for the first time, with severe pain and the other signs of inflammation, in the right great toe. Professor Riedel recognized the gouty nature of the attack, but, nevertheless, opened the affected joint, removed the urates, and extirpated the synovial sac, as well as an existing serous bursa. The operation wound healed perfectly. The patient lived eight years longer, and died of an affection of the aorta, without having had a second attack of gout in the foot.

Professor Riedel does not go so far as to declare that podagra should be handed over to the surgeon. He thinks that, as a gouty effusion into a joint is an aseptic arthritis, and the joint of the great toe is easily reached, a case of effusion into this joint might be treated by the knife. He even thinks that ablation of the capsule of the affected joint ought, *a priori,* to protect the patient from a relapse. Furthermore, even if a prolapse should occur, nothing, in his opinion, should prevent the surgeon from venturing on a fresh incision into the joint, inasmuch as this operation gives the patient a respite from podagra of several years' duration.

In Professor Riedel's first case, the fact that the patient did not have a recurrence of podagra, during the remaining fourteen years of his life, would seem to prove that he had been cured of gout. Although it is not mentioned in the record, a carefully regulated diet and other appropriate precautions may have helped to produce this result. However, the fact that the patient died of an arthritic disease of the spinal column requires explanation. The pathology of this attack is not mentioned, but the history of gouty disease in other patients induces one to surmise that it may have been of gouty origin. Thus Leube says, " Pains radiating from the vertebral column, as the results of gouty spondylitis (especially of the cervical vertebræ), or of a secretion of urates into the membranes of the spinal cord, have been noted in some rare cases."

In reference to Professor Riedel's female patient, who, after the arthrectomy had been done, lived eight years, without experiencing a second attack of podagra, and died of aortic disease, it is quite probable that the fatal disease was, also, in her case, of gouty origin. Leube states that " vascular changes of an atheromatous nature occur even in youthful persons who suffer from gout."

A surgeon adopting Professor Riedel's procedure would be obliged to attack the metatarso-phalangeal joints of both great toes, as gout appears in either foot, attacking the right foot when the left is relieved, and *vice versa.* Besides, although a painful affection, gout in a foot does not disable a patient for so long a period as a gouty neuritis of the lumbar plexus of nerves, and is less dangerous than a gouty arthritis of the spinal column.

Why the urate salts are attracted from the blood to the joints, etc., and deposited there, has not yet been explained. In atypical gout, affecting the stomach, heart, or brain, practitioners have endeavored, with more or less success, to relieve the patient by derivative measures, with the expectation of causing the malady to appear in a foot. Nature expels tophi to the helix of the ear, and sends urates to the foot, where they do not threaten the

sufferer's life. Were Professor Riedel's method generally adopted,
one metatarso-phalangeal joint would be safe from a second attack
of gout, at the expense of some mobility, but its fellow of the
opposite side would still be in peril, not to mention the ankle and
knee-joints, as well as the nobler organs of the body, the invasion
of which by gout leads to fatal results.

. It seems, therefore, that a gouty patient should seek safety
in a carefully regulated diet, methodical stimulation of the excre-
tory organs, and the avoidance of physical and mental over-work,
rather than in an operation which does not cure gout, although
it may prevent its reappearance in the joint upon which an
arthrectomy has been done.   J. J. C.

OLIPHANT NICHOLSON'S VIEWS ON THE TREATMENT OF PUERPERAL ECLAMPSIA.

THE views of Oliphant Nicholson on the cause and treatment of
puerperal eclampsia appeared in the *Journal of Obst. and Gyn.*,
July, 1902. The author contended that the principal symptoms
of the eclamptic state can be explained in terms of thyroid inadequacy. The thyroid gland is enlarged in normal pregnancy, but
this enlargement can be diminished or prevented by giving thyroid
extract. A larger supply of iodothyrin is needed in the pregnant than in the non-pregnant state. Lange observed that
albuminuria and eclampsia occurred in twenty out of twenty-
five cases in which the usual thyroid hypertrophy of pregnancy
did not occur. In the *International Medical Annual* for 1904,
p. 305, appears a *résumé* of Nicholson's views, as given by
Fothergill:

"It is generally agreed that the eclamptic symptoms are
dependent upon an autointoxication, and it may be assumed that
iodothyrin is essential to the efficient working of all the parts of
the defensive mechanism. Iodothyrin favors metabolism and
increases the excretion of urea. In eclampsia this is strikingly
diminished. Owing to a deficiency of iodothyrin, it is thought,
the metabolism of nitrogenous substances stops short of the formation of urea, at a point where the products are highly toxic.
The clinical features of a typical attack of eclampsia resemble

those of complete athyroidea, as caused by the removal of the thyroid gland in animals. Eclampsia may thus be regarded as a temporary athyroidea. The resulting toxemia may be slight or severe, short or prolonged. While the athyroidea lasts, the liver and the other organs cannot make urea for the kidneys to excrete, but instead, nitrogenous substances are only turned into toxins, which injure the kidney, and cause various other lesions and symptoms.

"Many cases, doubtless, occur, in which the poisons are formed, but in which the kidneys, though injured, remain able to defend the organism from profound intoxication. The principal way in which thyroid inadequacy may affect the renal function and produce eclampsia is by setting up a prolonged spasm of the renal blood vessels. Hence the curative effect of thyroid extract would be explained by its vaso-dilator and diuretic action. Thus iodothyrin may be regarded as a diuretic. Again, urea, for the formation of which an adequate supply of iodothyrin is necessary, may be regarded as the diuretic *par excellence*. It is evident that the real significance of the pre-eclamptic state is that it points to a breakdown of some part of the defensive mechanism. Furthermore, this breakdown is the result of some inadequacy of the thyroid and parathyroid glands, whereby the process of nitrogenous metabolism, instead of resulting in the formation of urea, ceases with the production of intermediate substances, which, when absorbed, excite the symptoms of a toxemia. In this way the degree of toxemia of pregnancy comes to be dependent, directly or indirectly, upon the quantity and activity of the thyroid secretion."

Nicholson treated successfully four cases of puerperal eclampsia with thyroid extract, artificial evacuation of the uterus not being required.

Dr. Baldowski reports two cases of puerperal eclampsia treated by him with thyroid extract, and he confirms the view that thyroid extract is an effective remedy for such cases (*Vratch Gazette,* 1904, t. xi., p. 31).

In his first case, an attack of eclampsia began in a multipara who was in the seventh month of pregnancy. On the first day of the attack, the doctor prescribed four tablets of thyroid extract (each containing 0.30 gm.), as well as narcotics. The convulsions ceased.   Treatment was continued for two days longer (two tablets a day), and the patient recovered.   After two weeks' time this patient had a return of the convulsions, which, however, yielded to the employment of thyroid extract.

In the second case, a primipara at full term, eclampsia appeared at the beginning of labor.   In this case Dr. Baldowski administered thyroid extract *alone*.   The convulsions ceased after two tablets (0.30 gm.) had been used, and before the rupture of the bag of waters had taken place.   The accouchement took place without any further casualty, and the after treatment presented nothing unusual.

Compressed tabloids of thyroid gland, each of which is equivalent to five grains (0.324 gm.), are procurable from the pharmacists. To men who have seen an undelivered primipara die of eclampsia, in spite of the efforts of several enlightened accoucheurs, Nicholson's views, as confirmed by Baldowski, are very instructive.

J. J. C.

" THESE ARE ALL HONORABLE MEN."

Havergal College, 354 Jarvis Street.
Toronto, October 24th, 1904.

Dr. MacCallum, 13 Bloor Street W., Toronto.

Dear Sir,—Mr. —— has asked that his daughter, ——, may be under your treatment twice a week for some time.   We can, I think, arrange this, subject to the usual condition that a discount of ten per cent. is deducted by the College off fees charged to the pupils.

Faithfully yours,
Edith A. Nainby.

Toronto, October 31st, 1904.

Dear Madame,—I have delayed answering your note *re* Miss ——, and what you term the usual condition.

I have never attended patients under any such condition. Will you be so good as to give me the names of some professional men who have attended the pupils of Havergal Hall under this condition, so that I may talk the matter over with them.

Yours truly,

Miss Edith A. Nainby,   James MacCallum.
Havergal Hall, Jarvis Street, City.

HAVERGAL COLLEGE, 350 JARVIS STREET.
TORONTO, NOVEMBER 1ST, 1904.

Dr. MacCallum, 13 Bloor Street W., Toronto.

DEAR SIR,—Your letter of the 31st ult. has been entered at the office. As Miss —— is the only pupil who will attend you from the College, your name will not be entered on the Staff of Specialists in connection with the College, and, therefore, the question of discount does not apply to your case.

Faithfully yours,
S. S. HENDERSON,
Bursar.

TORONTO, NOVEMBER 4TH, 1904.

S. S. Henderson, Esq., Bursar of Havergal Hall.

DEAR SIR,—Your note of November 1st received. Let me point out that it is a question not of discount to the pupil, but of commission demanded by Havergal College from physicians because the patient happens to be a pupil in that school.

No other school in Toronto—and I have had patients from them all—has made such a proposal. Of course, you inform the parents of your pupils that in case of illness the pupil will be sent to Dr. A——, because he gives Havergal College a commission, and that you do not recommend Dr. B——, because he does not give a commission.

No reputable physician will so far forget himself as to receive or give a commission, or employ runners or touts, even in the guise of the authorities of Havergal College.

I would have preferred to talk the matter over quietly with the physicians who have given commissions to the College, but your failure to give me their names forces me to make this matter public, and it now becomes my unpleasant duty to bring to the attention of the profession and of the College of Physicians and Surgeons of Ontario the fact that such unprofessional and reprehensible practices exist in connection with Havergal College and its staff of specialists.

Truly yours,
JAMES MACCALLUM.

The above correspondence is startling in the loudness with which it speaks for itself.

Only yesterday we read in a newspaper that the " tipping " system was going out of fashion in old London. Let us hope that the next good ship that ploughs the ocean may bring the tidings here, and that those who constitute themselves the Boards of management presiding over the instructors and instructresses of the sweet Toronto girl graduates may accept the dictum, retire from the gaze of the public and be replaced by others possessed of dignity unmarketable—others who have been long enough in their early days in the school of refinement where strictly ethical dealing was taught, and in whose spelling-book such old-fashioned words as " generosity " found a place. Even a strange old story about a costly box of ointment, broken and spilled by a maiden long ago, was deemed a commendable action, and gentlewomen reigned supreme at the heads of the young ladies' seminaries in the days of our mothers. Now, over many of these scholastic institutions, Boards of control, composed of all sorts of business men, preside, we understand, and in this strenuous age every effort is made to turn in money to the institutions. The motto seems to be: " Young ladies, make a dollar squeal, and we, your guardians educationally, will show you how we try to replenish the coffers of the college by getting a ' rake-off ' here and there—it's business, you know !"

This aspect of the question is hardly within our province to discuss, so we just make these few remarks, based on the policy pursued by the management of Havergal Hall, according to the letters printed above. But one point in this " pretty state of things " is very much our affair. As medical men, and as a medical journal that feels, as all our Canadian journals do, that we stand for the respectability of our noble profession, painful as our task is, we must ask, Who are the black sheep among our Toronto physicians who are accepting such an offer, and handing in a percentage of their fees to this seat of learning? From the correspondence in our hands we must infer, for we have to believe our eye-sight, that there are some of our medical men on a special staff of medical attendants, who charge the parents a regular fee and then hand out a portion of it as a " tip " to the College, who in its lofty capacity as bell-boy has rendered them the unthankable service of calling them in to see a patient.

Are any of our medical men in a state of starvation, that they have to resort to an almstaking of a half loaf? Physicians who compromise themselves by such exchange of bribes have no right to drag down the status of all others, and here we demand, for the sake of the gentlemen who worthily bear the insignia of Medical Doctors in our city, that these misguided men, who unthinkingly, or for want of innate refinement, have seen nothing amiss in their action of lowering themselves and accepting such an indignity, now make the *amende honorable* by sending in their names for publication (lest the innocent be left to suffer for the guilty), with the brief, but eloquent prefix, " We regret—."

W. A. Y.

EDITORIAL NOTES.

The Canada Thistle Causes Irritation of the Skin by Its Presence in Underwear.—In mid-October, when Canadians begin to put on heavy woollen underwear, physicians are consulted for sudden attacks of irritation of the skin. The parts of the body principally affected are the hypochondriac, lumbar, or umbilical regions. The affected skin is hyperemic, looking like the condition observed in erythema, and there are itching and burning sensations. In some individuals it resembles an eruption of hives limited to a certain' region. The limbs are not much affected, the greatest irritation being observed about the waist. The patient tries baths and soothing lotions; but, with each recurring morn, his skin irritation returns and the cure seems as distant as ever. Assuming that his gastro-intestinal system needs attention, he takes a few matutinal doses of Epsom salts, fortified by the cotemporaneous use of Psychine and the local application of Pond's Extract. All in vain. Finally he consults a physician. Recognizing from the history of the case the presence of a source of irritation, which is renewed during the day, the physician proceeds to scrutinize the victim's underwear. Placing the articles in a good light, he discovers a black, fine, hair-like body, closely wound around and dipping in among fibres of wool, offering a strong contrast to the latter on account of its color, and in new, unwashed garments, by its firm, straight outline. This body is the far-famed Canada thistle, the process of manufacture having failed to remove it from the fleece used in making the woollen yarn from which the underwear is manufactured. Found in expensive suits of woollen underwear, as well as in the cheaper kind, it plagues the wearer badly when first worn; not so badly if worn during a second season, because many of the thistle fibres become detached during the destructive operations of the machine laundry or the milder vibrations of the domestic one. As long, however, as the thistle remains in the underwear it is a hidden bur : " *Haeret lateri lethalis arundo.*" The cure of the patient's trouble consists in substituting cotton for the woollen article, or in carefully dissecting out the thistle fibres from the woollen underwear.

Notice Should be Given of Typhoid Fever.—The fact is being emphasized every month that there exists an almost entire disregard for those sections of the Ontario Public Health Act which require that notice should be given of each and every case of typhoid fever. By Section 86, the householder is required to give notification, and by Section 87, the physician is also required to notify. The local Board of Health, through either its Health Officer or Secretary, should provide each medical practitioner with six blank forms upon which to report any case. (See By-law 17, Ontario Health Act.) The placarding of houses infected with typhoid fever is not thought necessary, but notification of all cases of typhoid fever should be sent by the proper persons to the local Boards of Health, and the latter should advise the Provincial Board of Health, in order that early enquiries may be instituted to discover the cause of the outbreak, chiefly the investigation of water and milk supplies; that, preventive measures may be adopted ; and that intelligent statistical facts may be obtained as to prevalence, type, mortality, etc.

Tram-Cars as Hygienic Agents.—In the *Indian Lancet* of September 5th, we notice that a regularly-running electric tramway service has been established in Calcutta. The editor says: " It has been distinctly proved that the electric spark, which is so frequent an occurrence to the overhead trolley, and the emission of light from the car wheel when the rail is used for the return current, transforms the oxygen of the air into ozone. The high discharges, it is said, are frequent enough to influence greatly the atmospheric constituents. Especially where the line passes through narrow thoroughfares, they become antiseptic agents." In reading these lines commendatory of tram-cars, which we in Toronto merely regard as a convenience for rapid transportation, one is reminded of the fortunate hygienic circumstances which surround our lives in this northern land. We do not remember, in the course of our reading, to have seen any allusion to what the editor of the *Indian Lancet* says, although electric tram-cars have been running in this city for twelve years. Not that we doubt the truth of the assertion, that the electric sparks which fly from the trolley pole and car wheel tend to ozonize the air and thereby exercise an antiseptic power destructive of infectious microbes. A good system of street sweeping, and a regularly-working corps of scavengers, who with carts remove all refuse from lanes, streets and byways; a good system of house-cleaning and ventilation, with properly inspected plumbing; a pure water supply all seem to Canadians to be of the greatest importance in the conservation of public health and in preventing the inroads of infectious disease. So much so, indeed, that if these agencies were wanting, the swift-running electric tram-car, though it spurted sparks day and night, would not materially lessen the mortality roll in Toronto. From the melancholy fact that scarcely a week passes that we do not read of a death or severe injury, caused by the operation of these Toronto tram-cars—a child or an elderly person run over, a passenger thrown violently on to the pavement in alighting from a tram-car—many citizens do not look upon the trolley tram-car with favor. In counting up the undoubted advantages of the electric tram-car and offsetting them against the evils it inflicts, one should not forget the aseptic influence of the electric sparks.

Bulletin No. 99, Tea.—This bulletin, issued from the laboratory of the Inland Revenue Department, Ottawa, contains the cheering information that the tea used throughout Canada is genuine. There are slight differences in the specific gravity of ten per cent of each sample. For instance, sample of black tea, No. 25,182, purchased at Toronto, shows a specific gravity of 1.0125, while sample of black tea, No. 25,184, also purchased at Toronto, shows a specific gravity of 1.0117. No. 25,182 shows a total ash of 5.10 per cent, and No. 25,184, 5.80 per cent. The botanical examination, however, shows that both are genuine, the former containing large, broken tea-leaves, and the latter tea-leaves and stems. That out of seventy-five samples of tea purchased in different parts of Canada, over a range of territory extending from Halifax, N.S., to Winnipeg, Man., not one should be adulterated, is reassuring. The laboratory of the Internal Revenue Department, Ottawa, deserves great praise for its useful and instructive analysis.

Fatal Poisoning from Shoe-Blacking.—In the *Journal of the American Medical Association,* Oct. 1, 1904, W. J. Stone, B.Sc., M.D., reports a case of fatal poisoning due to skin absorption of liquid shoe-blacking. The patient had soaked the cloth uppers of his patent leather shoes with a polish in which pure nitrobenzol nearly equalled the total amount of blacking used, had put on the shoes before they were dry, and danced in them at a party the same evening. At 12.30 a.m. he began to feel ill, and died in collapse at 4.45 a.m. the same morning. Subsequent enquiry revealed the following facts: The young man on the evening of the dance above-mentioned, had applied a liquid shoe-blacking to the tan cloth uppers of a pair of shoes, which were black patent leather lowers with tan cloth tops. These shoes were worn at the dance. The cloth uppers absorbed enough of the blacking to entirely cover up the tan color, and, moreover, since the shoes were put on before the tops were dry, to stain his feet and ankles black. A chemical examination of three drams of the liquid shoe-blacking, secured from the coroner, showed an amount of pure nitrobenzol, nearly as much as the total amount of blacking received. The shoe tops were also extracted with solvents, and marked traces of nitro-benzol were obtained. Nitrobenzin (or nitrobenzol, $C_6H_5NO_2$) is used as a cheap solvent for anilin dyes and as a flavoring or odoriferous agent, under the name of "Essence de Mirbane," in cheap soaps, perfumes and confections. The conditions present in this case were such as to permit of absorption by the skin. The shoes were put on before the blacking was dry, and shortly afterwards the exercise incident to dancing probably aided its absorption. Nitrobenzol is probably used as a solvent for the anilin dyes in many liquid shoe-blackings on the market. Why fatal poisoning is comparatively so rare among shoe-blacks is not quite clear. Perhaps but extremely small quantities are absorbed, and the absorption extends over a considerable time. The use of nitrobenzol in shoe-blacking, in perfuming soap and as a flavoring agent should be prohibited.

Death from Asphyxia in the Sarnia Tunnel.—October 9th three train-men perished from asphyxia in the Sarnia Tunnel. They were endeavoring to get a broken freight train through the tunnel, and while doing so were exposed for a short time to the inhalation of noxious gases, which accumulate in the tunnel as the result of the combustion of coal in locomotives. A coroner's jury, having investigated the affair, brought in a verdict reflecting on the Grand Trunk Railway Company for its inadequate equipment to secure ventilation, and urging a more thorough investigation with a view to the prevention of like accidents hereafter. The medical evidence given at the inquest contended that the deaths were due to the effects of carbon dioxide. No post-mortems were performed, it being said that " the cause of death was obvious." This latter statement would require verification before it would carry conviction. How did the medical witnesses know that death had been caused by carbon dioxide? Might it not have resulted partly or wholly from carbon monoxide? A post-mortem would have thrown light on this chemical question.   " The blood of those asphyxiated by carbon monoxide is persistently bright red in color. . . . If a solution of caustic soda of sp. gr. 1.3 be added to normal blood, a black, slimy mass is formed, which, when spread on a white plate, has a greenish-brown color. The same reagent, added to blood altered by carbonic oxide, forms a firmly clotted mass, which, in thin layers upon a white surface, is bright red in color. (" General Medical Chemistry," Witthaus.) Both these gases result from the combustion of coal, only that carbon monoxide results when the access of air to the blood is limited, as in a confined place. If the deaths of the train-men were due to carbon monoxide, then the obvious influence would be that the supply of pure, new air to the St. Clair Tunnel is deficient in quantity, so much so that coal fires burn blue and give off the deadly carbon monoxide when trains are passing through the tunnel.   Carbon monoxide is an odorless gas, but exceedingly poisonous. Witthaus says that " An atmosphere containing but a small proportion of this gas produces asphyxia and death, even if the quantity of oxygen present be equal to or even greater than that normally existing in the atmosphere; 0.5 per cent. of carbon monoxide in air is sufficient to kill a small bird in a few moments, and one per cent. proves fatal to small animals." The presence of a large proportion of carbon dioxide gas in the Sarnia Tunnel would seriously modify the air there, not only by the addition of a deleterious gas, but by the simultaneous removal of an equal quantity of oxygen. As carbon dioxide and carbon monoxide are regularly produced by passing locomotives and imprisoned in the

Sarnia Tunnel, the escape of passengers using the tunnel from asphyxiation is probably due to the rapid transit of the trains. Arrest of a train in the tunnel through any cause would, therefore, be a serious misfortune. Probably the most thorough way of preventing a catastrophe in the future would be to provide electric motor cars at each end of the tunnel for the haulage of all trains, thus doing away with the production and retention of the deleterious gases of combustion in the tunnel. Should the use of ordinary coal-burning locomotives be continued, suitable ventilation of the tunnel, such, for instance, as is used in the ventilation of mines, should be provided and kept continuously in operation.

J. J. C.

PERSONAL.

DR. ALLAN SHORE has removed from 176 St. George Street to his new address, 425 Bloor Street West, corner Robert Street.

TYPHOID FEVER.

THE following comprises a circular recently sent out by the Secretary of the Ontario Provincial Board of Health as to the law compelling physicians to notify the local Board of Health as to any cases of typhoid fever under their care:

The fact is being more emphasized each month that there exists an almost entire disregard for those sections of the Public Health Act which requires that each and every case of typhoid fever (enteric) should be notified.

The sections of the Act relating to the notification of this disease are as follows:—

" 86. Whenever any householder knows that any person within his family or household has the smallpox, scarlet fever, diphtheria, cholera or typhoid fever, he shall (subject in each case of refusal or neglect to the penalties provided by sub-section 2 of section 115), within twenty-four hours give notice thereof to the local board of health, or to the medical health officer of the district in which he resides; and such notice shall be given either at the office of the medical health officer or by a communication addressed to him and duly mailed within the time above specified, and in case there is no medical health officer, then to the secretary of the local board of health, either at his office or by communication as aforesaid. R. S. O., 1887, c. 205, s. 77.

" 89. Whenever any physician knows that any person whom he is called upon to visit is infected with smallpox, scarlet fever, diphtheria, typhoid, or cholera, such physician shall (subject in each case of refusal or neglect to the penalties provided by sub-section 2 of section 115), within twenty-four hours give notice thereof to the local board of health, or medical health officer of the municipality in which such diseased person is, and in such manner as is directed by Rules 2 and 3 of Section 17 of Sched. B., R. S. O., 1887, c. 205, s. 80."

It is, therefore, quite evident that the Public Health Act requires that both the householder and physician in charge of a case of typhoid fever, shall notify the local health authorities of each case within twenty-four hours, and for this purpose it is the duty of each local Board of Health, through either its Health Officer or Secretary, to provide each medical practitioner with six blank forms upon which to report any case. See By-law 17.

The fact that it is statutory to report all cases of typhoid fever does not imply that it is necessary to placard the house in which it exists, for, according to the same By-law, Rule 4, placarding is only required for scarlet fever, diphtheria, smallpox, cholera or whooping-cough; and this precautionary measure is one that may not be resorted to by local Boards of Health—indeed, it is quite obvious that the Provincial Board of Health did not deem such to be necessary; but what it does desire is the systematic notification of all cases of typhoid fever, first to the local authorities, and second ·by the local boards to the central authority, for the following reasons:

First,—That enquiries may be instituted early to discover the cause, chiefly the investigation of water and milk supplies.

Second,—That preventative measures may be adopted.

Third,—That intelligent statistical facts may be obtained as to prevalence, type, mortality, etc.

Medical Health Officers, Boards of Health and physicians generally are reminded that samples of water are examined free in the provincial laboratory, and for this purpose properly sterilized bottles can be secured by application to Dr. J. A. Amyot, Bacteriologist of the Board; and to assist physicians in the early diagnosis of cases, samples of blood should be forwarded for the purpose of making the Widal test.

MEDICAL SCIENCE ADVANCE.

Dr. J. J. Cassidy spoke on the advancement of medical science before the Unitarian Club at their recent annual meeting at Webb's. President H. W. Brick was in the chair. Dr. Cassidy dealt entertainingly and informingly with the subject, and at the close of his address was plied with various questions on medical matters from the club, all of which he answered authoritatively.

Regarding the antiquated treatment of a wound received on the field of battle, the speaker traced the career of the great Ambroise Pare, who began life as a barber-surgeon, and before many years startled the savants of France with his works upon the treatment of wounds from arquebus, dart or arrow, published by the University of Paris. He dissented from the cauterizing of wounds with a hot poker, and from the treatment of plunging the injured member into boiling oil to allay hemorrhage. In 1552 he first used the ligature for this purpose, the usefulness of which was universally acknowledged.

Up to 1839 the search for surgical anesthesia was considered a chimerical pursuit. To Americans belonged the honor of the discovery of ether, the greatest anesthetic, the first practical demonstration of its efficacy being given by Dr. Morton, in 1846, at the Boston General Hospital.

Soporifics, such as belladonna, henbane and poppy, were used in early times. Mention is made of some such agents in Shakespearo's "Romeo and Juliet," in "Cymbeline," and in one of Middleton's tragedies. Alcohol may also have been used. Nitrous oxide—laughing gas—was successfully used as an anesthetic by Horace Wells, a dentist of Hartford, Connecticut, in 1844. Chloroform, discovered by Guthrie, at Sackett's Harbor, N.Y., in 1831, was first used as a surgical anesthetic by Sir James Simpson, an Edinburgh physician, in 1847. Although cocaine, which was introduced into medical practice by Karl Koller, in 1884, is a reliable local anesthetic, its use should always be surrounded by great restrictions.

The following officers were elected: President, H. W. Brick; Vice-President, D. J. Howell; Secretary-Treasurer, J. A. Wells; Executive Committee, A. Horton, A. W. Kinzinger, Dr. Swan (ex-officio), W. B. Campbell.

THE SANITARIUM BUILT AT WESTON.

THE Sanitarium for Consumptives which the National Association has created near Weston has been finished, and is now open for patients.

The situation is an ideal one, on a high bluff above the Humber River, approached from the Weston car route, and it includes about thirty-seven acres of land, which formed part of the extensive Buttonwood farm.

As you approach it by the long lane leading from the cars to the Humber and enter the gate, before you stands a large white rough-cast building, with a timbered tower at one corner, and a wide verandah in front, that is so imposing as to deserve the statelier name of "loggia," just as all our graperies since the World's Fair of 1894 have been called "pergolas." One is rather amazed to see about a dozen or so ex-street cars standing about in various places, having very evidently outlived their first use, but quite capable of an extended life in another capacity. Several of these are ranged parallel to the pavilion, a large one-storied dormitory for men, and are connected with it by a platform which runs the length of the building and cars. Each car will furnish a suite of two rooms to a patient. In the smaller of the two, which serves as bedroom, the windows have been replaced by canvas. The larger serves as a sitting room, and opens on to the platform. In winter each will be heated by a little stove, and the occupant will be " monarch of all he surveys."

The pavilion, which is a new structure, is spotless within, in green and white, and has its own lavatory and other appointments. Outwardly, it is white rough-cast, like the house, from which it is separated by a few feet of lawn. The house is the original farm house, with its French windows, old fireplaces, and thick walls, and it has been considerably added to for its present pur-poses. A large wing on the left provides a second men's dormi-tory, and above gives accommodation for the women's dormitory, and a number of single bedrooms. On the right the rooms added include downstairs the doctors' consulting room, the drug depart ment, and the throat room In the main and older part of the house downstairs there are two cheerful sitting-rooms, opening into one another, furnished with mission style furniture, the back one for the present also serving as office. The patients' dining-room, the staff dining-room, the pantries and kitchen, take up the remainder of the room downstairs; upstairs are rooms for the staff. Everywhere is the warm brown of bare floors, spotless white walls, and plenty of windows opening out on wide stretches of green in the front, or overlooking the lovely Humber valley at the back. The house is so placed that sunshine and air are on every side; the verandah accommodation is ample; for fresh air, good food, and rest play a most important part in the treatment.

Every attention has, of course, been paid to the sanitary con-ditions of the building. A windmill supplies abundance of water from the Humber, and is to be supplemented by an electric motor. A septic tank disposes in the most scientific way of the sewage. Electric light and telephone connection with the city go to make the appointments most complete.

The attention of the visitor is called to the old stone sundial on the lawn, not as having " anything to do with the case," but merely as an interesting reminder of days and ways long gone by. Perhaps, too, it will harmonize well with the occupation of those who come to this place, seemingly so remote from hurry and business. Here one may get the time freshly measured by the sun, instead of doled out automatically by a circular bit of mechanism. Sometimes, to be sure, the dial will get ahead of the little machine, and sometimes it will lag behind, but what of that, to one whose aim is not so much to accomplish a given task, as to so live that he may again feel the tide of life strong in his veins?

A remark of one of the officials struck the visitor very much when going through the building, and might be repeated for the benefit of others. Some one had said to him that there must be great danger in the hospital to those in good health, to all of which he quite agreed. " Yes, there is a good deal of danger in

a home of this kind," he said, slowly, " but there is a good deal
more outside of it. Here we take every possible care and pre
caution. Outside, in the city, the dust is laden with germs; you
are shut up with them in the street cars. You breathe them in
public assemblies, and those contaminated have no consideration,
often, for others. If there is danger here, it is doubled, quad-
rupled away from here."

PAN-AMERICAN MEDICAL CONGRESS.

THE Fourth Pan-American Médical Congress, which will convene
in Panama the first week in January next, bids fair to be a most
delightful mid-winter trip. The delegates will leave this country
by the Atlantic, Pacific and Gulf Coasts the last week in December.
They will return by the same routes, or will make round trips.

The Public Health Association will take place on the following week in Havana, and those desirous of attending both meetings
can arrange to do so.

There are two routes for the physicians to take from Panama
to Havana. The first is by way of Jamaica to Santiago de Cuba
by boat, and overland by rail to Havana. The second is by water
from Panama to Vera Cruz and from there to Havana. The
former will probably be the most pleasant trip.

From Havana, the return trip can be made directly north to
New York by water, or. *via* Miami or Tampa, Florida, or new
Orleans. The connections and dates of sailing are now being
arranged.

The Panamanian Government has appropriated $25,000 for
the Scientific Session and the entertainment. The Congress will
be held from the 2nd to the 6th of January. The afternoons will
be devoted to the Scientific Sessions and the mornings and evenings
to trips and social functions. So far as can be learned, the programme in Panama will be a reception on the first day by President Amador, of the Panama Republic, and the formal opening
session of the Congress the same evening. On the second day, an
excursion to the Canal in the morning, meeting of the various
sections in the afternoon, and a banquet in the evening. On the
third day, an excursion down the Bay to Taboga Island, where a
Panama breakfast will be served, scientific sessions in the afternoon, and a ball in the evening. On the fourth day. an excursion
to the U. S. Army barracks in the morning, section meetings in
the afternoon, and the formal closing session in the evening. On
the fifth day, an excursion to the plantation of the United Fruit
Company, and on the afternoon of this day, those of the con-
gresistas who'intend going to Cuba to attend the meeting of the

Public Health Association, will sail for Jamaica, while those who intend going by way of Vera Cruz, or returning home by way of New Orleans or New York, will remain until the following Tuesday.

The Secretaries of the Sections of the Congress for the United States are: Drs. A. II. Doty, of New York, Hygiene and Quarantine; Judson Daland, of Philadelphia, Medicine; R. Matas, of New Orleans, General Surgery; Bert Ellis, of Los Angeles, Eye; Hudson Maknen, of Philadelphia, Throat; Frederick Jack, of Boston, Ear; C. H. Hughes, of St. Louis, Nervous Diseases; Geo. Goodfellow, of San Francisco, Military Surgery; John Ridlon, of Chicago, Orthopedic Surgery; D. W. Montgomery, of San Francisco, Dermatology; C. G. Kerley, of New York, Pediatrics; Noble P. Barnes, of Washington, Therapeutics; Walter Chase, of Boston, Pathology.

Communications from physicians in the United States, interested in these branches, can be sent directly to these different Secretaries. Delegates intending to attend the Congress, desirous of obtaining information concerning it, should communicate with the Secretary of the International Executive Committee in the United States.

THE GYNECOLOGICAL IMPORTANCE OF PROLAPSED KIDNEY.

In a paper presented at the annual meeting of the New York State Medical Association, October 17th to 20th (*Medical Record,* October 22nd, 1904), Dr. Augustin H. Goelet, of New York, shows conclusively that the prolapsed kidney is an important etiological factor in producing and maintaining pelvic congestion and diseases of the female pelvic organs arising therefrom. He points out that constriction of the waist by the corset or clothing forces the misplaced kidney back upon the ovarian vein, as it ascends along the spine, causing compression and hence obstruction to the return circulation from the pelvis. The importance of recognizing this condition in gynecological cases is emphasized, and the diagnosis must be incomplete otherwise.

He cites cases to show that many needless operations on the pelvic organs may be done if this condition and its relations thereto is not recognized.

Restoration of the kidney to its normal position is, he believes, the essential object of the operation for fixing the kidney, and unless this is accomplished, the patient is often left in a worse condition than before.

Patients, he finds, are often given an erroneous idea of the gravity of the operation by those who do not understand it. He contends that the operation has no mortality, since he has completed a series of 197 consecutive nephropexies, without a death, in 47 cases fixing both kidneys at the same time.

THE WELLCOME PHYSIOLOGICAL RESEARCH LABORA- TORIES AT THE ST. LOUIS EXPOSITION, 1904.

THE anti-serums exhibited in the upper portion of the case form part of a long series. Diphtheria Antitoxic Serum and Anti-Streptococcus Serum had their beginnings in the earliest days of serum therapy. These laboratories were pioneers in the production of these serums in the British Empire, and it is believed that the first anti-diphtheritic serum used in America was produced in this institution.

The series includes, as a special feature, an anti-serum for a particular case of malignant endocarditis. It was prepared by injecting under the skin of a donkey cultures of a streptococcus obtained from the blood of a woman suffering from this disease. The patient was subsequently treated by subcutaneous injections of the serum, which was produced to meet her particular case. This course was taken in view of the special difficulty in the case of bactericidal serums of knowing whether the microbe in the tissues of the patient belongs to the same variety as that used in obtaining the serum.

As a further special feature in connection with anti-serums, products are shown, in another part of the case, obtained by fractionation of diphtheria antitoxic serum. Comparing equal bulks, these fractions contain not more than the quantity of proteid in the original serum, but twice the quantity of antitoxin. The importance of these products lies in the fact that the toxic effects sometimes observed after the injection of horse serum are due not to the antitoxin, but to products which are found in normal serum.

An Anti-Typhoid Serum is shown which has some special features described in the *Lancet* of October 3rd, 1903. The particular point of interest is that the normal bactericidal power of the blood is used to dissolve the bacteria, and thus, if possible, liberate any intracellular toxins. The toxins so prepared are then used for the immunisation of a horse.

A series of preparations is shown illustrating a research on the lesions produced in animals by the micrococcus obtained from patients suffering from acute rheumatism. The research is described in the *Journal of Pathology and Bacteriology* for December, 1903. The preparations shown illustrate the fact that the lesions occurring in man can be reproduced in animals by inoculation with this micrococcus.

The following is a list of the specimens in the case illustrating the various lesions:

62	Acute rheumatism—endocarditis, aortic and mitral valves—heart		rabbit
66	"	endocarditis, right ventricle	"
67	"	endocarditis, mitral valve	"
68	"	early endocarditis, mitral valve	"
69	"	mitral valve and left auricle	
70	"	hemorrhagic nephritis	
71	"	extensive endocarditis, mitral valve	"
72	"	early endocarditis	
73	"	dilation, right ventricle	
74	"	knee joint	
75	"	shoulder and elbow joints	
76	"	knee joint	
77	..	"	early nutmeg liver	..

This series of products is a representative collection of the constituents of blood and their chief decomposition products. It seemed desirable to make this collection complete in order to bring out the relations of its most noteworthy specimens, the various proteid constituents of blood. These proteid bodies are in a state of great purity and represent distinct compounds in the blood when tested by their physical properties.

Seventeen specimens in the case illustrate these bodies; they are numbered:

22 Fibrin, clot, in water
23 Fibrin, similar clot, dried
24 Fibrinogen solution, coagulated
25 Fibrinogen, solution
26 Fibrinogen, powdered
27 Fibrinogen, flakes
28 Fibrinogen, suspension in water
37 Electrolytic proteid, dried
38 Electrolytic proteid, suspension in water
39 Albumin solution, coagulated by heat
40 Albumin, solution in water
41 Albumin, crystalline
42 Globulin solution, coagulated by heat
43 Globulin, dried powder
44 Globulin, dried, flakes
45 Globulin solution, in sodium chloride
46 Globulin, suspension in water

The various pigments are also interesting, and in the series exhibited it is possible to trace the chemical connection between the hemoglobin of the blood, the bile pigments of the liver, and the urochrome of the urine.

Specimens of thyroid and suprarenal bodies are shown. The well-known physiological action of the internal secretion of these organs is further illustrated by " Hemisine," a preparation of the active principle of the suprarenal bodies.

"Hemisine" is a derivative of the suprarenal gland, possessing powerful hemostatic and other properties. This product is dry, stable and soluble.

Tracings are shewn illustrating the extraordinary potency of "Hemisine." When only 1-20000 gramme of "Hemisine" is injected into the circulation of one of the smaller mammalia a well marked rise of blood pressure takes place. "Hemisine" also has a local constricting action when directly applied to the smaller blood vessels.

Tracings are exhibited showing the physiological properties of the active principle of these drugs. Attention is drawn to the marked slowing action of strophanthus on the rhythm of the heart.

Often, in pharmacological research, the amount of active principle which is available is very small. This method is peculiarly useful owing to the fact that the determination can be carried out with very moderate quantities of the substance. It differs considerably from existing methods, and depends on the comparison of the vapor-pressures of two solutions, one of which is prepared from a standard substance of known molecular weight, while the other is that of the substance under investigation.

It possesses the following advantages:

a. It can be carried out at the ordinary temperature, or at a higher or lower one.

b. The solvent employed need not have either a definite boiling point or a definite melting point; hence it need not be pure.

c. Determinations can be made with very small quantities of the substance (50 milligrammes or less).

The margin of error is slightly greater than with the Beckmann method (usually 5-10 per cent; yet the method is sufficiently accurate for the selection of the proper formula from among those suggested by the results of analysis.

The Committee on Awards at the Exposition conferred upon the Wellcome Chemical Research Laboratories a grand prize and three gold medals in recognition of the educational value of the researches conducted in these Laboratories. The Committee also awarded Messrs. Burroughs, Wellcome & Co. two additional grand prizes for their exhibit of "Wellcome" brand chemicals, "Tabloids," and other pharmaceutical products and medical equipments.

ITEMS OF INTEREST.

An Honor Conferred upon W. R. Warner & Co.—The Grand Prize for pharmaceutical preparations exhibited at the Louisiana Exposition, St. Louis, Mo., which closed on November 30th, was awarded to the well-known firm, W. R. Warner & Co., Philadelphia, Pa., an honor which we feel sure was but deserved.

Do You Wish to Sell Your Practice?—When a physician desires to sell his property and practice, it is of first importance that it should be done with as little publicity as possible; hence, the sale and purchase of medical practices forms an important department of medical affairs, and one that nearly all physicians find necessary to use at some time or other. Appreciating the needs of the profession in this line, Dr. W. E. Hamill has for ten years been perfecting a system which we consider almost faultless as to efficiency, promptness and secrecy, and we cordially recommend Dr. Hamill as an expert in this line, and advise our readers to take advantage of his ripe experience when they think of selling their practices. See list of practices for sale by Dr. Hamill among our advertising pages.

Postponement of Historical Medical Exhibition.—Mr. Henry S. Wellcome, of London, England, writes us as follows: The response to the announcement of the proposed Historical Medical Exhibition has been beyond my expectations, and this, together with the many valuable suggestions received from leading members of the profession and the trade, at home and abroad, has prompted me to considerably widen its scope. The extent of the work involved renders it impossible to fix a definite date for the exhibition until a later period, announcement of which will be duly made. Although in one sense I regret this delay, it will, on the other hand, enable me to make the exhibit more comprehensive and complete, and to include many objects of exceptional interest that have been promised me from different quarters of the globe.

The New York School of Clinical Medicine announces the following changes in faculty: General Medicine—Professors Wm. Brewster Clark and Henry Lawrence Schively; Associate Professors Thos. M. Acken and Edw. L. Kellogg. General Surgery—Professor Simon J. Walsh and Associate Professor J. Cameron Anderson. Gynecology—Professors Augustin H. Goelet and A. Ernest Gallant. Pediatrics—Professors Dillon Brown and Henry Comstock Hazen. Nervous and Mental Diseases—Professors J. Arthur Booth and Emmet C. Dent. Gastro-Intestinal Diseases—Professor Robert Coleman Kemp. Ophthalmology and Otology—Professors John L. Adams and Geo. Ash Taylor. Dermatology—Professor Robert J. Devlin. Laryngology and Rhinology—Professor Max J. Schwerd. Orthopedic Surgery—Professor Homer Gibney. Hydrotherapeutics—Professor Alfred W. Gardiner. Genito-Urinary Diseases—Professors Wm. K. Otis, Walter Brooks Bronner and John von Glahn. Pathology—Professor E. H. Smith. The facilities of the School have been materially enlarged.—John L. Adams, M.D., Secretary.

The Physician's Library.

BOOK REVIEWS.

Encyclopedia Medica. Vol. XIV. Index volume. Under the general editorship of CHALMERS WATSON, M.D. Edinburgh and London: William Green & Sons. Canadian agents: J. A. Carveth & Co., Toronto.

The editor and publishers are to be congratulated on the completion of this very useful work. As has been said in the review of the various volumes as they appeared, many of the articles are exceedingly good, and none of them are below a fair standard.

There are very few omissions to be noted in the work, so that one may consult it with pretty fair assurance that he will find something on the subject on which he is seeking light. The work is especially useful to the general practitioner, as it deals with the practice of medicine and surgery generally.

This volume consists of over 280 pages of indices that are very full, rendering reference to any subject quite easy. One need have no hesitation in recommending it to any practitioner.

A. M'P.

A Hand-Book of Surgery. For Students and Practitioners. By FREDERIC R. GRIFFITH, M.D., Surgeon to the Bellevue Dispensary, New York City; Assistant Surgeon at the New York Polyclinic School and Hospital. 12mo volume of 579 pages, containing 417 illustrations. Philadelphia, New York, London: W. B. Saunders & Co. 1904. Flexible leather, $2.00, net. Canadian agents: J. A. Carveth & Co., 434 Yonge St., Toronto.

Dr. Griffith has given us a little work of some merit. It is a brief outline of the principles and practice of surgery, written as concisely as is possible with clearness. We are sure it will be of some value, alike to the student and the practitioner, because the entire subject of surgery is covered, including all the specialties, as diseases of the eye, ear, nose and throat; genito-urinary diseases; diseases of women, etc. There are also articles on life insurance, rape, sexual perversion, microscopy, and on many other subjects of great importance to the practising surgeon. There are 417 illustrations, selected for their clearness, accuracy and general usefulness. The book-making is excellent, and the publishers are to be congratulated upon the style and general get-up of the work.   F. N. G. S.

Saunders' Question Compends, No. 7.—Essentials of Materia Medica, Therapeutics and Prescription Writing. Arranged in the form of questions and answers. Prepared especially for students of medicine by HENRY MORRIS, M.D., Fellow of the College of Physicians of Philadelphia; Associate Member of the Association of Military Surgeons of the United States; Member of the American Medical Association, etc.   Sixth edition. Thoroughly revised by W. A. BASTEDO, PH.G., M.D., Tutor in Materia Medica and Pharmacology at Columbia University (College of Physicians and Surgeons) New York; Assistant Attending Physician to the Roosevelt Hospital Dispensary and to the Vanderbilt Clinic.   Philadelphia, New York, London: W. B. Saunders & Co.   1904.

That the " Question Compends " are invaluable to the student of medicine is beyond dispute, as, since the issue of the first volume of the " Saunders' Question Compends " over 240,000 copies of these unrivalled publications have been sold.   The present, or sixth, edition, although retaining the original classification and arrangement, has been brought up-to-date, and some of the chapters have been re-written and much useful information added on the action of opium, alcohol, antipyrin, mercury, formaldehyde, etc.   A. J. H.

Medical Electricity.   A Practical Hand-book for Students and Practitioners. By H. LEWIS JONES, M.A., M.D., Fellow of the Royal College of Physicians; Medical Officer in charge of the Electrical Department in St. Bartholomew's Hospital, London; President of the British Electro-therapeutic Society; Honorary Fellow of the American Electro-therapeutic Association; Member of the Société Francaise d'Electrotherapie et de Radiologie. Fourth edition, with illustrations.   London: H. K. Lewis, 136 Gower Street, W.C.   1904.

We have frequently referred, and with advantage, to the pages of the third edition of Dr. Jones' book on medical electricity, which appeared in 1900, and now feel agreeably surprised at the evidences of increased growth in the fourth edition of the same work.   In addition to the revision of the subject-matter, much new material has been added.

As the author says, " Medical electricity will continue to advance with the advance of general electrical knowledge.   To those who have followed its developments, the progress achieved in the past decade is enormous. The house-to-house distribution of electricity, by electric light companies, has called into existence a large number of new instruments and methods, by providing a constant and steady supply of current without the need of batteries."

The general effect of static treatment is interestingly described, the statement being made, on the authority of Vigouroux, that this kind of treatment is useful even in certain forms of insanity and morbid mental states, particularly in melancholia. In the nervous disturbances which occur about the time of the menopause, decided benefit may be obtained from simple static charging with the use of the negative breeze. Even if a physician should not employ electrical apparatus in his practice, such a book affords, at a small outlay, very instructive reading. The book is well printed and bound. J. J. C.

The Practical Application of the Roentgen Rays in Therapeutics and Diagnosis. By WILLIAM ALLEN PUSEY, A.M., M.D., Professor of Dermatology in the University of Illinois, and EUGENE WILSON CALDWELL, B.S., Director of the Edward N. Gibbs X-ray Laboratory, University and Bellevue Hospital Medical College, New York. Second edition, thoroughly revised and enlarged. Octavo volume of 690 pages, 182 illustrations, including four colored plates. Philadelphia, New York, London: W. B. Saunders & Co. 1904. Canadian agents: J. A. Carveth & Co., Limited, 434 Yonge St., Toronto. Cloth, $5.00 net; sheep or half-morocco, $6.00 net.

That a second edition of this work should be necessary in little more than a year from the appearance of the first, speaks well for the popularity of the book and attests a widespread and earnest quest for authentic and authoritative teaching concerning the X-ray. The literature of the past year has been reviewed, histories of cases have been extended to the present year, and much new matter added, so that about one hundred pages additional appear in this volume. The copious use of photographs illustrating different stages of treatment is a very valuable feature. A fair and conservative estimate of the present status of the X-ray in diagnosis and therapy is given. The statement that there is nothing thus far to give us any inkling as to whether the induction of artificial fluorescence of tissues in connection with raying, as suggested by Morton, is of any value or not will be challenged by many observers, and will probably be modified in a future edition. The description of apparatus and its management is very full and satisfactory. This handsome volume should find its way to the library of every practitioner interested in the X-ray and its developments. C. R. D.

Old Gorgon Graham. More Letters from a Self-Made Merchant
to His Son. By GEORGE HORACE LORIMER. Toronto: Wm.
Briggs, Publisher.

Those who read the first letters of Old Gorgon Graham to his
son have been awaiting the " some more " now published. Sound
philosophy, in the guise of humor, abounds throughout the series
of letters.

The reader has the added pleasure of a former acquaintance
with the old man's style of diction, the reading of the letters is
a few hours' amusement that should not be missed.

Just a quotation or two that may remind one of a friend of
auld lang syne: " Some men are like oak leaves that don't know
when they are dead, but still hang right on." Who does this cap
fit among the notables of our profession? " A broad-gauged merchant is a good deal like our friend Doc Graver, who'd cut out
the washerwoman's appendix for five dollars, but would charge
a thousand for showing me mine—he wants all the money that's
coming to him, but he really doesn't give a cuss how much it is,
just so he gets the appendix."   W. A. Y.

Guide to the Examination of the Throat, Nose and Ear. For
Senior Students and Junior Practitioners. By WM. LAMB,
M.D., C.M., Honorary Surgeon, Birmingham Ear and Throat
Hospital. London: Bailliére, Tindall & Cox. 1904. Crown
8vo. 5s. net.

The title gives a very good idea of the scope of this little book,
but it is full of just the things which the beginner needs. It is
a judicious mixture of methods of examination, gross appearances and diagnosis.   J. M.

*Essentials of Nervous Diseases and Insanity: Their Symptoms
and Treatment.* By JOHN C. SHAW, M.D., late Clinical Pro-
fesser of Diseases of the Mind and Nervous System, Long
Island College Hospital Medical School. Fourth edition,
thoroughly revised. By SMITH ELY JELLIFFE, PH.G., M.D.,
Clinical Assistant, Columbia University, Department of
Neurology; Visiting Neurologist, City Hospital, New York.
12mo volume of 196 pages, fully illustrated. Philadelphia,
New York, London: W. B. Saunders & Co. 1904. Canadian
agents: J. A. Carveth & Co., Limited, 434 Yonge St., Toronto.
Cloth, $1.00 net.

This is the fourth edition of one of those valuable little books
that contain so much in such a small space. The whole edition
has been revised in such a way that it has been found necessary
to recast the work completely. In this way our present knowledge

of this important subject is thoroughly brought out. The subjects are grouped in such a way as to show the natural relations which exist between certain nervous disorders. This arrangement should overcome to a great extent many of the difficulties which present themselves to every student in the study of neurology.

In the section on disorders of the mind, the general views of such leading psychologists as Ziehen, Weygandt, Kraepelin, Berkeley and Petersen have been carefully weighed.

The book is one well worthy of recommendation and will be found exceedingly valuable to the general practitioner as well as to the student. A. J. J.

The Nutrition of the Infant. By RALPH VINCENT, M.D., Member of the Royal College of Physicians of London; Physician to the Infants' Hospital; late Senior Medical Officer, Queen Charlotte's Lying-in Hospital. Second edition, revised and enlarged. London: Bailliére, Tindall & Cox, 8 Henrietta St., Covent Garden.

The work is carefully prepared, showing wide reading and careful observation on the part of the author. "The Bacteriology of Milk," and "The Functions of Bacteria in Relation to Digestion," are exceedingly interesting and instructive chapters. The gastro-intestinal diseases are dealt with fully, concisely and rationally, and with the subjects, marasmus, rachitis and scurvy the work is a valuable one on infant dietetics. It is well bound, the type good, and the work altogether very acceptable. A. R. G.

Lectures on Clinical Psychiatry. By DR. EMIL KRAEPELIN. Authorized translation from the German. Revised and edited by THOMAS JOHNSTONE, M.D., M.R.C.P.(Lond.). London: Bailliére, Tindall & Cox. Canadian agents: J. A. Carveth & Co., Limited, 434 Yonge St., Toronto, and Chandler & Massey Limited, Toronto.

These most excellent studies in clinical psychiatry will be warmly welcomed by all interested in mental diseases, and as a genuine aid to the busy general practitioner, they deserve the highest commendation.

Dr. Kraepelin, who is known to all alienists as one of the brightest minds in the particular branch of medicine to which he has devoted himself, has given to the profession in this book an extremely scientific and well-written treatise in the form of clinical lectures.

There is no wide variation from the grouping of mental diseases, as laid down by many of the authorities of the present day, but what strikes one is the evident desire of the author to so study the symptomatology of these morbid conditions that each one stands out as an almost pathological, as well as clearly defined (in most cases), clinical entity.

The history of each case is succinctly given, the diagnosis and prognosis are carefully discussed, and, what is eminently to be admired, the further progress of the case for some years noted, and the condition at this time recorded.

The practical importance of the study of mental diseases to the general physician has induced the author to consider the subject in the form he has chosen, and the remark in the introduction that insanity, even in its mildest forms, involves the greatest suffering that physicians have to meet, is now being fully recognized by the profession in general.

The translation has been well done, and the printing and binding reflect every credit on the publishers. D. C. M.

Elementary Practical Physiology. By JOHN THORNTON, M.A., author of " Elementary Physiography "; Head-master of the Municipal Secondary School, Bolton. With 187 illustrations. London, New York and Bombay: Longmans, Green & Co., 39 Paternoster Row. 1904.

This work has been prepared for the use of beginners in the study of anatomy and physiology. It is adapted for senior pupils in Public Schools and for pupils in High Schools. It contains a large number of illustrations, some of them in colors, and many of them are excellent.

Directions are given for practical exercises in examining the organs, such as the heart, lungs, kidneys and so on, of the sheep, rabbit and other small animals. These exercises should be very helpful where the teachers and pupils prepare the specimens properly and study them carefully. On the whole, it is a very excellent little work for beginners. The price of this book is 3s. 6d. A. E.

The Art of Compounding. A Text-Book for Students and a Reference Book for Pharmacists at the Prescription Counter. By WILBUR L. SCOVILLE, PH.G., formerly Professor of Theory and Practice of Pharmacy in the Massachusetts College of Pharmacy; Member of the Committee of Revision of the United States Pharmacopeia. Third edition, revised and enlarged. Philadelphia: P. Blakiston's Son & Co., 1012 Walnut St. 1904.

While this book is intended for students and pharmacists, and to whom it must prove invaluable, it will be a very welcome addition to the library of the country doctor who is forced to do his own dispensing. We speak from long experience of this kind, and many times would have been thankful for the information and help found in this volume. The whole subject of compounding is very carefully considered in sixteen chapters. Every form of mixture, powder, emulsion, confection, pill, capsule, lozenge, suppository, ointment or external preparation is considered, and minute instructions given so as to produce the best result, both from a therapeutic and esthetic standpoint. We have no hesitation in recommending this work to the student, the pharmacist, or the dispensing physician.   w. j. w.

Blakiston's Quiz Compends. A Compend of Medical Latin Designed Expressly for Elementary Training of Medical Students. By W. T. St. Clair, A.M., Professor of the Latin Language and Literature in the Male High School of Louisville, Kentucky; author of "Cæsar for Beginners," "Notes to Cæsar's Gallic War, Book Three," etc. Second edition, revised. Philadelphia: P. Blakiston's Son & Co., 1012 Walnut Street. 1904.

This will prove a very useful little book to the student of medicine, and, in fact, to many practitioners, as well, giving, as it does, the "fundamental principles upon which the medical language is built." It is absolutely essential for everyone intending to study medicine to have first a minute knowledge of Latin, as so many of the terms and phrases used are in, or derived from, that language. This compend will be most useful towards this end.

Diseases of the Nervous System. By F. Savary Pearce, M.D. New York and London: D. Appleton & Co.

This little work, written for the medical student and general practitioner, is nothing if not comprehensive. Consisting of less than four hundred pages, it covers the immense field of organic and functional nervous disorders, and space is still found to devote a large share to the treatment of functional diseases, which is of much value in some of these very perplexing cases.

Hydro-therapeutic measures, as well as the movements in massage, are so fully detailed that the student, for whom the text is intended, can easily grasp the main essentials. The therapeutic worth of faradic, galvanic and static electricity also receives careful consideration.

The book is divided into sections, and briefly covers the ground very well. It should find favor with the busy practitioner as a handy book of reference, and its brevity and lucid description of nervous disease will commend it to all.

The illustrations, many of which are colored, are excellent, both in regard to their selection and finish, and the entire work makes one keenly regret that the author, at so early an age, has been prevented from continuing the good work he so ably began, as he had intended publishing a similar treatise on mental diseases.

The publishers have performed their share of this book in a most creditable manner.   D. C. M.

Saunders' Question Compends, No. 3: Essentials of Anatomy. Including the Anatomy of the Viscera, arranged in the form of Questions and Answers, prepared especially for Students of Medicine. By CHARLES B. NANCREDE, M.D., Professor of Surgery and of Clinical Surgery in the University of Michigan; Emeritus Professor of General and Orthopedic Surgery, Philadelphia Polyclinic; Senior Vice-President of the American Surgical Association; Corresponding Member of the Royal Academy of Medicine, Rome, Italy; Member of the American Academy of Medicine, etc. Seventh edition thoroughly revised. Philadelphia, New York, London: W. B. Saunders & Co. 1904.

The fact that this small work has reached its seventh edition indicates that there must be a large demand for a condensed treatise on anatomy, from which all but essential descriptive matter has been judiciously eliminated. The book must be regarded as one particularly adapted for the use of students who desire to review their work as rapidly as possible and to memorize only what is absolutely necessary. It does not pretend to replace the larger anatomical works. As an aid to the student in mastering the more important facts of anatomy, and especially for the purpose of making very rapid review possible, this book must prove to be decidedly useful.   H. P. H. G.

International Clinics. A Quarterly of Illustrated Clinical Lectures and Especially Prepared Original Articles on Treatment, Medicine, Surgery, Neurology, Pediatrics, Obstetrics, Gynecology, Orthopedics, Pathology, Dermatology, Ophthalmology, Otology, Rhinology, Laryngology, Hygiene, and other topics of interest to students and practitioners. By leading members of the medical profession throughout the world. Edited by A. O. J. KELLY, M.D., Philadelphia, U.S.A., with the collaboration of Wm. Osler, M.D., Baltimore, U.S.A.; John H. Musser, M.D., Philadelphia; Jas. Stewart, M.D., Montreal; J. B. Murphy, M.D., Chicago, A. McPhedran, M.D., Toronto; Thos. M. Rotch, M.D., Boston; J. G. Clark, M.D., Philadelphia; Jas. J. Walsh, M.D., New York; J. W. Ballantyne, M.D., Edinburgh; John Harold, M.D., London; Edmund

Landolt, M.D., Paris,. and Richard Kretz, M.D., Vienna. With regular correspondents in Montreal, London, Paris, Berlin, Vienna, Leipsic, Brussels and Carlsbad. Vol. III. Fourteenth Series. Price, cloth, $2.00 net. 1904. Philadelphia: J. B. Lippincott Co. Canadian agent: Chas. Roberts, Montreal.

We find among the contributors to Volume III., Dr. W. H. Allchin, London; Dr. J. W. Ballantyne, Edinburgh; Dr. Chanffard, Paris; Dr. W. S. Gottheil, New York; Dr. Alfred Fournier, of Paris Faculty of Medicine; Dr. T. S. Stuart, of the Vanderbilt Clinic, New York; Dr. T. H. Manley, New York, and Mr. Campbell Williams, London, Eng.

The first section of the book consists of twelve clinics by various authors, on syphilis, syphilitic inoculation, fever, headache, laryngeal, fetal syphilis, syphilis and suicide, treatment of chancre and treatment by calomel injections. This alone makes the volume one of value. The balance of the book is devoted to treatment, surgery, medicine, gynecology and neurology. Dr. T. H. Manley contributes' an article on umbilical hernia in the female that possesses a great deal of merit, and is well worthy of careful perusal.

Malignant Disease of the Larynx—Carcinoma and Sarcoma. By
PHILIP DE SANTI, F.R.C.S., Surgeon to the Throat, Nose
and Ear Departments, Westminster Hospital. London:
Baillière, Tindall & Cox. 1904. Pp. 106.

Fortunately, malignant disease of the larynx is rare. In this country patients have usually been recommended to get their estates in order, for there is no hope for them. In England and Germany there has been a greater disposition to offer operation to the patient. In Germany the operation has usually been extirpation of the larynx; in England it has been thyrotomy and, if need be, extirpation of part or all of the larynx, as operation showed necessary. The English results have been very good, and De Santi's monograph is really a plea for this operation as offering the greatest measure of hope to the patient. J. M.

Regional Minor Surgery. By GEORGE GRAY VAN SCHAICK,
Consulting Surgeon to French Hospital, N.Y. Second edition, enlarged and revised. 228 pages, bound in cloth. Profusely illustrated. Price, $1.50. International Journal of
Surgery Co., N.Y.

The practicability and usefulness of this book is best indicated by the demand, necessitating a second edition in an unusually short time. This edition has been subjected to a thorough revision, and additional chapters have been added.

8

The author's object, to furnish the general practitioner with such practical information on minor surgery conditions as will be of the greatest service to him in his daily practice, has been well accomplished. Subjects of a technical character have been avoided, and only the most applicable methods demonstrated by twenty years' private and hospital experience are presented. The book is liberally illustrated with original sketches and is so eminently practical and useful, we believe it will be run through many more editions.

Minor surgery is minor in name only, since the most trivial injury may be followed by disastrous results.

A ready reference, free from technicalities and theories, is of great advantage in emergency work, for the busy practitioner as well as for the student, and while in a small work like this much cannot be included, still there is a reasonable share of what is necessary for such purposes.   E. H. A.

A Text-Book of Physiological Chemistry. For Students of Medicine and Physicians. By CHARLES E. SIMON, M.D., of Baltimore, Md. Second edition, revised and enlarged. Philadelphia and New York: Lea Brothers & Co.

" The subject-matter has been arranged in such a manner that in the first section of the work a general survey is given of the origin and the chemical nature of the three great classes of foodstuffs, and also of the most important products of their decomposition. The second section deals essentially with the processes of digestion, resorption and excretion. The third and last portion is devoted to the chemical study of the elementary tissues and the various organs of the animal body, the specific products of their activity, and their relation to physiological function."

In this second edition, many important additions have been made, while some of the chapters have been almost entirely rewritten in order to include in them the advances in chemical research that are rapidly taking place.

The style adopted by the author is very clear, the subject-matter is thoroughly treated, and we are sure that the work will be exceedingly popular with all those who are interested in this most fascinating subject.   A. E.

Text-Book of Human Physiology. Including Histology and Microscopical Anatomy, with Especial Reference to the Practice of Medicine. By DR. L. LANDOIS, Professor of Physiology and Director of the Physiological Institute in the University of Griefswald. Tenth revised and enlarged edition. Edited by ALBERT P. BRUBAKER, M.D., Professor of Physiology and Hygiene in the Jefferson Medical College. Translated by

Augustus A. Eshner, M.D., Professor of Clinical Medicine in the Philadelphia Polyclinic. With 394 illustrations. Philadelphia: P. Blakiston's Son & Co., 1012 Walnut Street. 1904.

This is a translation of the tenth and last German edition of Landois' well-known text-book of human physiology. In the preparation of this work the author says that he has tried to provide for physicians and students a book that should supply the needs of the practising physician in larger measure than is done by the majority of similar works. In every section a brief outline of the usual pathological variations follows the description of the normal processes. This linking together of the normal and abnormal, physiology and pathology, cannot fail to help both students and practitioners in their efforts to recognize and interpret the significance of clinical symptoms in any departure from normal conditions.

Many new illustrations have been added, and some of the old ones have been replaced by better ones.

It would be hard to find a more complete or more useful work on physiology, and we think the improvements in this edition will add even still more to its popularity.   A. E.

A Text-Book of Histology. By Frederick R. Bailey, A.M., M.D., Adjunct Professor of Normal Histology, College of Physicians and Surgeons, Medical Department, Columbia University, New York City. Profusely illustrated. New York: Wm. Wood & Co. 1904.

In those days when medical teaching is almost entirely conducted on the laboratory system, a book written along the line of Dr. Bailey's will be found especially useful for both teacher and student. It is practical and concise, all unnecessary material having been culled out, without the value of the book having been in any way sacrificed. As a text-book of histology, it will not be easy to find one to excel it.

The Physician's Visiting List for 1905. Fifty-fourth year of its publication. Philadelphia: P. Blakiston's Son & Co., 1012 Walnut Street.

Blakiston's " Visiting List " for the coming year is practically the same as for 1904. It contains some useful, practical information on incompatibility of drugs, poisoning, the metric system, dose table, asphyxia and apnea, comparison of thermometers, and a table for calculating the period of utero gestation. It can be procured for from twenty-five to one hundred patients per week, or in perpetual form. The leather cover, with pocket and pencil, sells at $1.00. Blakiston's list is excelled by none.

"General Catalogue of Medical Books." P. Blakiston's Son & Co., Philadelphia, Pa. This is a useful list of the most recent works in all branches of medicine and surgery, arranged alphabetically. The book is interleaved.

The Medical News' Visiting List for 1905 has come to hand. It varies little from that for the year now closing, but will be found by physicians who like to carry a daily visiting list, to be exceedingly compact and handy. It contains a lot of memoranda and data, that will be found most useful to the busy practitioner, and can be procured in four styles, a weekly, monthly, perpetual, and one undated, for sixty patients weekly. The List is published by Wm. Wood & Co., New York, N.Y.

"Visiting and Pocket Reference Book for 1905." The following is a comprehensive contents: Table of signs and how to keep visiting accounts, obstetrical memoranda, clinical emergencies, poisons and antidotes, dose table, blank leaves for weekly visiting list, memorandum, nurses' addresses, clinical, obstetrical, birth, death and vaccination records, bills rendered, cash received, articles loaned, money loaned, miscellaneous, calendar 1905. 126 pages, lapel binding, red edges. This very complete call book will be furnished by the Dios Chemical Co., of St. Louis, Mo., on receipt of 10 cents for postage.

The December *Delineator,* with its message of good cheer and helpfulness, will be welcomed in every home. The fashion pages are unusually attractive, illustrating and describing the very latest modes in a way to make their construction during the busy festive season a pleasure instead of a task, and the literary and pictorial features are of rare excellence. A selection of Love Songs from the Wagner Operas, rendered into English by Richard de Gallienne and beautifully illustrated in colors by *J. C.* Leydendecker, occupies a prominent place, and a chapter in the Composers' Series, relating the Romance of Wagner and Cosima, is an interesting supplement to the lyrics. A very clever paper, entitled "The Court Circles of the Republic," describes some unique phases of Washington social life, is from an unnamed contributor, who is said to write from the inner circles of society. There are short stories from the pens of F. Hopkinson Smith, Robert Grant, Alice Brown, Mary Stewart Cutting and Elmore Elliott Peake, and such interesting writers as Julia Magruder, L. Frank Baum and Grace Mac-Gowan Cooke hold the attention of the children. Many Christmas suggestions are given in needlework, and the Cookery pages are redolent of the Christmas feast. In addition, there are the regular departments of the magazine, with many special articles on topics relating to woman's interests within and without the home.

The Canadian journal of
medicine and surgery